Protein–Ligand Interactions

Protein–Ligand Interactions: Target Identification and Drug Discovery

Editor

Fabio Altieri

MDPI • Basel • Beijing • Wuhan • Barcelona • Belgrade • Manchester • Tokyo • Cluj • Tianjin

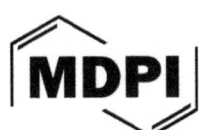

Editor
Fabio Altieri
La Sapienza University
Italy

Editorial Office
MDPI
St. Alban-Anlage 66
4052 Basel, Switzerland

This is a reprint of articles from the Special Issue published online in the open access journal *Biomedicines* (ISSN 2227-9059) (available at: https://www.mdpi.com/journal/biomedicines/special_issues/protein_ligand_drug).

For citation purposes, cite each article independently as indicated on the article page online and as indicated below:

LastName, A.A.; LastName, B.B.; LastName, C.C. Article Title. *Journal Name* **Year**, *Volume Number*, Page Range.

ISBN 978-3-0365-1050-7 (Hbk)
ISBN 978-3-0365-1051-4 (PDF)

© 2021 by the authors. Articles in this book are Open Access and distributed under the Creative Commons Attribution (CC BY) license, which allows users to download, copy and build upon published articles, as long as the author and publisher are properly credited, which ensures maximum dissemination and a wider impact of our publications.

The book as a whole is distributed by MDPI under the terms and conditions of the Creative Commons license CC BY-NC-ND.

Contents

About the Editor vii

Preface to "Protein–Ligand Interactions: Target Identification and Drug Discovery" ix

Evangelia Sereti, Chrisiida Tsimplouli, Elisavet Kalaitsidou, Nikos Sakellaridis and Konstantinos Dimas
Study of the Relationship between Sigma Receptor Expression Levels and Some Common Sigma Ligand Activity in Cancer Using Human Cancer Cell Lines of the NCI-60 Cell Line Panel
Reprinted from: *Biomedicines* **2021**, *9*, 38, doi:10.3390/biomedicines9010038 1

Bashir Lawal, Yen-Lin Liu, Ntlotlang Mokgautsi, Harshita Khedkar, Maryam Rachmawati Sumitra, Alexander T. H. Wu and Hsu-Shan Huang
Pharmacoinformatics and Preclinical Studies of NSC765690 and NSC765599, Potential STAT3/CDK2/4/6 Inhibitors with Antitumor Activities against NCI60 Human Tumor Cell Lines
Reprinted from: *Biomedicines* **2021**, *9*, 92, doi:10.3390/biomedicines9010092 23

Nidal Zeineh, Nunzio Denora, Valentino Laquintana, Massimo Franco, Abraham Weizman and Moshe Gavish
Efficaciousness of Low Affinity Compared to High Affinity TSPO Ligands in the Inhibition of Hypoxic Mitochondrial Cellular Damage Induced by Cobalt Chloride in Human Lung H1299 Cells
Reprinted from: *Biomedicines* **2020**, *8*, 106, doi:10.3390/biomedicines8050106 45

Gabriel Zazeri, Ana Paula Ribeiro Povinelli, Marcelo de Freitas Lima and Marinônio Lopes Cornélio
Detailed Characterization of the Cooperative Binding of Piperine with Heat Shock Protein 70 by Molecular Biophysical Approaches
Reprinted from: *Biomedicines* **2020**, *8*, 629, doi:10.3390/biomedicines8120629 63

Sherif T. S. Hassan
Brassicasterol with Dual Anti-Infective Properties against HSV-1 and *Mycobacterium tuberculosis*, and Cardiovascular Protective Effect: Nonclinical In Vitro and In Silico Assessments
Reprinted from: *Biomedicines* **2020**, *8*, 132, doi:10.3390/biomedicines8050132 79

Suresh Velnati, Sara Centonze, Federico Girivetto, Daniela Capello, Ricardo M. Biondi, Alessandra Bertoni, Roberto Cantello, Beatrice Ragnoli, Mario Malerba, Andrea Graziani and Gianluca Baldanzi
Identification of Key Phospholipids That Bind and Activate Atypical PKCs
Reprinted from: *Biomedicines* **2021**, *9*, 45, doi:10.3390/biomedicines9010045 91

Jinhwan Cho, Junyong Park, Giyoong Tae, Mi Sun Jin and Inchan Kwon
The Minimal Effect of Linker Length for Fatty Acid Conjugation to a Small Protein on the Serum Half-Life Extension
Reprinted from: *Biomedicines* **2020**, *8*, 96, doi:10.3390/biomedicines8050096 109

Pitchayakarn Takomthong, Pornthip Waiwut, Chavi Yenjai, Bungon Sripanidkulchai, Prasert Reubroycharoen, Ren Lai, Peter Kamau and Chantana Boonyarat
Structure–Activity Analysis and Molecular Docking Studies of Coumarins from *Toddalia asiatica* as Multifunctional Agents for Alzheimer's Disease
Reprinted from: *Biomedicines* **2020**, *8*, 107, doi:10.3390/biomedicines8050107 121

Annamaria Sandomenico, Lorenzo Di Rienzo, Luisa Calvanese, Emanuela Iaccarino, Gabriella D'Auria, LuciaFalcigno, Angela Chambery, Rosita Russo, Guido Franzoso, Laura Tornatore, Marco D'Abramo, Menotti Ruvo, Edoardo Milanetti and Domenico Raimondo
Insights into the Interaction Mechanism of DTP3 with MKK7 by Using STD-NMR and Computational Approaches
Reprinted from: *Biomedicines* **2021**, *9*, 20, doi:10.3390/biomedicines9010020 . . . . **137**

Margarida Lorigo, Carla Quintaneiro, Luiza Breitenfeld and Elisa Cairrao
UV-B Filter Octylmethoxycinnamate Alters the Vascular Contractility Patterns in Pregnant Women with Hypothyroidism
Reprinted from: *Biomedicines* **2021**, *9*, 115, doi:10.3390/biomedicines9020115 . . . . **153**

About the Editor

Fabio Altieri obtained a masters degree in Biology from Sapienza University of Rome (Italy) in 1981, and a Ph.D. in Biochemistry from Sapienza University of Rome (Italy) in 1986. Since 2000, he has been Professor of Biochemistry at the Department of Biochemical Sciences "A. Rossi Fanelli", Sapienza University of Rome. For several years, he was involved in research projects on the characterization of non-histone chromosomal proteins. Subsequently, he focused the attention on nuclear protein purification and characterization, and protein–protein and protein–DNA interactions. His particular interests are related to the analysis of PDIA3, a protein disulfide isomerase, and its cellular functions. His current research covers the analysis of proteins involved in signal transduction, cancer onset and progression, and oxidative stress responses, as well as the screening of bioactive compounds and their impact on protein functionality.

Preface to "Protein–Ligand Interactions: Target Identification and Drug Discovery"

Bioactive compounds and drugs are designed and screened on the basis of specific molecular targets as well as via the identification of active ingredients from traditional medicine or by serendipitous discovery. The development of novel therapeutic strategies not only requires a deep knowledge of the molecular processes and the cellular pathways involved in each pathological condition and disease, but also the specific protein targets and the effects of drug binding on protein conformation and activity. Understanding of how drugs can modify and modulate specific cellular pathways and functions will be helpful during the process of drug development and clinical trials.

Fabio Altieri
Editor

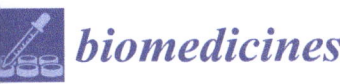

Article

Study of the Relationship between Sigma Receptor Expression Levels and Some Common Sigma Ligand Activity in Cancer Using Human Cancer Cell Lines of the NCI-60 Cell Line Panel

Evangelia Sereti [1,2], Chrisiida Tsimplouli [1], Elisavet Kalaitsidou [1], Nikos Sakellaridis [1] and Konstantinos Dimas [1,*]

[1] Department of Pharmacology, Faculty of Medicine, University of Thessaly, 41500 Larissa, Greece; evangelia.sereti@med.lu.se (E.S.); xrisida@med.uth.gr (C.T.); e.kalaitsidou@students.uu.nl (E.K.); nsakella@uth.gr (N.S.)

[2] Department of Translational Medicine, Division of Urological Cancers, Lund University, SE 205 02 Malmö, Sweden

* Correspondence: kdimas@med.uth.gr

Abstract: Sigma (σ) receptors have attracted great interest since they are implicated in various cellular functions and biological processes and diseases, including various types of cancer. The receptor family consists of two subtypes: sigma-1 (σ1) and sigma-2 (σ2). Both σ receptor subtypes have been proposed as therapeutic targets for various types of cancers, and many studies have provided evidence that their selective ligands (agonists and antagonists) exhibit antiproliferative and cytotoxic activity. Still, the precise mechanism of action of both σ receptors and their ligands remains unclear and needs to be elucidated. In this study, we aimed to simultaneously determine the expression levels of both σ receptor subtypes in several human cancer cell lines. Additionally, we investigated the in vitro antiproliferative activity of some widely used σ1 and σ2 ligands against those cell lines to study the relationship between σ receptor expression levels and σ ligand activity. Finally, we ran the NCI60 COMPARE algorithm to further elucidate the cytotoxic mechanism of action of the selected σ ligands studied herein.

Keywords: sigma receptors; sigma ligands; cancer; SIGMAR1; PGRMC1; TMEM97; NCI60 COMPARE analysis

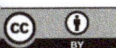

1. Introduction

Sigma receptor is a class of receptors that have been the subject of intensive pharmacological research since their discovery in 1976 by Martin et al. [1]. Since then, considerable progress has been made, especially in the last years. It is now known that the family consists of two members: the sigma-1 (σ1) and sigma-2 (σ2) receptors, which are substantially different from each other. Sigma-1 has been cloned by two different groups independently [2,3] and is now widely accepted as a membrane receptor and a chaperone protein with multiple cellular functions [4]. Until recently, the identification of sigma-2 receptor was a matter of debate. In 2011, it was proposed that the PGRMC1 may harbor binding sites for sigma ligands [5]. A few years later in 2017, Alon et al. published evidence showing that the sigma-2 receptor is in fact identical to TMEM97 [6], which is now the prevailing theory. Sigma-2/TMEM97, a member of the insulin-like growth factor binding proteins, is a protein that is reported to be increased in several types of cancer [7]. To complicate things even more, a 2018 study reported that σ2/TMEM97 forms a trimeric complex with PGRMC1 and the low-density lipoprotein receptor (LDLR), which is responsible for the rapid internalization of the low-density lipoprotein (LDL) in HeLa cells, a human cervical cancer cell line [8]. That work suggested that both PGRMC1 and TMEM97 could in fact be part of a more complex receptor that can bind σ2-ligands.

Interestingly, both sigma subtypes have been proposed as therapeutic targets for several diseases and pathological conditions, with various types of cancer being amongst them [9]. However, the precise mechanism of their action is still a matter of debate, even though many independent studies have provided evidence of antiproliferative and cytotoxic activity for both the sigma-1 and sigma-2 receptor ligands [10].

In this study, we try to shed some light on the relationship of the σ1 and σ2 receptors and the anticancer activity of sigma ligands. To this aim, we used Western blot (WB) to study the expression levels of σ1, PGRMC1, and σ2/TMEM97 receptors in several human cancer cell lines, representing nine different cancer types. Most of the tested cell lines included in this study are also included in the NCI60 cell line panel list that is widely used for the in vitro testing of potential anticancer drugs [11]. In addition to the WB studies, we further addressed the in vitro antiproliferative activity of some commonly used σ1 and σ2 ligands against those cell lines to (a) test the efficacy of these ligands against various human cancer types, (b) compare their activity under the same experimental conditions, and (c) assess if there whether any correlation of their activity in relation to the expression of the receptors.

2. Materials and Methods

2.1. Cell Culture

All cell lines used were purchased from the National Cancer Institute (National Institutes of Health, Bethesda, MD, USA), and were cultured in RPMI 1640 (Roswell Park Memorial Institute 1640) medium (Cat. No. 31870025; Thermo Fisher Scientific, Waltham, MA, USA) supplemented with 5% fetal bovine serum (Cat. No. 1001G; Biosera, Nuaille, France), 2 mM L-glutamine (Cat. No. XC-T1715; Biosera, Nuaille, France), and 100 U/mL penicillin and 100 µg/mL streptomycin (Cat. No. XC-A4122; Biosera, Nuaille, France). Cell cultures were maintained at 37 °C in a humidified incubator with a 5% CO_2 air atmosphere.

2.2. Western Blot Analysis

Cell lysis was performed in T-PER tissue protein extraction reagent (Cat. No. 78510; Thermo Fisher Scientific, Waltham, MA, USA) supplemented with 1% protease and phosphatase inhibitor cocktail (Cat. No. 5872; Cell Signaling Technology, Beverly, MA, USA). Cell lysates were then sonicated (3 cycles, 10 s/cycle) and centrifuged at 13,000 rpm for 30 min at 4 °C, and supernatants were then collected. Protein concentration was determined using a Pierce BCA Protein Assay Kit (Cat. No. 23227; Thermo Fisher Scientific, Waltham, MA, USA). Lysates containing equal amount of protein (20 µg) were run on a 10% acrylamide gel and transferred to a 0.22 µm pore size polyvinylidene difluoride (PVDF) membrane, Immobilon-P^{SQ} Transfer Membrane (Cat. No. ISEQ85R; Merck, Millipore, Darmstadt, Germany). Membranes were blocked for 1 h at room temperature with the appropriate blocking buffer, according to each antibody's specific protocol, and then incubated overnight at 4 °C with rabbit anti-SIGMA1 antibody (Cat. No. 61994; Cell Signaling Technology, Beverly, MA, USA), rabbit anti-PGRMC1 antibody (Cat. No. 13856; Cell Signaling Technology, Beverly, MA, USA), or rabbit anti-TMEM97 antibody (Cat. No. NBP1-30436; Novus Biologicals, Centennial CO, USA). All antibodies were used at a 1:1000 dilution. Finally, membranes were incubated with the secondary horseradish peroxidase-conjugated anti-rabbit antibody (Cat. No. 7074; Cell Signaling Technology, Beverly, MA, USA) at 1/6000 dilution, developed with Clarity Western enhanced chemiluminescence (ECL) Substrate (Cat. No. 170-5060; Bio-Rad Laboratories, Hercules, CA, USA) and detected with Uvitec Cambridge chemiluminescence imaging system with the help of Alliance Software (ver. 16.06) (Uvitec Cambridge, Cambridge, UK).

2.3. Cell Viability Assay

The cytotoxic effect of the sigma ligands Siramesine (kindly offered by H. Lundbeck A/S), PB28 dihydrochloride (Cat. No. sc-204834; Santa Cruz Biotechnology, Dallas, TX, USA), rimcazole dihydrochloride (Cat. No. 1497; Tocris, Abingdon, United Kingdom), BD1047 dihydrobromide (Cat. No. 0956; Tocris, Abingdon, United Kingdom), and SM-21 maleate (Cat. No. sc-204289; Santa Cruz Biotechnology, Dallas, TX, USA) was determined using sulforhodamine B (SRB) colorimetric assay. Cell viability was determined at the beginning of each experiment by trypan blue dye exclusion method and was always greater than 97%. Cells were seeded into a flat bottom 96-well plate at a density of 5000 cells per well, 24 h before treatment. Sigma ligands were dissolved in dimethyl sulfoxide (DMSO) and were serially diluted in culture medium to acquire the desired concentrations. The final concentration of DMSO in each cell culture was no higher than 0.1%. After 48 h treatment, cells were fixed by gentle addition of 50% (v/v) trichloroacetic acid (TCA) (Cat. No. A1431; Applichem, Darmstadt, Germany) to each well and stained for 1 h at 4 °C. Cells were washed (three times) with slow running tap water; excess water was removed by gentle tapping onto a paper towel and the plates were allowed to air-dry at room temperature (RT). A solution of 0.04% (w/v) SRB (Cat. No. S9012; Sigma-Aldrich, St Louis, MO, USA) in 1% (v/v) acetic acid (Cat. No. 45731; Fluka, Buchs, Switzerland) was subsequently used to dye cells for 10 min at RT. After incubation, the excess dye was removed by repeated rinses with 1% (v/v) acetic acid (Cat. No. 45731; Fluka, Buchs, Switzerland) and cell monolayers were allowed to dry at RT. The protein-bound dye was dissolved in 10 mM Tris base solution by incubation for 10 min at 37 °C followed by solubilization in an orbital shaker for 10 min. Absorbance was measured at 540 nm in a BioTek EL311 microplate reader (BioTek Instruments, Winooski, VT, USA). From the generated dose-response curves, we determined the GI_{50} (50% cell growth inhibition), TGI (total growth inhibition), and LC_{50} (50% lethal concentration) parameters. Growth inhibition of 50% (GI_{50}) is calculated from ((Ti-Tz)/(C-Tz)) x 100 = 50. The drug concentration resulting in total growth inhibition (TGI) is calculated from Ti = Tz. The LC_{50} indicating a net loss of cells following treatment is calculated from ((Ti-Tz)/Tz) x 100 = − 50. In these formulas Tz represents a measurement of the cell population for each cell line at the time of drug addition, Ti is a measurement representing the growth of cells in the presence of a given concentration of the drug and C the measurement of the control cells at the end of the 48 h incubation period.

Following standardization, the GI_{50} z-scores were defined and cell lines were categorized, with z-scores ≥ 0.8 categorized as being resistant and z-scores ≤ 0.8 as being sensitive to the compounds tested.

2.4. Statistical Analysis

All data are presented as the mean ± SD of at least 3 independent experiments. A two-tailed Student's t-test was used to calculate the statistical significance between sigma receptors' expression levels in the cancer cell lines tested versus cell lines with the lowest protein expression levels. A two-way ANOVA with either Bonferroni's or Tukey's post hoc test was used to determine statistical significance of sigma ligands' antiproliferative activity within cell lines of the same cancer type. Data normalization was performed by z-score analysis. Pearson's linear correlation coefficient (r) was calculated to measure the strength of the linear relationship between the antiproliferative efficacy of the selected sigma ligands to the expression levels of sigma receptors. The NCI60 COMPARE algorithm was used to calculate the Pearson correlation coefficient (PCC) of the sigma ligands against compounds with known mechanism of action (MoA) in the National Cancer Institute (NCI) database. Differences were considered significant (rejection of the null hypothesis) when $p \leq 0.05$.

3. Results

3.1. σ1 Receptor, PGRMC1, and σ2/TMEM97 Were Heterogeneously Expressed in 23 Human Cancer Cell Lines

For the first time in the literature, the expression levels of σ1 receptor, PGRMC1, and σ2/TMEM97 were studied simultaneously by Western blot analysis in 23 human cancer cell lines. The cell lines used represent nine different types of cancer: lung, colon, CNS, melanoma, ovarian, breast, renal, prostate, and pancreatic ductal adenocarcinoma (PDAC). Figure 1a shows that σ1, PGRMC1, and σ2/TMEM97 receptors were expressed with different expression patterns in the studied cell lines. Sigma-1 receptor showed the highest expression levels in NCI-H460 (lung cancer) and HCT-15 (colon cancer) cell lines, while the lowest expression levels were reported in CAKI-1, SN12C (kidney cancer), OVCAR-3, OVCAR-5 (ovarian cancer), HCT-116 (colorectal cancer), and MCF7 (breast cancer) cell lines (Figure 1b). Sigma-2/TMEM97 receptor was found to be highly expressed in NCI-H460 (lung cancer), HCT-15 (colorectal cancer), and MCF7 (breast cancer) cell lines, with low expression levels in MDA-MB-435 (melanoma), SF268 (CNS cancer), and MDA-MB-231 (breast cancer) cell lines. Regarding PGRMC1 receptor, BxPC-3 (pancreatic cancer) and MCF-7 (breast cancer) cell lines expressed the highest levels, while the lowest levels were observed in NCI-H23 (lung cancer), HCT15, HCT116 (colon cancer), MDA-MB-231 (triple negative breast cancer), and T-47D (breast cancer) cell lines (Figure 1c). Despite the different profiles reported above, it seemed that there were few exceptions where the σ receptors did share similarities in terms of their expression levels. Specifically, in NCI-H460 and HCT-15 cell lines, both σ1 and σ2/TMEM97 showed the highest expression levels among all the cell lines studied. Moreover, MCF7 cell line expressed high levels of both σ2/TMEM97 and PGRMC1 receptors. However, σ1, PGRMC1, and σ2/TMEM97 were generally expressed differentially, even between cell lines of the same cancer type. Examples of this were σ1 expression in ovarian and breast cancer, PGRMC1 expression in lung and breast cancer, and σ2/TMEM97 in melanoma and breast cancer cell lines.

3.2. In Vitro Antiproliferative Efficacy of Sigma Ligands

The in vitro antiproliferative efficacy of five common sigma ligands was investigated in the same panel of the 23 human established cancer cell lines in which we earlier investigated the expression levels of σ1, PGRMC1, and σ2/TMEM97 receptors. The selected sigma ligands were siramesine and PB28 dihydrochloride, referred to in the literature as σ2 agonists with high σ2 receptor affinities [12,13], and rimcazole [14], SM-21 maleate [15], and BD-1047 dihydrobromide [16], referred to as σ1/σ2 antagonists. The chemical structures of the sigma ligands tested are shown in Figure 2.

Twenty-three established human cancer cell lines were treated with the sigma ligands for 48 h at various concentrations (100, 10, 1, and 0.1 μM), and a cell viability assay (SRB) was performed. Dose–response curves were generated after incubation with different concentrations of the various sigma ligands (Figure 3).

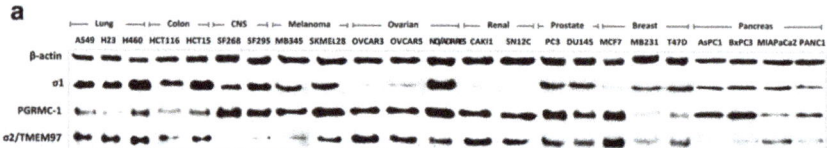

Figure 1. *Cont.*

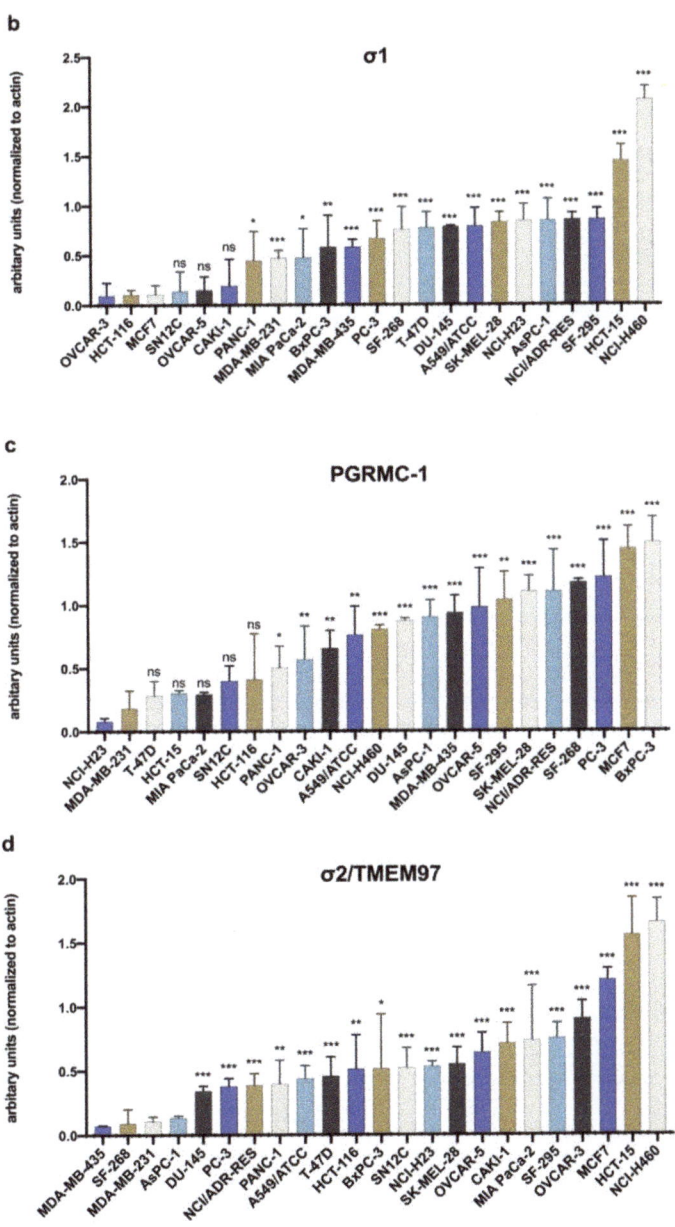

Figure 1. Expression levels of σ1, PGRMC1, and σ2/TMEM97 in the 23 human cancer cell lines. (**a**) Western blot analysis of σ1, PGRMC1, and σ2/TMEM97 expression in 23 human cancer cell lines representing nine different cancer types. β-Actin was used as a loading control. Bar graphs of σ1 (**b**), PGRMC1 (**c**), and σ2/TMEM97 (**d**) relative expression levels normalized to β-actin. Results are expressed as mean ± SD of at least three independent experiments. Statistical significance was calculated versus cell lines with the lowest protein expression levels: OVCAR-3, HCT-116, MCF-7 (**b**); NCI-H23, MDA-MB-231 (**c**); and MDA-MB-435, SF-268, MDA-MB-231, AsPC-1 (**d**). * $p \leq 0.05$; ** $p \leq 0.01$; *** $p \leq 0.001$; ns: not significant.

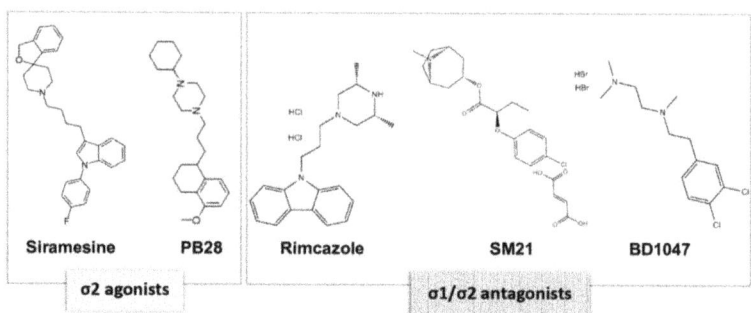

Figure 2. Chemical structures of the selected sigma receptors agonists and antagonists siramesine, PB28 dihydrochloride (PB28), rimcazole, SM21 maleate (SM21), and BD1047 dihydrobromide (BD1047).

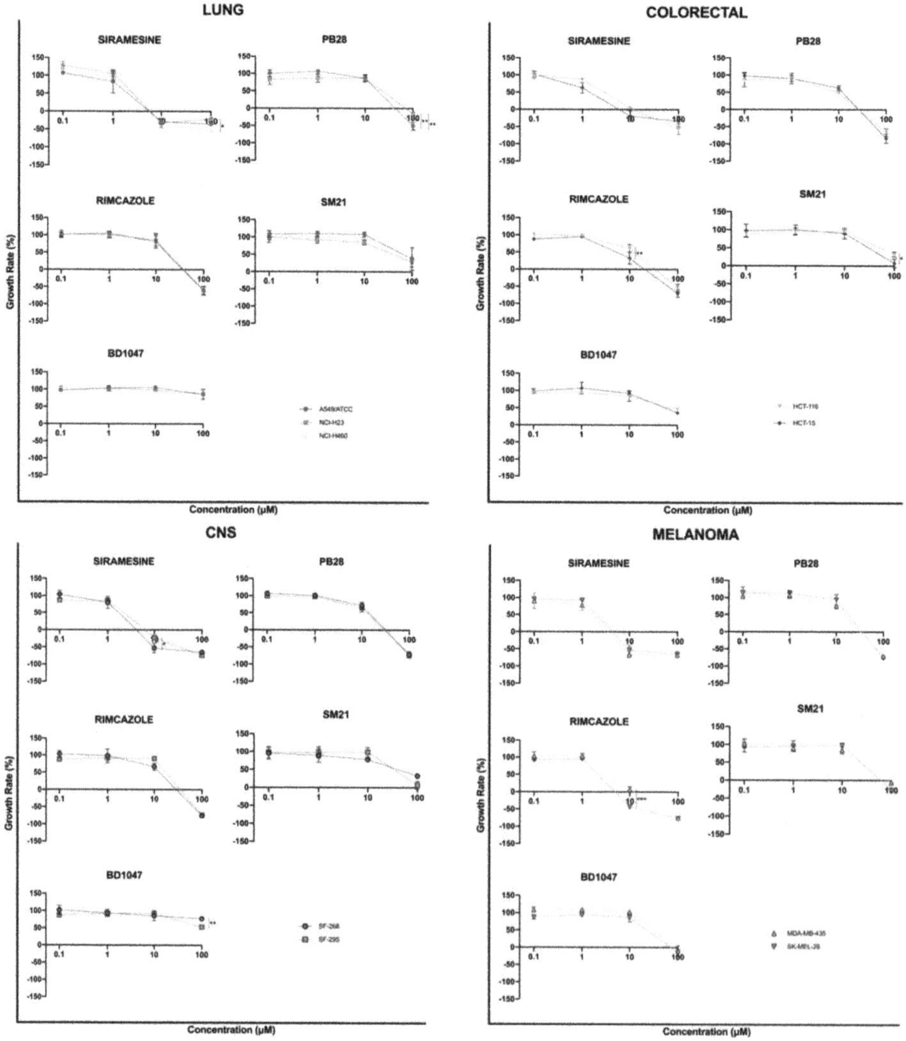

Figure 3. Cont.

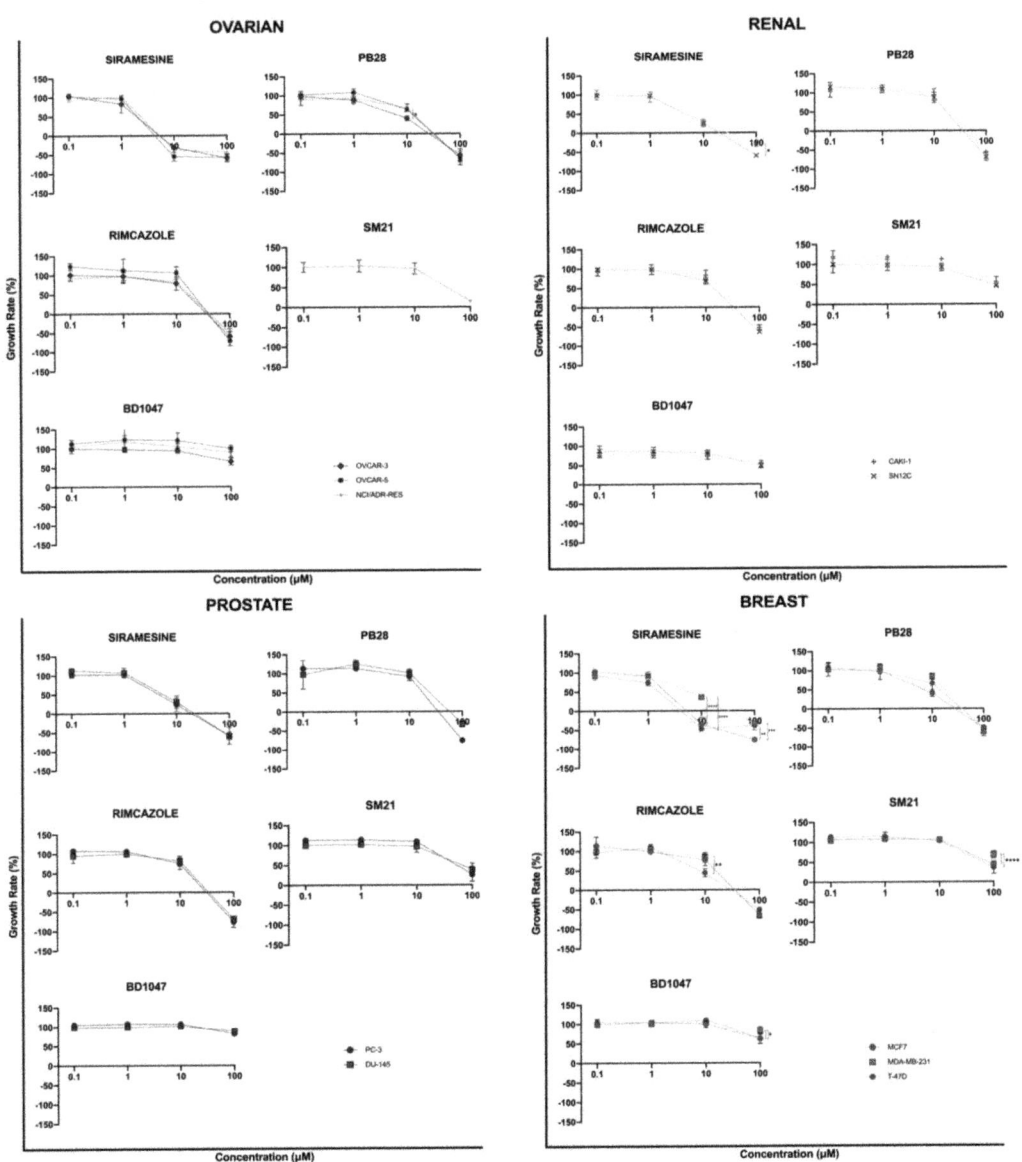

Figure 3. *Cont.*

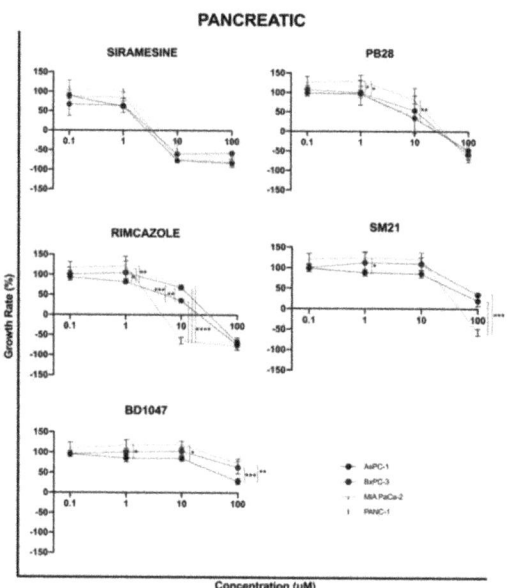

Figure 3. Dose–response effect of the selected sigma ligands siramesine, PB28 dihydrochloride (PB28), rimcazole, SM21 maleate (SM21) and BD1047 dihydrobromide (BD1047) in 23 human cancer cell lines. Cells were exposed to different concentrations of the compounds for 48 h and growth rates were calculated with sulforhodamine B (SRB) assay. All compounds were tested at four concentrations (one log serial dilutions from 10^{-4} M to 10^{-7} M). The results are the average of three independent experiments; each one ran in triplicate. * $p \leq 0.05$; ** $p \leq 0.01$; *** $p \leq 0.001$; **** $p \leq 0.0001$.

From the dose–response curves, GI_{50}, TGI, and LC_{50} parameters were calculated for each cell line, representing the antiproliferative, cytostatic, and cytotoxic effects, respectively. Therapeutic index (TI) was also calculated as LC_{50} to GI_{50} ratio, determining the relative safety of the compounds (Table 1).

Table 1. GI$_{50}$ (50% cell growth inhibition), TGI (total cell growth inhibition), LC$_{50}$ (50% lethal concentration), and therapeutic index (TI) parameters for each cell line and compound tested as calculated by the graphs shown in Figure 3. Dots (•) mean not tested. For more details on the three parameters see M&M under "2.3 Cell viability assay". Note: In cases where GI$_{50}$ and LC$_{50}$ were higher than the highest tested concentration (100 μM), the TI was calculated using GI$_{50}$ and LC$_{50}$ at 100 μM.

CANCER TYPE	CELL LINES	SIRAMESINE				PB28				RIMCAZOLE				SM21				BD1047			
		GI$_{50}$	TGI	LC$_{50}$	TI	GI$_{50}$	TGI	LC$_{50}$	TI	GI$_{50}$	TGI	LC$_{50}$	TI	GI$_{50}$	TGI	LC$_{50}$	TI	GI$_{50}$	TGI	LC$_{50}$	TI
NSCL	A549/ATCC	3.6	7.7	11.7	3.3	34.2	66.8	99.3	2.9	29.2	61.0	92.7	3.2	84.2	100.0	100.0	1.2	>100	>100	>100	1.0
	NCI-H23	4.7	7.9	11.2	2.4	42.9	87.0	>100	2.3	31.9	62.8	93.7	2.9	65.2	100.0	100.0	1.5	>100	>100	>100	1.0
	NCI-H460	4.3	7.7	83.1	19.3	27.5	62.6	97.7	3.6	31.6	63.6	95.6	3.0	88.9	100.0	100.0	1.1	>100	>100	>100	1.0
Colon	HCT-116	5.0	15.9	90.5	18.1	9.6	48.0	87.4	9.1	18.5	57.5	96.5	5.2	74.5	100.0	100.0	1.3	89.9	>100	>100	1.1
	HCT-15	2.4	7.9	13.5	5.6	17.9	48.6	79.4	4.4	7.5	38.5	82.1	10.9	53.7	100.0	100.0	1.9	77.8	>100	>100	1.3
CNS	SF-268	3.1	6.4	9.8	3.2	24.0	55.5	86.9	3.6	20.1	51.9	83.7	4.2	65.5	100.0	100.0	1.5	>100	>100	>100	1.0
	SF-295	4.0	8.2	58.6	14.7	19.9	52.5	85.0	4.3	31.9	59.4	86.9	2.7	57.7	100.0	100.0	1.7	>100	>100	>100	1.0
Melanoma	MDA-MB-435	2.8	5.9	9.0	3.2	25.6	56.6	87.7	3.4	6.0	10.7	72.5	12.1	44.0	94.2	100.0	2.3	51.7	10.1	>100	1.9
	SK-MEL-28	3.6	6.7	0.8	2.7	33.4	59.9	86.3	2.6	3.9	7.2	28.4	7.2	44.6	80.1	100.0	2.2	42.6	86.8	>100	2.3
Ovarian	OVCAR-3	3.6	7.6	71.9	20.0	8.2	47.5	94.0	11.5	28.8	61.3	93.8	3.3	•	•	•	•	>100	>100	>100	1.0
	OVCAR-5	3.8	6.7	9.7	2.6	19.5	54.4	89.3	4.6	38.7	64.0	89.2	2.3	•	•	•	•	>100	>100	>100	1.0
	NCI/ADR-RES	4.3	7.6	>100	23.3	22.3	56.3	90.2	4.0	32.4	65.9	99.3	3.1	86.3	100.0	100.0	1.2	>100	>100	>100	1.0
Kidney	CAKI-1	6.8	50.7	>100	14.7	36.4	66.5	96.5	2.7	31.8	64.8	97.8	3.1	100.0	100.0	100.0	1.0	>100	>100	>100	1.0
	SN12C	6.9	36.2	89.3	13.0	31.5	60.2	89.0	2.8	22.6	56.3	90.0	4.0	91.9	100.0	100.0	1.1	98.5	>100	>100	1.0
Prostate	PC-3	7.0	35.9	90.5	12.9	32.5	59.3	86.0	2.6	24.6	31.2	84.3	3.4	73.9	100.0	100.0	1.4	>100	>100	>100	1.0
	DU-145	7.7	40.6	90.8	11.8	44.3	77.9	>100	2.3	28.8	58.7	88.5	3.1	82.3	100.0	100.0	1.2	>100	>100	>100	1.0
Breast	MCF7	4.0	7.5	42.3	10.7	8.6	49.8	98.8	11.5	27.1	58.8	90.5	3.3	91.8	100.0	100.0	1.1	>100	>100	>100	1.0
	MDA-MB-231	7.7	55.9	>100	13.0	31.3	62.3	93.4	3.0	31.2	60.8	90.4	2.9	100.0	100.0	100.0	1.0	>100	>100	>100	1.0
	T-47D	2.8	6.5	10.2	3.6	22.8	61.8	>100	4.4	9.2	51.9	99.1	10.8	81.8	100.0	100.0	1.2	>100	>100	>100	1.0
Pancreas	AsPC-1	1.7	5.0	8.3	4.9	7.8	47.6	>100	13.1	7.2	39.2	80.4	11.2	58.6	100.0	100.0	1.7	65.7	>100	>100	1.5
	BxPC-3	2.0	5.6	9.3	4.7	12.8	53.1	93.4	7.3	22.1	55.2	88.3	4.0	81.5	100.0	100.0	1.2	>100	>100	>100	1.0
	MIAPaCa-2	3.1	5.9	8.7	2.8	28.8	58.5	88.1	3.1	4.5	6.9	9.3	2.1	45.8	71.1	96.4	2.1	>100	>100	>100	1.0
	PANC-1	4.0	7.0	6.3	1.6	•	•	•	•	22.6	52.9	83.3	3.7	•	•	•	•	•	•	•	•
MEAN		4.3	15.3	45.0	9.2	24.6	58.8	92.4	5.0	22.3	49.6	83.3	4.9	73.6	97.3	99.8	1.4	92.1	361.1	100.0	1.1

Siramesine was found to exhibit the best in vitro antiproliferative activity among the sigma ligands tested, as indicated by the low GI_{50} values in all studied cell lines (mean GI_{50} = 4.3 µM). Rimcazole (mean GI_{50} = 22.3 µM) and PB28 (mean GI_{50} = 24.6 µM) demonstrated moderate antiproliferative efficacy, while SM21 (mean GI_{50} = 73.6 µM) and BD1047 (mean GI_{50} = 92.1 µM) showed no significant cell growth inhibition efficacy. Siramesine exhibited the best cytostatic and cytotoxic efficacy, as indicated by the low TGI mean parameter of 15.3 µM and low LC_{50} mean parameter of 45 µM.

GI_{50}, TGI, and LC_{50} parameters of the selected sigma ligands against the 23 established human cancer cell lines were further visualized by heat correlation maps (Figure 4). The parameter values were coded on a warm-to-cool color spectrum in which the warmer color (red) corresponds to the lowest values, while the colder color (light green) corresponds to the highest values. Low parameter values indicate better sigma ligands activity. Figure 4 shows that the GI_{50} parameter values for siramesine were in the warm range of the color scale (red, light red) in all the tested cancer cell lines, which contrasted with GI_{50} parameter values for the other tested sigma ligands, which were in the cold color region (green, light green). The same pattern was observed for TGI and LC_{50} parameters, as siramesine was in the warm region of the color scale in several cell lines, in contrast to the rest of the sigma ligands tested. This indicates that among the sigma ligands studied, the σ2 agonist siramesine exhibited the best antiproliferative, cytostatic, and cytotoxic activity. Unlike siramesine, PB28 was found to exhibit significant antiproliferative activity against only four cell lines (HCT116—colorectal cancer, OVCAR3—ovarian cancer, MCF7—breast cancer, and AsPC1—pancreatic cancer). Interestingly, rimcazole's highest activity was observed against the two melanoma cell lines tested and two out of the four pancreatic cancer cell lines (AsPC1 and MiaPaCa2) tested.

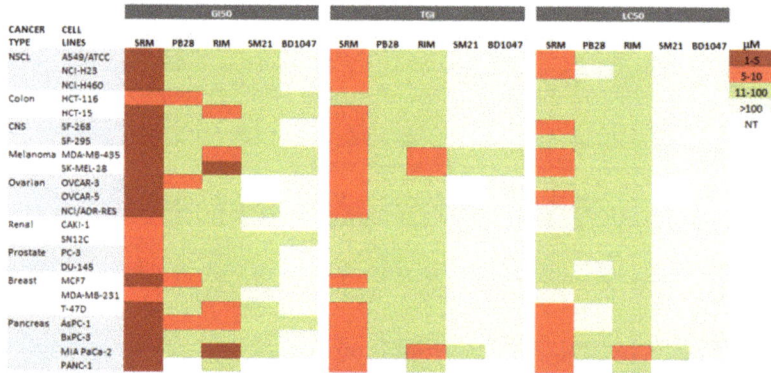

Figure 4. Heat maps representing GI_{50}, TGI, and LC_{50} parameters of the sigma ligands tested against 23 human cancer cell lines. A warm-to-cool color spectrum (red > light red > green > light green) is used to represent the parameter value range (1–5 µM, 5–10 µM, 10–100 µM, >100 µM), respectively. White color stands for not tested (NT) cell lines. SRM: siramesine; RIM: rimcazole.

The therapeutic index (TI) of the selected ligands was also calculated as an LC_{50} to GI_{50} ratio as an indicator of the relative safety of a substance (Figure 5). High TI values indicate a more favorable safety profile. Figure 5 shows that the σ2 agonist siramesine has a very good therapeutic index (>10) in many of the cell lines studied in comparison to the other sigma ligands tested.

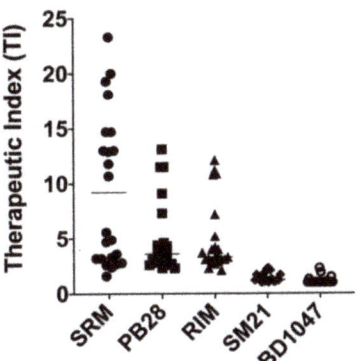

Figure 5. Therapeutic index (TI) values of the selected sigma ligands (SRM, PB28, RIM, SM21, and BD1047) for the 23 human cancer cell lines tested in this study. SRM: siramesine; RIM: rimcazole. Note: In cases where GI_{50} and LC_{50} were higher than the highest tested concentration (100 µM), the TI was calculated using GI_{50} and LC_{50} at 100 µM.

3.3. Sigma Ligands' Sensitivity Was Not Correlated to Their Activity as Either Agonists or Antagonists

We next sought to identify possible patterns in the sigma ligands' sensitivity profiles that could be related to the sigma ligands activity as either agonists or antagonists. GI_{50} values were normalized using the z-score statistical parameter and grouped by cancer type (Figure 6). The z-score normalization reflects the GI_{50} deviation from the mean, in terms of standard deviation. Positive and negative values were plotted along a vertical line that represents the mean GI_{50} value of all the cell lines against the tested sigma ligand. Negative values, projected to the right, represent cellular sensitivities that exceed the mean (i.e., more sensitive cell lines), while positive values, projected to the left, represent cell lines less sensitive to the mean (i.e., more resistant cell lines). Figure 6 shows that there was no distinct sensitivity pattern of the sigma ligands studied herein, regardless of their receptor specificity or the agonistic/antagonistic classification. Instead, it seemed that there was a general sensitivity/resistance pattern, discrete for each cell line, against the effect of the selected sigma ligands. These distinct responses may reflect a cell line or, in some cases, tissue-dependent sigma ligand effect. Indeed, our data suggest that all the lung, renal, and prostate cancer cell lines tested are resistant against all the studied sigma ligands, whereas all colorectal, melanoma, and pancreatic cancer cell lines appeared to be sensitive against the effect of all sigma ligands studied. Focusing on siramesine, which our data indicates has the best in vitro anticancer efficacy, it appears that pancreatic cancer cell lines are more sensitive against siramesine's activity, suggesting that siramesine should be further investigated as a novel putative therapeutic approach in the treatment of pancreatic cancer.

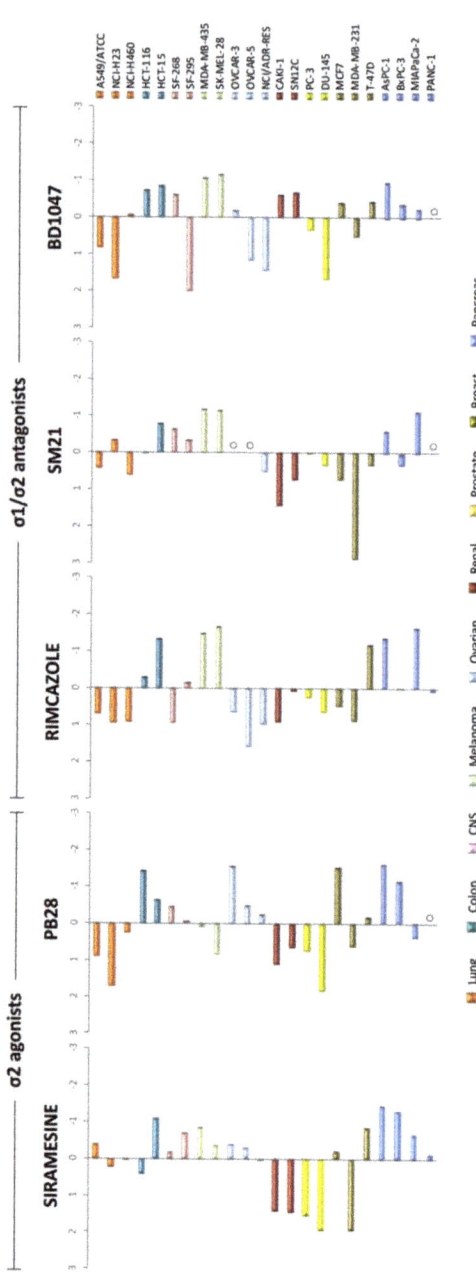

Figure 6. Distribution of z-score-normalized GI$_{50}$ parameter values for each sigma ligand against 23 human cancer cell lines. Cell lines are color-coded to represent different cancer types. The vertical line represents the mean response. Sigma ligand-sensitive cell lines are projected to the right of the vertical line while sigma ligands-resistant cell lines are projected to the left of the vertical line. Open circle (○) means not tested.

3.4. Sigma Receptors Expression Levels Did Not Appear to Correlate with the Sigma Ligands' Antiproliferative Effect

Pearson's linear correlation coefficient (r) was calculated to investigate the relationship between the antiproliferative efficacy of the selected sigma ligands to the expression levels of sigma receptors. The Pearson's r is a statistical measure of the strength of the linear relationship between two variables and is constrained between values $-1 \leq r \leq 1$. Positive r values denote positive linear correlation while negative values denote negative linear correlation. An r of -1 indicates a perfect negative linear relationship, an r of 0 indicates no linear relationship, and an r of 1 indicates a perfect positive linear relationship. Scatter plots of the tested sigma ligands' antiproliferative effect (GI_{50}) versus σ1 expression levels (Figure 7a), PGRMC1 expression levels (Figure 7b), and σ2/TMEM97 expression levels (Figure 7c) were generated, and the Pearson's r was calculated for each relationship. Figure 7a shows that there was a weak negative linear correlation ($r = -0.24$) between siramesine antiproliferative effect and σ1 expression levels, while no other significant correlation was reported between the other tested sigma ligand efficacies and the σ1 expression levels. Figure 7b shows that there was a weak negative linear correlation between siramesine and PB28 antiproliferative effect and PGRMC1 expression levels ($r = -0.2$ and $r = -0.3$, respectively), while no other significant correlation was reported between the other tested sigma ligand efficacies and the PGRMC1 expression levels. Figure 7c shows that there was a weak negative linear correlation between PB28 antiproliferative effect and σ2/TMEM97 expression levels ($r = -0.22$), while no other significant correlation was reported between the other tested sigma ligand efficacies and the σ2/TMEM97 expression levels.

3.5. Putative Sigma Ligands' Mechanism of Action: Prediction Using the COMPARE Algorithm

Sigma ligands' possible mechanism of action (MoA) was investigated using the COMPARE algorithm. The COMPARE algorithm from the Developmental Therapeutics Program, NCI, was used at the GI_{50} level in order to identify compounds from the standard agent database sharing similar mechanisms of growth inhibition with the sigma ligands studied herein. Pairwise correlation coefficients of greater than 0.6 were used as the cut-off for assessing whether two agents were likely to share a similar MoA [17,18]. The NCI anticancer screen employs 60 human tumor cell lines (NCI60 panel) that have been grouped in cancer type subpanels. Since pancreatic cancer is not included in the NCI60 panel, COMPARE analysis was performed on 19 of the 23 human cancer cell lines included in this study. Dose–response curves for each cell line assessed against the tested sigma ligands were converted into "endpoint" patterns, thus giving a snapshot of sigma ligands' activity. GI_{50} values for each of the 19 cell lines plotted against the tested sigma ligands were calculated from the dose–response curves (Figure 3) and converted to their log10 GI_{50} values. Log10 GI_{50} values were averaged, and each value was subtracted from the average to create positive and negative values, referred to as deltas. Plotted delta values along a vertical line represent the mean response of each cell lines in the panel to the test agent. The "mean graph" pattern was unique for each sigma ligand (Figure 8). Positive values project to the right of the vertical line and represent cellular sensitivities to the tested sigma ligand that exceed the mean, while negative values project to the left of the vertical line and represent cell line sensitivities to the tested sigma ligand that were less than the average value. Consistent with our previous observations on the z-score-normalized GI_{50} parameter values for each cell line (Figure 6), the mean graph display showed little similarities between the sigma ligands tested.

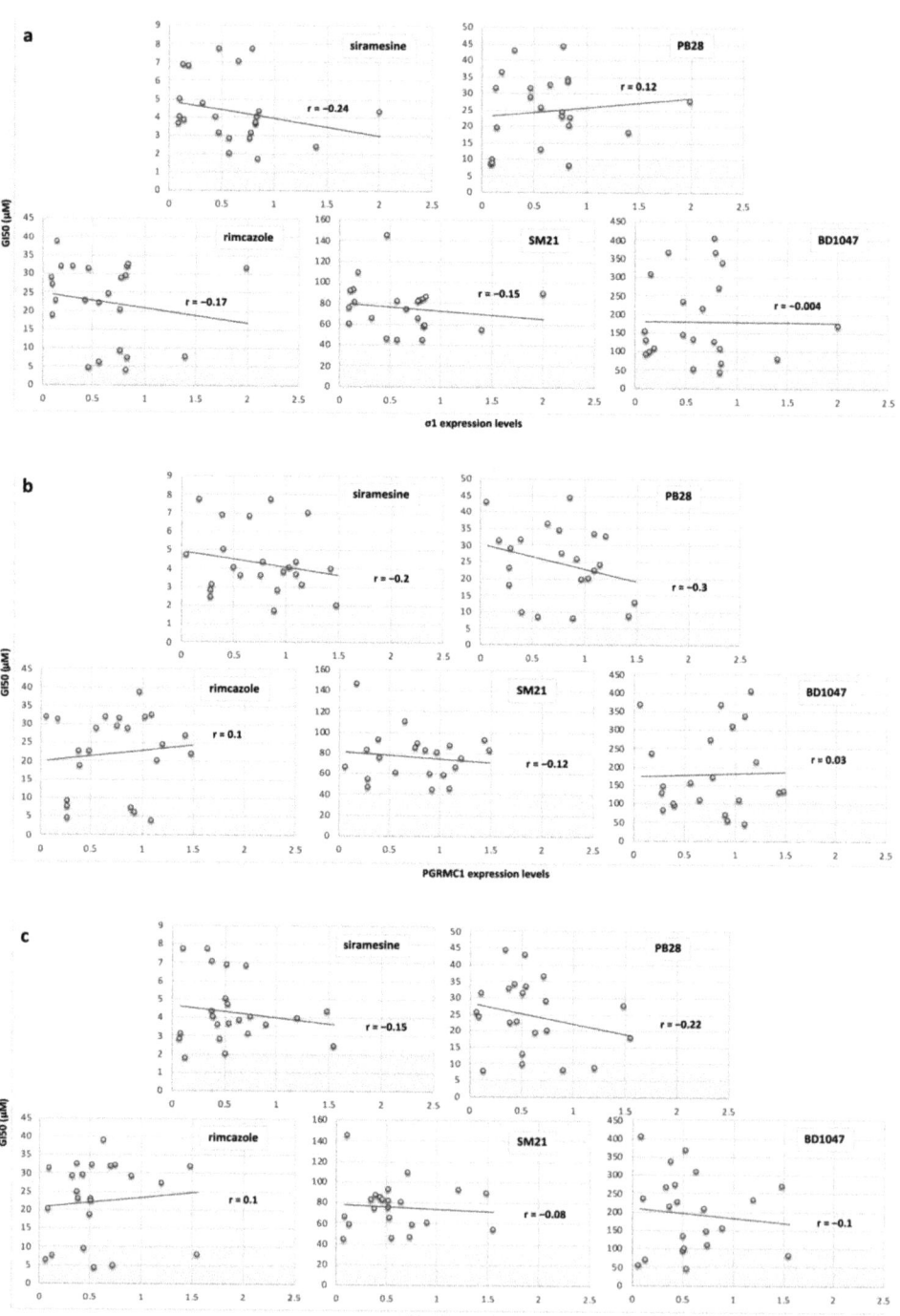

Figure 7. Scatter plots correlating sigma ligand antiproliferative efficacy (GI$_{50}$) versus σ1 expression levels (**a**), PGRMC1 expression levels (**b**), and σ2/TMEM97 expression levels (**c**).

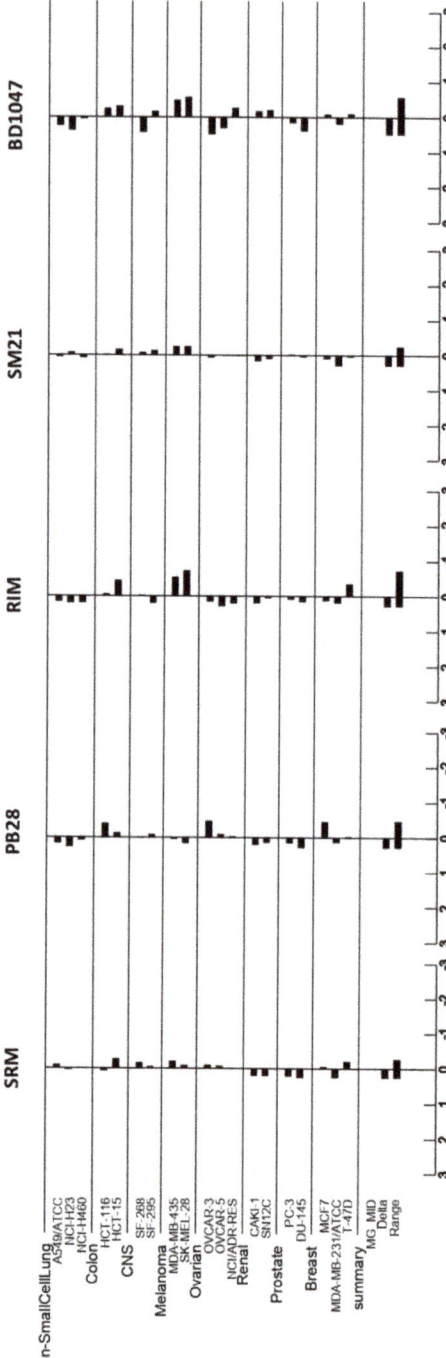

Figure 8. Mean graph plots generated from the National Cancer Institute (NCI, National Institutes of Health, Bethesda, MD, USA) database for the tested sigma ligands siramesine (SRM), PB28 dihydrochloride (PB28), rimcazole (RIM), SM21 maleate (SM21), and BD1047 dihydrobromide (BD1047). Sensitive cell lines are projected to the right of the vertical line, while resistant cell lines are projected to the left of the vertical line. The mean graphs for each of the sigma ligands studied were further used to run the COMPARE algorithm and calculate the Pearson correlation coefficient (PCC) against compounds in the NCI database with known mechanism of action (MoA). The PCC is a measurement of pattern similarity and as such, substances with similar mean graphs show high similarity (high PCC) in their anticancer mechanisms in vitro. The highest similarity between two compounds is expressed with a PCC value approaching 1. A PCC of −1.0 denotes a perfect mirror image, while a PCC of 0 means that there is no correlation between the two compounds [19]. Table 2 shows data retrieved after running the COMPARE algorithm against the NCI standard agents' database and presents the five substances with the highest correlation to the selected sigma ligands, as proposed by the algorithm.

The highest PCC (0.884) was reported for rimcazole to thalicarpine. Thalicarpine (or thaliblastine) is a natural vinca alkaloid with antineoplastic activity, which induces single strand breaks in DNA and arrests cancer cells at the G2/M and G1 phase of the cell cycle. It is also reported to exhibit RNA- and protein synthesis-inhibiting activities [20]. Interestingly, spirogermanium, the second most related compound to rimcazole (PCC 0.687), is also related to protein synthesis inhibition (Table 2, [4]). The second highest correlation, as determined by the PCC, was PB28 with pibenzimol hydrochloride (PCC 0.724), an agent known to inhibit DNA replication by inhibiting topoisomerase I and DNA polymerase. BD1047 and siramesine showed only weak correlations with the tested agents from the standard agents' database (Table 2). BD1047 showed a weak correlation (PCC 0.618) with spirogermanium, which, as mentioned above, is a protein synthesis inhibitor and tamoxifen that reduces DNA synthesis and cellular response to estrogen [21]. Finally, siramesine was found to be weakly associated with dihydro-5-azacytidine (PCC 0.601). Dihydro-5-azacytidine is a synthetic nucleoside analogue of deoxycytidine that inhibits DNA methyltransferase, thereby interfering with abnormal DNA methylation patterns that are associated with genetic instability in some tumor cells consequently acting as an epigenetic modifier drug.

Table 2. The five substances with the highest correlation (PCC) to the selected sigma ligands as proposed by the COMPARE algorithm and their mechanism of action.

Ligand	PCC	Target Vector	Mechanism of Action (MoA)
Siramesine	0.601	dihydro-5-azacytidine	DNA damage [21]
	0.519	cyanomorpholino-ADR	Alkylating agent [22]
	0.507	cytembena	Inhibition of DNA and protein synthesis [23]
	0.487	anguidine	Inhibition of protein synthesis [21]
	0.462	caracemide	Inhibition of DNA synthesis [23]
PB28 dihydrochloride	0.724	pibenzimol hydrochloride	Inhibition of DNA replication [21]
	0.561	cytembena	Inhibition of DNA and protein synthesis [23]
	0.514	chloroquinoxaline sulfonamide	DNA damage [21]
	0.501	tamoxifen	Inhibition of DNA synthesis [23]
	0.46	6-mercaptopurine	Inhibition of DNA synthesis [23]
Rimcazole dihychloride	0.884	thalicarpine	Inhibition of DNA, RNA, and protein synthesis [24]
	0.687	spirogermanium	Inhibition of protein synthesis [25]
	0.541	caracemide	Inhibition of DNA synthesis [21]
	0.516	tetrocarcin A sodium salt	Inhibition of mitochondrial function [26]
	0.513	semustine (methyl-CCNU)	Alkylating agent [21]
SM21 maleate	0.585	anguidine	Inhibition of protein synthesis [21]
	0.523	caracemide	Inhibition of DNA synthesis [21]
	0.490	rhizoxin	Antimitotic agent [21]
	0.485	tetrocarcin A sodium salt	Inhibit mitochondrial function [26]
	0.466	didemnin B	Inhibition of protein synthesis [21]
BD1047 dihydrobromide	0.618	spirogermanium	Inhibition of DNA, RNA, and protein synthesis [25]
	0.618	tamoxifen	Inhibition of DNA synthesis [21]
	0.575	chloroquinoxaline sulfonamide	DNA damage [21]
	0.566	thalicarpine	Inhibition of DNA, RNA, and protein synthesis [24]
	0.543	flavoneacetic acid	Change the permeability of the tumor vasculature [21]

4. Discussion

Sigma receptors have attracted increased research interest over the last few decades, as reflected in the growing number of extensive and complex literature published in this rapidly evolving field. It is now undisputed that σ1 receptor is an allosteric modulator of multiple cellular signaling systems that, in the context of cancer, act as a chaperone protein, which is a component of the cancer cell support machinery [27]. Until recently, σ2 receptor was considered to be related to the progesterone receptor membrane component

1 (PGRMC1) [5]. More recently, studies have revealed the molecular identification of σ2 receptor as TMEM97 [6], thereby elucidating a longstanding pharmacological mystery and paving the way to applying modern molecular biology tools and techniques to mechanistic studies of this receptor. However, the function of σ2 receptor remains a mystery and to make things more complex, recent studies show that PGRMC1 and TMEM97 may co-operate and form a ternary complex of LDLR–PGRMC1–TMEM97 that results in the rapid internalization of LDL by LDLR in HeLa cells [8].

Several studies report overexpression of σ receptors in cancer; however, these studies mainly involved the indirect detection of σ receptors by radio-binding of their selectively labeled ligands [28–31]. In this study, we determined for the first time the expression levels of σ receptors by direct detection of their protein expression via Western blotting, investigating the expression levels of the σ1, σ2/TMEM97, and PGRMC1 receptors simultaneously in 23 human cancer cell lines, representing nine different types of cancer. Our data suggest that σ1, PGRMC1, and σ2/TMEM97 receptors are expressed in the majority of the 23 cell lines tested, exerting different expression patterns without showing any selectivity to a particular cancer type. However, we should emphasize that both σ1 and σ2/TMEM97 showed the highest expression levels in NCI-H460 (non-small cell lung cancer) and HCT-15 (colorectal cancer) cell lines. Of note, several reports suggest overexpression of TMEM97, otherwise known as MAC30, and a correlation with poor outcome in lung and colorectal cancer [32–34]. Moreover, even though the expression of these receptors was diverse, the breast cancer cell line MCF7 expressed high levels (as compared to the majority of the rest of the cancer cell lines tested herein) of both σ2/TMEM97 and PGRMC1 receptors. These findings are to an extent in agreement with data in the literature reporting high expression levels of σ1 receptor in lung cancer [35] and high expression levels of σ2 [36] and PGRMC1 [37] in MCF7 breast cancer cell line. Further, in agreement with the work published by Vilner et al. based on radio-ligand assays [36], sigma-1 receptor was found to be expressed at very low levels in the MCF7 cell line. Overall, we here provide novel data regarding expression—especially of PGRMC1 and σ2/TMEM97, for which very little is known [9]—in different human cancer types and cell lines included in a significant tool for anticancer drug development, the NCI60 cell line panel. Additionally, in light of the putative interaction between these two receptors reported previously [8], it seems that their interrelationship is far more complex as this is judged from the differences in their expression levels in the cell lines tested herein.

On the basis of our data showing that σ1, PGRMC1, and σ2/TMEM97 receptors are highly expressed in many of the cell lines tested, we further explored whether sigma receptors mediate the in vitro anticancer activities of five commonly used sigma ligands. In this context, we investigated the in vitro antiproliferative efficacy of siramesine, PB28 dihydrochloride, rimcazole dihydrochloride, BD1047 dihydrobromide, and SM-21 maleate under the same experimental conditions and against the same panel of the 23 human established cancer cell lines in which the expression levels of σ1, PGRMC1, and σ2/TMEM97 receptors were previously studied. The selected sigma ligands were representative sigma agonists and antagonists with high affinities for σ1 and/or σ2 receptor. It is worth noting that in the literature, the classification of sigma ligands as agonists or antagonists is based on the recapitulation of the σ1 gene overexpression or knockdown phenotypes [38]. First, we attempted to identify possible patterns in the sigma ligands' sensitivity profiles that could be related to the sigma ligands activity as either agonists or antagonists. We must underline that this is the first report where the anticancer activity of those agents is tested under the same experimental conditions and following the guidelines and requirements of the NCI Developmental Therapeutics Program (National Cancer Institute, National Institutes of Health, Bethesda, MD, USA; https://dtp.cancer.gov/), the most successful and comprehensive program worldwide established since 1955 and dedicated to the discovery and development of anticancer drugs. Through this program, many important anticancer drugs such as taxanes, vinca alkaloids, and even more advanced anticancer approaches such as sipeulucel-T have entered clinics. Our data suggest that under the experimental conditions tested in this study, there was no distinct sensitivity pattern between the sigma receptor agonists compared to the sigma receptor antagonists studied. Pearson's linear correlation coefficient (r) was calculated to further investigate the relationship between the antiproliferative efficacy of the selected sigma ligands and the expression levels of sigma receptors. Our data confirmed that there was no significant relationship between sigma receptor expression levels and the sigma ligands' antiproliferative effect ($-0.3 < r < 0.22$). These results indicate that the compounds tested in this study exert their effect mainly through mechanisms that do not involve the σ receptors, even though they show in vitro anticancer activity. A recent study by the group of Mach et al. reported that sigma-2 receptor/TMEM97 and PGRMC1 do not mediate sigma-2 ligand cytotoxicity [39], supporting this assumption. Among the tested σ ligands, the σ2 agonist siramesine was found to exhibit the best antiproliferative, cytostatic, and cytotoxic activity, and thus appears to be the most promising compound. It is also worth noting that, among the nine cancer types studied, pancreatic cancer appears to be the most sensitive cancer type against siramesine. Moreover, of interest is the finding that whilst rimcazole was, in general, found to exert weak anticancer efficacy, the two melanoma cell lines tested were found to be very sensitive to the activity of this compound, even though the σ1 levels in these cell lines were not the highest amongst the 23 cell lines tested herein.

An essential missing element in sigma receptor biology in cancer is a clear definition of the underlying molecular MoA that translates into the cellular response of the sigma receptor ligand effect. In the literature, many potential mechanisms of action have been proposed to mediate sigma ligands' anticancer efficacy, including apoptosis [40,41], autophagy [42], lysosomal destabilization [43], mitochondria destabilization [44], and ferroptosis [45,46]. The diversity in the mechanisms of action show that ligand binding of sigma receptors is a multistep process that may be ligand- or cancer type-dependent, thus underlining the significant need to further validate and expand our knowledge in this field. In this context, we attempted to investigate the potential mechanisms of action of the selected sigma ligands using, for the first time in the field, the COMPARE NCI60 anticancer drug screening algorithm. Consistent with our previous observations, the mean graph displays of the NCI60 cell line screening for the selected sigma ligands, showing only minor similarities between the sigma ligands tested. Interestingly, the most common MoA was found to be related to either the synthesis of DNA or the integrity of DNA followed by protein and RNA synthesis inhibition, as judged by the PCC of the sigma ligands and the standard agents returned after running the COMPARE algorithm. It is also important to note that siramesine, which was found to be the most potent agent, appeared to have the highest degree of association with the DNA damage substance dihydro-5-azacytidine, followed by the alkylating agent cyanomorpholino-ADR, although, in general, these are considered to be moderate-to-low associations on the basis of the corresponding PCC. Thus, an interaction of this compound with DNA might be a part of its MoA.

In conclusion, we show that sigma receptors are indeed expressed in the majority of the 23 human cancer cell lines assessed in this study. We provided evidence that sigma receptor expression does not follow a cancer-type pattern or (with some exceptions) a pairwise expression pattern and that it may not mediate the antiproliferative efficacy of a panel of some very common σ ligands studied in this report. Among the ligands tested, the σ2 receptor ligand siramesine showed the most promising anticancer activity, especially against pancreatic cancer. These findings also provide a platform that rationally warrants the further evaluation of siramesine as a potential anticancer compound, especially against pancreatic cancer.

Author Contributions: Conceptualization, E.S. and K.D.; methodology, E.S., C.T., and E.K.; software E.S.; validation, E.S., C.T., and E.K.; formal analysis, E.S. and K.D.; writing—original draft preparation E.S., N.S., and K.D.; writing—review and editing, E.S., N.S., and K.D.; supervision, K.D.; project administration, K.D.; funding acquisition, K.D. All authors have read and agreed to the published version of the manuscript.

Funding: This research has been co-financed by the European Union and Greek national funds through the Operational Program Competitiveness, Entrepreneurship and Innovation, under the call RESEARCH–CREATE–INNOVATE (project code: T1EDK-01612 and T1EDK-01833).

Institutional Review Board Statement: Not applicable.

Informed Consent Statement: Not applicable.

Data Availability Statement: The data presented in this study are available within the article. For any further request contact the corresponding author.

Acknowledgments: The authors would like to thank Susan Evans-Axelsson for her great help in critically reading and editing the manuscript.

Conflicts of Interest: The authors declare no conflict of interest.

References

1. Martin, W.R.; Eades, C.G.; Thompson, J.A.; Huppler, R.E.; Gilbert, P.E. The effects of morphine- and nalorphine-like drugs in the nondependent and morphine-dependent chronic spinal dog. *J. Pharmacol. Exp. Ther.* **1976**, *197*, 517–532. [PubMed]
2. Hanner, M.; Moebius, F.F.; Flandorfer, A.; Knaus, H.G.; Striessnig, J.; Kempner, E.; Glossmann, H. Purification, molecular cloning, and expression of the mammalian sigma1-binding site. *Proc. Natl. Acad. Sci. USA* **1996**, *93*, 8072–8077. [CrossRef] [PubMed]
3. Kekuda, R.; Prasad, P.D.; Fei, Y.-J.; Leibach, F.H.; Ganapathy, V. Cloning and Functional Expression of the Human Type 1 Sigma Receptor (hSigmaR1). *Biochem. Biophys. Res. Commun.* **1996**, *229*, 553–558. [CrossRef] [PubMed]
4. Hayashi, T.; Su, T.P. Sigma-1 receptor chaperones at the ER-mitochondrion interface regulate Ca(2+) signaling and cell survival. *Cell* **2007**, *131*, 596–610. [CrossRef] [PubMed]
5. Xu, J.; Zeng, C.; Chu, W.; Pan, F.; Rothfuss, J.M.; Zhang, F.; Tu, Z.; Zhou, D.; Zeng, D.; Vangveravong, S.; et al. Identification of the PGRMC1 protein complex as the putative sigma-2 receptor binding site. *Nat. Commun.* **2011**, *2*, 380. [CrossRef]
6. Alon, A.; Schmidt, H.R.; Wood, M.D.; Sahn, J.J.; Martin, S.F.; Kruse, A.C. Identification of the gene that codes for the sigma2 receptor. *Proc. Natl. Acad. Sci. USA* **2017**, *114*, 7160–7165. [CrossRef]
7. Schmit, K.; Michiels, C. TMEM Proteins in Cancer: A Review. *Front. Pharm.* **2018**, *9*, 1345. [CrossRef]
8. Riad, A.; Zeng, C.; Weng, C.-C.; Winters, H.; Xu, K.; Makvandi, M.; Metz, T.; Carlin, S.; Mach, R.H. Sigma-2 Receptor/TMEM97 and PGRMC-1 Increase the Rate of Internalization of LDL by LDL Receptor through the Formation of a Ternary Complex. *Sci. Rep.* **2018**, *8*, 16845. [CrossRef]
9. Schmidt, H.R.; Kruse, A.C. The Molecular Function of sigma Receptors: Past, Present, and Future. *Trends Pharm. Sci.* **2019**, *40*, 636–654. [CrossRef]
10. Georgiadis, M.O.; Karoutzou, O.; Foscolos, A.S.; Papanastasiou, I. Sigma Receptor (sigmaR) Ligands with Antiproliferative and Anticancer Activity. *Molecules* **2017**, *22*, 1408. [CrossRef]
11. Covell, D.G.; Huang, R.; Wallqvist, A. Anticancer medicines in development: Assessment of bioactivity profiles within the National Cancer Institute anticancer screening data. *Mol. Cancer Ther.* **2007**, *6*, 2261–2270. [CrossRef]
12. Søby, K.K.; Mikkelsen, J.D.; Meier, E.; Thomsen, C. Lu 28-179 labels a sigma(2)-site in rat and human brain. *Neuropharmacology* **2002**, *43*, 95–100. [CrossRef]
13. Berardi, F.; Colabufo, N.A.; Giudice, G.; Perrone, R.; Tortorella, V.; Govoni, S.; Lucchi, L. New sigma and 5-HT1A receptor ligands: Omega-(tetralin-1-yl)-n-alkylamine derivatives. *J. Med. Chem.* **1996**, *39*, 176–182. [CrossRef]
14. Ferris, R.M.; Tang, F.L.; Chang, K.J.; Russell, A. Evidence that the potential antipsychotic agent rimcazole (BW 234U) is a specific, competitive antagonist of sigma sites in brain. *Life Sci.* **1986**, *38*, 2329–2337. [CrossRef]
15. Ghelardini, C.; Galeotti, N.; Gualtieri, F.; Bellucci, C.; Manetti, D.; Giotti, A.; Malmberg-Aiello, P.; Galli, A.; Bartolini, A. Antinociceptive profile of 3-alpha-tropanyl 2-(4-Cl-phenoxy)butyrate (SM-21) [corrected]: A novel analgesic with a presynaptic cholinergic mechanism of action. *J. Pharm. Exp.* **1997**, *282*, 430–439.
16. Matsumoto, R.R.; Bowen, W.D.; Tom, M.A.; Vo, V.N.; Truong, D.D.; De Costa, B.R. Characterization of two novel sigma receptor ligands: Antidystonic effects in rats suggest sigma receptor antagonism. *Eur. J. Pharm.* **1995**, *280*, 301–310. [CrossRef]
17. Developmental Therapeutics Program. Available online: https://dtp.cancer.gov/databases_tools/compare.htm (accessed on 24 March 2020).
18. Mahaira, L.G.; Tsimplouli, C.; Sakellaridis, N.; Alevizopoulos, K.; Demetzos, C.; Han, Z.; Pantazis, P.; Dimas, K. The labdane diterpene sclareol (labd-14-ene-8, 13-diol) induces apoptosis in human tumor cell lines and suppression of tumor growth in vivo via a p53-independent mechanism of action. *Eur. J. Pharmacol.* **2011**, *666*, 173–182. [CrossRef]
19. Holbeck, S.L.; Collins, J.M.; Doroshow, J.H. Analysis of Food and Drug Administration-approved anticancer agents in the NCI60 panel of human tumor cell lines. *Mol. Cancer* **2010**, *9*, 1451–1460. [CrossRef]
20. Allen, L.M.; Creaven, P.J. Inhibition of Macromolecular Biosynthesis in Cultured L1210 Mouse Leukemia Cells by Thalicarpine (NSC 68075). *Cancer Res.* **1973**, *33*, 3112–3116.
21. NCI Drug Dictionary. Available online: https://www.cancer.gov/publications/dictionaries/cancer-drug (accessed on 26 December 2020).

2. Wilson, J.J.; Lippard, S.J. In vitro anticancer activity of cis-diammineplatinum(II) complexes with β-diketonate leaving group ligands. *J. Med. Chem.* **2012**, *55*, 5326–5336. [CrossRef]
3. Jackson, R.C.; Taylor, G.A.; Harrap, K.R. Aspects of the biochemical pharmacology of cytembena. *Neoplasma* **1975**, *22*, 259–268.
4. Isah, T. Anticancer Alkaloids from Trees: Development into Drugs. *Pharm. Rev.* **2016**, *10*, 90–99. [CrossRef]
5. Slavik, M.; Blanc, O.; Davis, J. Spirogermanium: A new investigational drug of novel structure and lack of bone marrow toxicity. *Investig. New Drugs* **1983**, *1*, 225–234. [CrossRef]
6. Fang, J.; Zhang, Y.; Huang, L.; Jia, X.; Zhang, Q.; Zhang, X.; Tang, G.; Liu, W. Cloning and Characterization of the Tetrocarin A Gene Cluster from *Micromonospora chalcea* NRRL 11289 Reveals a Highly Conserved Strategy for Tetronate Biosynthesis in Spirotetronate Antibiotics. *J. Bacteriol.* **2008**, *190*, 6014–6025. [CrossRef]
7. Mori, T.; Hayashi, T.; Hayashi, E.; Su, T.P. Sigma-1 receptor chaperone at the ER-mitochondrion interface mediates the mitochondrion-ER-nucleus signaling for cellular survival. *PLoS ONE* **2013**, *8*, e76941. [CrossRef]
8. Leithner, K.; Wohlkoenig, C.; Stacher, E.; Lindenmann, J.; Hofmann, N.A.; Gallé, B.; Guelly, C.; Quehenberger, F.; Stiegler, P.; Smolle-Jüttner, F.M.; et al. Hypoxia increases membrane metallo-endopeptidase expression in a novel lung cancer ex vivo model—role of tumor stroma cells. *BMC Cancer* **2014**, *14*, 40. [CrossRef]
9. Spruce, B.A.; Campbell, L.A.; McTavish, N.; Cooper, M.A.; Appleyard, M.V.; O'Neill, M.; Howie, J.; Samson, J.; Watt, S.; Murray, K.; et al. Small molecule antagonists of the sigma-1 receptor cause selective release of the death program in tumor and self-reliant cells and inhibit tumor growth in vitro and in vivo. *Cancer Res.* **2004**, *64*, 4875–4886. [CrossRef]
10. Schrock, J.M.; Spino, C.M.; Longen, C.G.; Stabler, S.M.; Marino, J.C.; Pasternak, G.W.; Kim, F.J. Sequential cytoprotective responses to Sigma1 ligand-induced endoplasmic reticulum stress. *Mol. Pharm.* **2013**, *84*, 751–762. [CrossRef]
11. Brune, S.; Schepmann, D.; Lehmkuhl, K.; Frehland, B.; Wünsch, B. Characterization of Ligand Binding to the σ1 Receptor in a Human Tumor Cell Line (RPMI 8226) and Establishment of a Competitive Receptor Binding Assay. *Assay Drug Dev. Technol.* **2011**, *10*, 365–374. [CrossRef]
12. Han, K.Y.; Gu, X.; Wang, H.R.; Liu, D.; Lv, F.Z.; Li, J.N. Overexpression of MAC30 is associated with poor clinical outcome in human non-small-cell lung cancer. *Tumour Biol.* **2013**, *34*, 821–825. [CrossRef]
13. Moparthi, S.B.; Arbman, G.; Wallin, A.; Kayed, H.; Kleeff, J.; Zentgraf, H.; Sun, X.F. Expression of MAC30 protein is related to survival and biological variables in primary and metastatic colorectal cancers. *Int. J. Oncol.* **2007**, *30*, 91–95. [CrossRef] [PubMed]
14. Ding, H.; Gui, X.H.; Lin, X.B.; Chen, R.H.; Cai, H.R.; Fen, Y.; Sheng, Y.L. Prognostic Value of MAC30 Expression in Human Pure Squamous Cell Carcinomas of the Lung. *Asian Pac. J. Cancer Prev.* **2016**, *17*, 2705–2710. [PubMed]
15. Aydar, E.; Onganer, P.; Perrett, R.; Djamgoz, M.B.; Palmer, C.P. The expression and functional characterization of sigma (sigma) 1 receptors in breast cancer cell lines. *Cancer Lett.* **2006**, *242*, 245–257. [CrossRef]
16. Vilner, B.J.; John, C.S.; Bowen, W.D. Sigma-1 and sigma-2 receptors are expressed in a wide variety of human and rodent tumor cell lines. *Cancer Res.* **1995**, *55*, 408–413. [PubMed]
17. Neubauer, H.; Adam, G.; Seeger, H.; Mueck, A.O.; Solomayer, E.; Wallwiener, D.; Cahill, M.A.; Fehm, T. Membrane-initiated effects of progesterone on proliferation and activation of VEGF in breast cancer cells. *Climacteric* **2009**, *12*, 230–239. [CrossRef] [PubMed]
18. Nguyen, L.; Lucke-Wold, B.P.; Mookerjee, S.A.; Cavendish, J.Z.; Robson, M.J.; Scandinaro, A.L.; Matsumoto, R.R. Role of sigma-1 receptors in neurodegenerative diseases. *J. Pharm. Sci.* **2015**, *127*, 17–29. [CrossRef]
19. Zeng, C.; Weng, C.-C.; Schneider, M.E.; Puentes, L.; Riad, A.; Xu, K.; Makvandi, M.; Jin, L.; Hawkins, W.G.; Mach, R.H. TMEM97 and PGRMC1 do not mediate sigma-2 ligand-induced cell death. *Cell Death Discov.* **2019**, *5*, 58. [CrossRef]
20. Crawford, K.W.; Bowen, W.D. Sigma-2 receptor agonists activate a novel apoptotic pathway and potentiate antineoplastic drugs in breast tumor cell lines. *Cancer Res.* **2002**, *62*, 313–322.
21. Kashiwagi, H.; McDunn, J.E.; Simon, P.O.; Goedegebuure, P.S.; Xu, J.; Jones, L.; Chang, K.; Johnston, F.; Trinkaus, K.; Hotchkiss, R.S.; et al. Selective sigma-2 ligands preferentially bind to pancreatic adenocarcinomas: Applications in diagnostic imaging and therapy. *Mol. Cancer* **2007**, *6*, 48. [CrossRef]
22. Zeng, C.; Rothfuss, J.; Zhang, J.; Chu, W.; Vangveravong, S.; Tu, Z.; Pan, F.; Chang, K.C.; Hotchkiss, R.; Mach, R.H. Sigma-2 ligands induce tumour cell death by multiple signalling pathways. *Br. J. Cancer* **2012**, *106*, 693–701. [CrossRef]
23. Ostenfeld, M.S.; Fehrenbacher, N.; Høyer-Hansen, M.; Thomsen, C.; Farkas, T.; Jäättelä, M. Effective tumor cell death by sigma-2 receptor ligand siramesine involves lysosomal leakage and oxidative stress. *Cancer Res.* **2005**, *65*, 8975–8983. [CrossRef] [PubMed]
24. Hafner Česen, M.; Repnik, U.; Turk, V.; Turk, B. Siramesine triggers cell death through destabilisation of mitochondria, but not lysosomes. *Cell Death Dis.* **2013**, *4*, e818. [CrossRef] [PubMed]
25. Ma, S.; Henson, E.S.; Chen, Y.; Gibson, S.B. Ferroptosis is induced following siramesine and lapatinib treatment of breast cancer cells. *Cell Death Dis.* **2016**, *7*, e2307. [CrossRef] [PubMed]
26. Bai, T.; Wang, S.; Zhao, Y.; Zhu, R.; Wang, W.; Sun, Y. Haloperidol, a sigma receptor 1 antagonist, promotes ferroptosis in hepatocellular carcinoma cells. *Biochem. Biophys. Res. Commun.* **2017**, *491*, 919–925. [CrossRef]

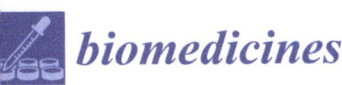

Article

Pharmacoinformatics and Preclinical Studies of NSC765690 and NSC765599, Potential STAT3/CDK2/4/6 Inhibitors with Antitumor Activities against NCI60 Human Tumor Cell Lines

Bashir Lawal [1,2,†], Yen-Lin Liu [3,4,5,6,†], Ntlotlang Mokgautsi [1,2], Harshita Khedkar [1,2], Maryam Rachmawati Sumitra [1,2], Alexander T. H. Wu [6,7,8,9,*] and Hsu-Shan Huang [1,2,9,10,11,*]

1. PhD Program for Cancer Molecular Biology and Drug Discovery, College of Medical Science and Technology, Taipei Medical University and Academia Sinica, Taipei 11031, Taiwan; d621108004@tmu.edu.tw (B.L.); d621108006@tmu.edu.tw (N.M.); d621108005@tmu.edu.tw (H.K.); maryamrachma60@gmail.com (M.R.S.)
2. Graduate Institute for Cancer Biology and Drug Discovery, College of Medical Science and Technology, Taipei Medical University, Taipei 11031, Taiwan
3. Department of Pediatrics, Taipei Medical University Hospital, Taipei 11031, Taiwan; yll.always@gmail.com
4. Taipei Cancer Center, Taipei Medical University, Taipei 11031, Taiwan
5. Department of Medicine, School of Medicine, College of Medicine, Taipei Medical University, Taipei 11031, Taiwan
6. TMU Research Center of Cancer Translational Medicine, Taipei Medical University, Taipei 11031, Taiwan
7. The PhD Program of Translational Medicine, College of Science and Technology, Taipei Medical University, Taipei 11031, Taiwan
8. Clinical Research Center, Taipei Medical University Hospital, Taipei Medical University, Taipei 11031, Taiwan
9. Graduate Institute of Medical Sciences, National Defense Medical Center, Taipei 11490, Taiwan
10. School of Pharmacy, National Defense Medical Center, Taipei 11490, Taiwan
11. PhD Program in Biotechnology Research and Development, College of Pharmacy, Taipei Medical University, Taipei 11031, Taiwan
* Correspondence: chaw1211@tmu.edu.tw (A.T.H.W.); huanghs99@tmu.edu.tw (H.-S.H.)
† These authors contributed equally to this work.

Abstract: Signal transducer and activator of transcription 3 (STAT3) is a transcriptional regulator of a number of biological processes including cell differentiation, proliferation, survival, and angiogenesis, while cyclin-dependent kinases (CDKs) are a critical regulator of cell cycle progression. These proteins appear to play central roles in angiogenesis and cell survival and are widely implicated in tumor progression. In this study, we used the well-characterized US National Cancer Institute 60 (NCI60) human tumor cell lines to screen the in vitro anti-cancer activities of our novel small molecule derivatives (NSC765690 and NSC765599) of salicylanilide. Furthermore, we used the DTP-COMPARE algorithm and in silico drug target prediction to identify the potential molecular targets, and finally, we used molecular docking to assess the interaction between the compounds and prominent potential targets. We found that NSC765690 and NSC765599 exhibited an anti-proliferative effect against the 60 panels of NCI human cancer cell lines, and dose-dependent cytotoxic preference for NSCLC, melanoma, renal, and breast cancer cell lines. Protein–ligand interactions studies revealed that NSC765690 and NSC765599 were favored ligands for STAT3/CDK2/4/6. Moreover, cyclization of the salicylanilide core scaffold of NSC765690 mediated its higher anti-cancer activities and had greater potential to interact with STAT3/CDK2/4/6 than did NSC765599 with an open-ring structure. NSC765690 and NSC765599 met the required safety and criteria of a good drug candidate, and are thus worthy of further in-vitro and in-vivo investigations in tumor-bearing mice to assess their full therapeutic efficacy.

Keywords: protein-ligand interaction; molecular docking simulation; target identification; small-molecule derivatives of salicylanilide; drug discovery; drug development

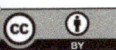

1. Introduction

Despite advances in biomedical research, cancer remains a public health concern and is currently ranked the second leading cause of global mortality [1,2]. The etiology of cancer is often multifactorial, involving an interplay between genetic and epigenetic factors which amount to dysregulation of molecular networks, proteins, RNA, and DNA in favor of cell growth and proliferation [3,4]. The survival, growth, and metastasis of tumor cells depend on cellular differentiation, proliferation, angiogenic, and apoptotic mechanisms [5], which are controlled by a range of protein kinases and signal transduction pathways [6,7]. Cyclin-dependent kinases (CDKs) are a family of serine/threonine protein kinases with catalytic and regulatory subunits [8]. Out of the nine CDKs so far identified, four (CDK1, CDK2, CDK4, and CDK6) play important regulatory roles in the cell cycle; CDK4/D-cyclin, CDK2/E-cyclin, and CDK6/D-cyclin regulate the G_1 to S phase of the cell cycle transition, while the complex of CDK1 or CDK2 with cyclin A regulates the S to G_2 transition [9]. Under physiological conditions, the catalytic and regulatory (cyclin) subunits of CDKs remain dissociated. However, periodic complexation of a cyclin with its catalytic unit leads to its activation and phosphorylation of a variety of downstream target proteins required for cell cycle progression [10,11]. CDKs regulate cell cycle transitions via phosphorylation and subsequent inactivation of the retinoblastoma (Rb) protein, a tumor suppressor that prevents cell cycle transition [12]. Thus, the inactivation of this Rb protein allows the free flow and progression of cells into the cell cycle, leading to multi-cell cycles, cell proliferation, and eventual development into cancer cells [12].

A number of key oncogenic abnormalities, including amplification of cyclin D; inactivation of CDKN2A (p16); and deletions/mutations upstream of cyclin D, such as activating mutations of phosphatidylinositol 4,5-bisphosphate 3-kinase catalytic subunit alpha (PIK3CA)/the B-raf proto-oncogene, serine/threonine kinase (BRAF), and phosphatase and tensin homolog (PTEN) deletion [13,14], were identified as contributing factors to hyperactive CDKs and consequently deregulated the cell cycle. Therefore, since dysfunctional cell cycle regulation via oncogenic aberrations of CDKs is a hallmark of all human cancers [15], pharmacological targeting of CDKs will undoubtedly affect cancer proliferation and survival [16,17]. Hence, CDK inhibitors have been developed and evaluated; however, disappointingly, while first-generation inhibitors of CDK were non-selective and besieged with toxicity [18,19], second-generation CDK4/6 inhibitors, although showing promising outcomes, are plagued with acquired resistance, which develops in almost all cases [20] due to the activation of other oncogenic pathways, including c-Myc, signal transducer and activator of transcription 3 (STAT3), and phosphatidylinositol 3-kinase (PI3K)/AKT/mammalian target of rapamycin (mTOR) signaling pathways [21,22].

STAT3 is a cytoplasmic transcription factor involved in a number of biological processes including cell differentiation, proliferation, survival, and angiogenesis [23]. Overexpression of STAT3 is associated with poor clinical prognoses of cancer patients [24]. It is therefore not surprising that the STAT3 signaling axis has long been explored in cancer therapy owing to its roles in tumor formation, metastasis, and therapeutic failure [25,26]. Preclinical studies revealed that aberrant STAT3 expression mediates immunosuppression of tumor cells [27,28], while inhibition of STAT3 re-sensitizes therapy-resistance breast cancer cells to palbociclib treatment [29]. Summing up the above clinical and preclinical evidence, it is convincing that identifying and validating novel CDK inhibitors capable of simultaneously targeting STAT3 signaling may open up new windows for long-lasting and multilayered tumor control [30].

The translational value of knowledge of cancer biology into developing effective prognostic/diagnostic and therapeutic strategies for clinical practice remains disappointing [31]. However, increasing knowledge of the molecular basis of tumorigenesis, applications of multi-omics approaches, and molecular simulations based on a structural analysis of receptor–ligand interactions have jointly contributed to the identification of more-reliable predictive markers and the discovery of novel, less-toxic, and target-specific anticancer agents [31–34]. At present, substantial attention is being focused on small molecules for targeted therapy in cancer treatments [35].

NSC765599 and NSC765690 are small molecule derivatives of salicylanilides (PubChem CID: 60202556; NDMC101), which were previously synthesized and evaluated for biological activities in our Lab [36]. We had previously conducted a series of chemical modifications of the lead molecule, NDMC101, to yield the open ring (NSC765599) [37] and close ring (NSC765690) [38] derivatives. Herein we demonstrated that both NSC765690 and NSC765599 exerted antitumor activities in vitro against panels of NCI60 human tumor cell lines. We further identified and validated CDK2/4/6 and STAT3 as druggable candidates for the compounds, through in silico and molecular simulation of ligand–receptor interaction studies. Hence, our data provide evidence that expressions of CDK2/4/6 and STAT3 can be directly regulated by NSC765690 and NSC765599 with consequent antitumor implications in multiple cancer types.

2. Materials and Methods

2.1. In Vitro Anticancer Screening against 60 Full NCI Cell Panels of Human Tumor Cell Lines

NSC765690 and NSC765599 (Figure 1) were submitted to the National Cancer Institute (NCI) for the screening of its panel of NCI60 cancer cell lines. The preliminary single-dose screening of the two compounds was conducted against 60 full NCI cell line panels comprising melanomas, leukemia, central nervous system (CNS) cancers, NSCLC, renal cancer, breast cancer, ovarian cancer, and prostate cancer in agreement with the protocol of the NCI. Following single-dose testing at 10 µM, the two compounds were selected for five-dose screening against the same panels of cancer cell lines. As described previously [39,40], protocols for NCI60 cell five-dose screening involved seeding of about 5000~40,000 cells/well (depending on the doubling time of individual cell lines) in 96-well plates, followed by treatment with NSC765690 or NSC765599 at concentrations of 0.01, 0.1, 1.0, 10, and 100 µM and incubation at 37 °C in 5% humidified CO_2 for 48 h. Cells were fixed with a sulforhodamine B (SRB) solution [41] followed by a series of washing and staining to determine their viability. Growth inhibition was calculated relative to cells without drug treatment and time-zero control. Results of the five-dose assay are represented in terms of a dose-dependent curve, tumor growth inhibition (TGI), LC_{50} (concentration needed to kill 50% of cells by cytotoxic activity) for each cell line tested, and GI_{50} (concentration needed to inhibit 50% of cancer cell growth) [42]. Results were presented as cell growth relative to the untreated cell control and to the time zero number of cells. Growth inhibitions were indicated by values between 0 and 100, while lethality (cytotoxic effect) was indicated by values less than 0.

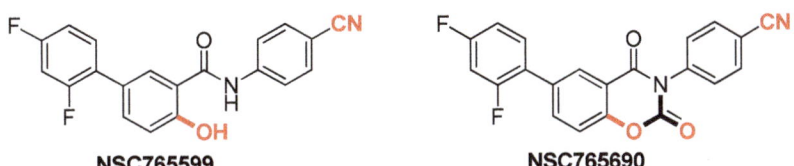

Figure 1. Chemical structures of NSC765599 (N-(4-cyanophenyl)-2′,4′-difluoro-4-hydroxy-[1,10-biphenyl]-3-carboxamide) and NSC765690 (4-(6-(2,4-Difluorophenyl)-2,4-dioxo-2H-benzo[e][1,3]-oxazin-3(4H)-yl) benzonitrile).

2.2. Identifying the Molecular Targets and Therapeutic Classes of NSC765599 and NSC765690

NSC765599 and NSC765690 were screened for potential drug target using SwissTarget prediction algorithm, which predicts potential drug target based on the principle of similarity [43]. In addition, we also employ the computer-aided Prediction of Biological Activity Spectra (PASS) web resources to predict the potential drug targets [44]. The activity patterns (fingerprints) of both NSC765599 and NSC765690 were correlated to NCI synthetic compounds, standard agents and molecular targets using the DTP-COMPARE algorithms [45]. The NSC numerical IDs were used as "seed" while GI_{50}, TGI and LC_{50} were set as the endpoints.

2.3. In Silico Molecular Docking Analyses

The three-dimensional (3D) structure of palbociclib (CID: 5330286) and SH-4-54 (CID 72188643) were retrieved in SDF file format from the PubChem database, while the 3D structures of NSC765690 and NSC765599 were drawn out in sybyl mol2 format using the Avogadro molecular builder and visualization tool vers. 1.XX [46] and were subsequently transformed into the protein data bank (PDB) format using the PyMOL Molecular Graphics System, vers. 1.2r3pre (Schrödinger, LLC). The PDB file of the 3D structure of the receptors and crystal structures of apo CDK2 (PDB; 4EK3), CDK4/cyclin D3 (PDB 3G33), CDK6/cyclin (PDB; 1JOW), and STAT3 (PDB; 4ZIA), were retrieved from the Protein Data Bank. The PDB file formats of the ligands (NSC765690, NSC765599, and palbociclib) and the receptors (STAT3; CDK2, 4, and 6) were subsequently converted into the Auto Dock Pdbqt format using AutoDock Vina (vers. 0.8, The Scripps Research Institute, La Jolla, CA, USA) [47]. Pre-docking preparation of the receptors followed the removal of water molecules, while hydrogen atoms and Kolmman charges were added accordingly. Molecular docking studies were performed using Autodock VINA software and by following the protocols described in our previous study [3]. The docking results based on hydrogen bonds and electrostatic and hydrophobic interactions of the best pose of the ligand–receptor complexes were expressed as binding energy values (kcal/mol). PyMOL software was used to visualize H-bond interactions, binding affinities, interacting amino acid residues, binding atoms on the ligands and receptors, and 3D graphical representations of ligand-receptor complexes, while 2D graphical illustrations of ligand-binding interactions were further visualized using Discovery studio visualizer vers. 19.1.0.18287 (BIOVIA, San Diego, CA, USA) [48].

2.4. Pharmacokinetics, Drug-Likeness, Toxicity and Medicinal Chemical Analyses

The drug-likeness, medicinal chemistry, and pharmacokinetics, including the adsorption, distribution, metabolism, excretion, and toxicity (ADMET) properties of NSC765690 and NSC765599 were analyzed using SwissADME software developed by the Swiss Institute of Bioinformatics [49]. The drug-likeness properties were analyzed in terms of Ghose (Amgen), Egan (Pharmacia), and Veber (GSK), and more importantly, the Lipinski (Pfizer) rule-of-five, as well as cLogP, molecular mass, hydrogen acceptor, hydrogen donor, and molar refractive index [50] for drug-likeness and drug discovery. The Abbot Bioavailability Score was calculated based on the probability of the compound to have at least 0.1 (10%) oral bioavailability in rats or measurable Caco-2 permeability [51], while gastrointestinal absorption and brain penetration properties were analyzed using the Brain Or IntestinaL EstimateD permeation (BOILED-Egg) model [52]. The acute toxicity (LD_{50}) in rats and environmental toxicity were predicted using GUSAR software [53].

2.5. Data Analysis

Spearman's rank correlation was used to assess the correlations of NSC765599 and NSC765690 fingerprints with NCI synthetic compounds, standard agents, and molecular targets. The COMPARE correlation threshold was set to ≥ 45 common cell lines, ≥ 0.1 correlation coefficient, and ≥ 0.05 standard deviation. The growth inhibition by NSC765690 and NSC765599 in single-dose assay was obtained by subtracting the positive value on the plot from 100, i.e., a value of 40 would mean 60% growth inhibition.

3. Results

3.1. NSC765690 and NSC765599 Exhibited Anti-Proliferative Effects on NCI60 Human Cancer Cell Lines

Both NSC765690 and NSC765599 exhibited anti-proliferative effect against all the 60 panels of NCI human cancer cell lines (Figure 2). Furthermore, single-dose treatment with NSC765690 and NSC765599 also demonstrated cytotoxic effects against some cell lines. As indicated by the percentage growth altered by treatment, melanoma (SK-MEL-5, SK-MEL-2, and MALME-3M), renal (A498, UO-31, and CAKI-1), leukemia (HL-60, molt-4, and RPMI-8226), and breast (MDA-MB-468, T-47D, and HS 578T) cancer cell lines were the most responsive to NSC765690 treatment. For NSC765599, melanoma, renal cancer, leukemia, and the breast cancer cell line were also sensitive to cytotoxic effects of NSC765599 at 10 µM. However, panels of prostate, ovarian, and colon cancer cell lines were less responsive to NSC765690 and NSC765599 treatment (Figure 2). These primary single dose screening results clearly indicated the anti-proliferative activities of NSC765690 and NSC765599 against different kinds of human cancer cell lines, and thus are worthy of further evaluation for dose-dependent activities.

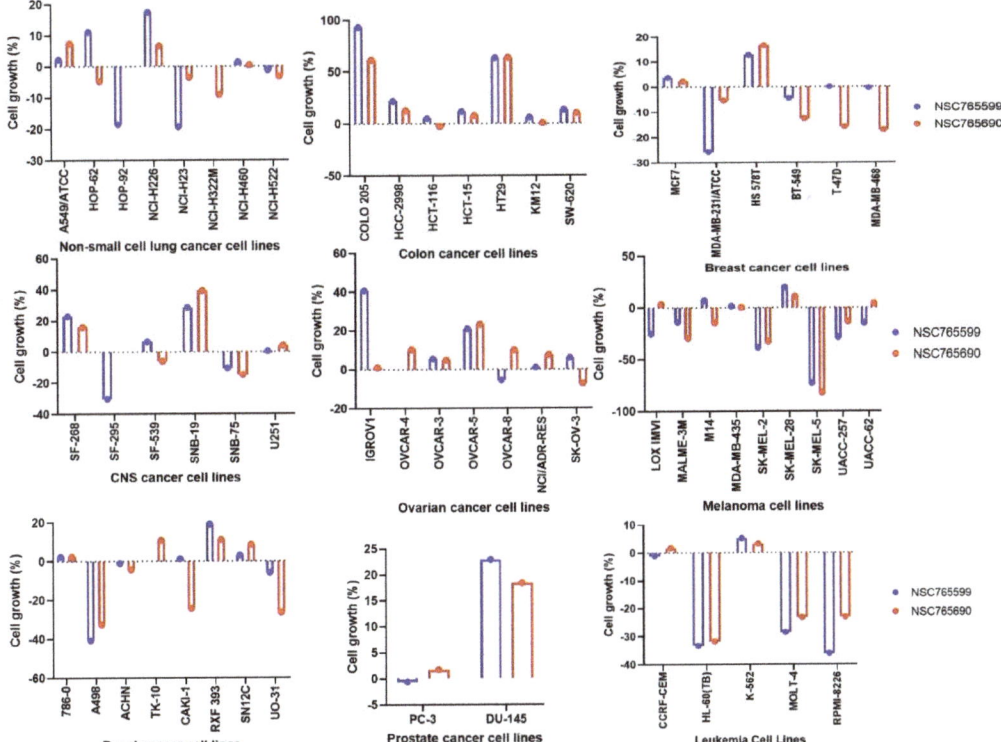

Figure 2. Anti-proliferative effect of NSC765690 and NSC765599 against panels of 60 human cancer cell lines. Each cell line was treated with a single dose of (10 µM) of each compound. The zero points denote the mean percentage of cell growth. The percentage growth inhibition of each cell line relative to the mean is represented by values under 100, whereas those values below 0 indicate cell death.

3.2. NSC765690 and NSC765599 Exhibited Dose-Dependent Cytotoxic Effects against NCI 60 Human Cancer Cell Lines

Both NSC765690 and NSC765599 exhibited dose-dependent cytotoxic activities against melanoma (SK-MEL-5, SK-MEL-2, and MALME-3M), NSCLC (HOP-92, A549/ATCC, NCI-H23, NCI-H522, and NCI-H522), CNS (SF-268, SNB-19, and U251), renal (A498, UO-31, and CAKI-1), leukemia (HL-60, molt-4, and RPMI-8226), and breast (MDA-MB-468, T-47D, and HS 578T) cancer cell lines (Figures 3 and 4). The GI_{50} values ranged from 0.14~2.79 µM in NSC76569-treated cell lines and 0.219~5.55 µM in NSC765599-treated cell lines. Consistent with the activities demonstrated in single-dose treatments, the NSCLC, melanoma, renal, and breast cancer cell lines were most sensitive to NSC765690 treatment, while leukemia, CNS, ovarian, and colon cancer cell lines were the least sensitive to NSC765690 (Table 1). Analysis of LC_{50} values also indicated that the melanoma cell lines were the most sensitive to drug treatments, with NSC765690 being the most active (Table 1).

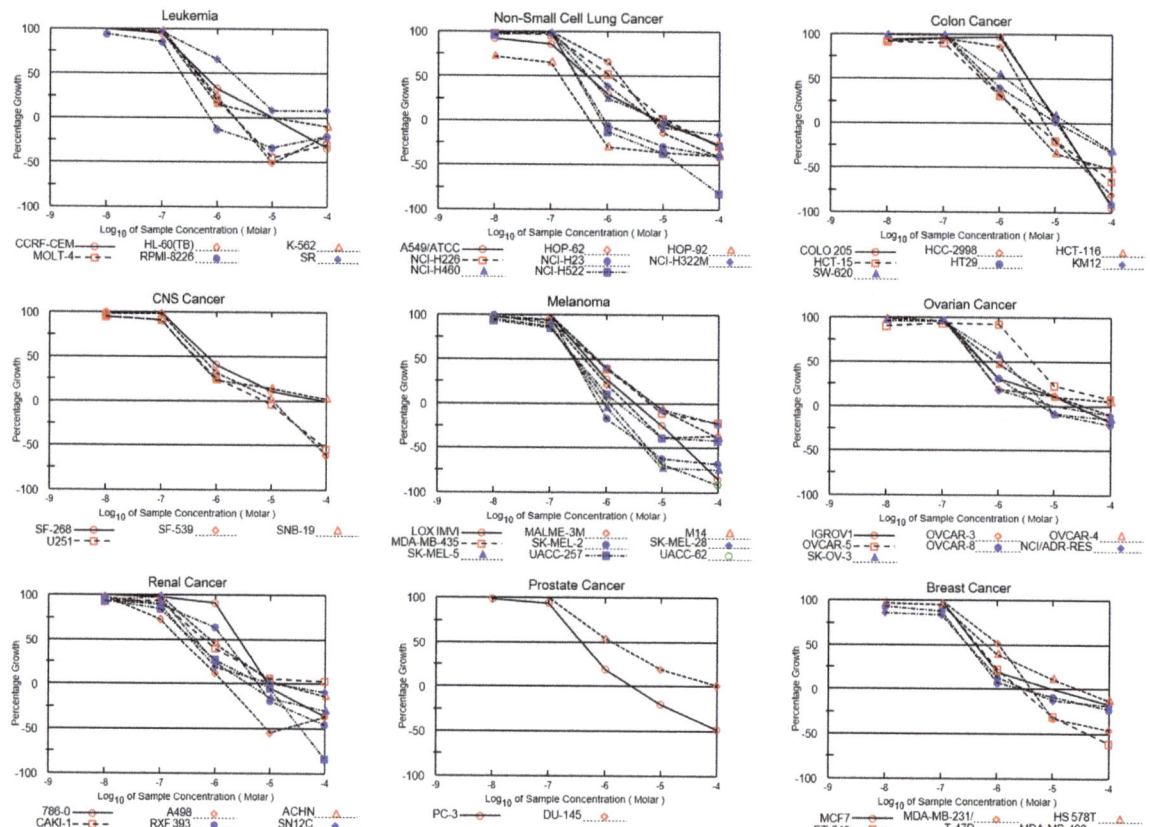

Figure 3. Dose–cytotoxic response curves of NSC765690 against panels of 60 NCI human cancer cell lines. The growth percentage value of +100 on the Y-axis represents the growth of untreated cells, the 0 value represents no net growth, while −100 represents the complete death of cells.

3.3. NSC765599 and NSC765690 Shared Similar NCI Anti-Cancer Fingerprints and Molecular Targets of Cell Cycle Transition Proteins

DTP-COMPARE analysis results showed that the 10 NCI synthetic compounds that are most correlated with NSC765690 and NSC765599 anti-cancer fingerprints are small molecules (MW: 168.19~506.5 g/mol), with p values in the range of 0.44~0.62. In addition, NSC765690 (p-value range of 0.33~0.74) and NSC765599 (p-value range of 0.15~0.36) shared anticancer mechanism with a number of standardized drugs in the NCI database (Table 2). The molecular target fingerprints generated also showed that both compounds shared a similar positive correlation (p = 0.1~0.3) with the expression of multiple genes, most of which are proteins involved in cell cycle progressions (Table 3).

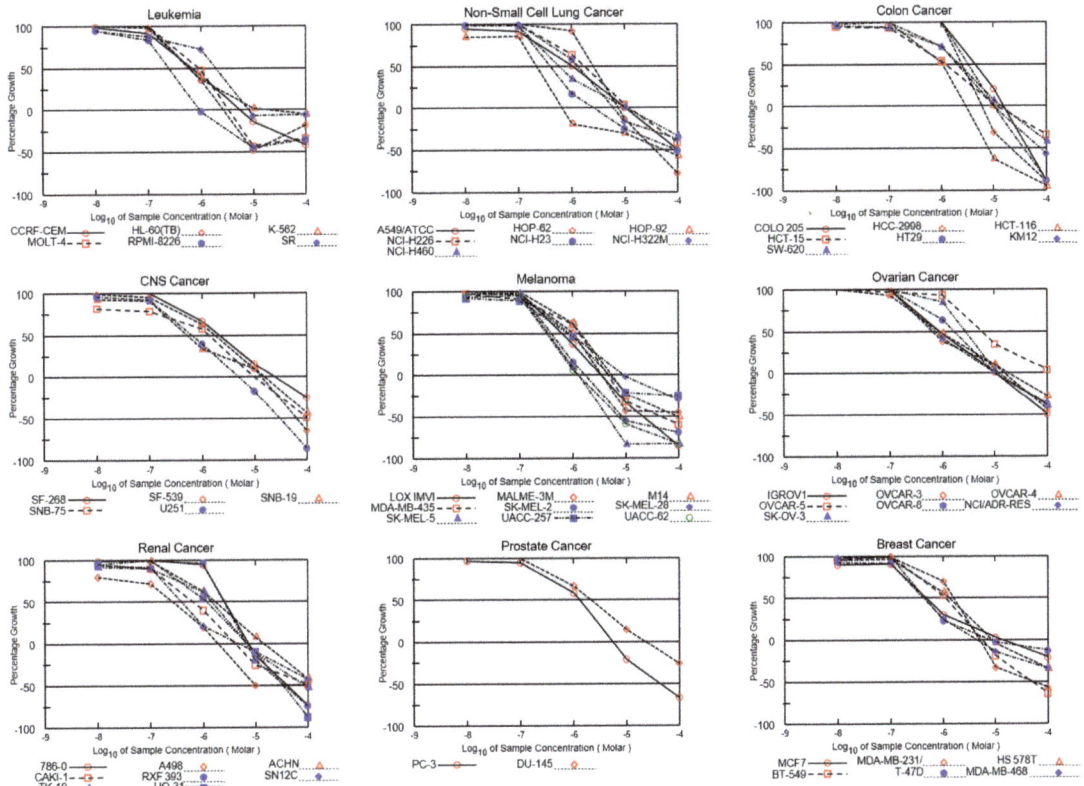

Figure 4. Dose–cytotoxic response curves of NSC765599 against panels of 60 NCI human cancer cell lines. The growth percentage value of +100 on the Y-axis represents the growth of untreated cells, the 0 value represents no net growth, while −100 represents the complete death of cells.

Table 1. Anti-proliferative and cytotoxic activities of NSC765690 and NSC765599 against panels of NCI60 human cancer cell lines.

Cancer Type	Panel/Cell Line	GI_{50} (µM)		TGI (µM)		LC_{50} (µM)	
		NSC765690	NSC765599	NSC765690	NSC765599	NSC765690	NSC765599
Leukemia	CCRF-CEM	0.53	0.703	9.73	5.6	>100	>100
	HL-60(TB)	0.51	0.586	2.09	2.68	>100	>100
	K-562	0.37	0.628	10.2	19.1	>100	>100
	MOLT-4	0.46	0.928	2.05	3.39	>100	>100
	RPMI-8226	0.23	0.248	0.74	0.951	>100	>100
	SR	1.91	1.95	>100	8.27	>100	>100
NSCLC	A549/ATCC	0.44	1.05	7.96	10.6	>100	99.4
	HOP-62	1.61	2.51	6.78	7.48	>100	37
	HOP-92	0.14	0.219	0.48	0.655	>100	53.7
	NCI-H226	1.07	1.73	11.2	12	>100	>100
	NCI-H23	0.29	0.395	0.88	2.54	>100	94.2
	NCI-H322M	0.68	1.3	6.7	6.13	>100	>100
	NCI-H460	0.45	0.569	8.78	10.7	>100	>100
	NCI-H522	0.28		0.77		19.4	

Table 1. Cont.

Cancer Type	Panel/Cell Line	GI$_{50}$ (µM)		TGI (µM)		LC$_{50}$ (µM)	
		NSC765690	NSC765599	NSC765690	NSC765599	NSC765690	NSC765599
Colon Cancer	COLO 205	3.23	4.48	11.2	15.6	35.8	44.4
	HCC-2998	2.16	2.42	6.31	5.83	30.6	21.2
	HCT-116	0.55	1.05	3.1	2.84	93.1	7.7
	HCT-15	0.48	1.22	4.05	11.4	45.9	>100
	HT29	3.63	3.43	10.6	9.93	36.5	36.6
	KM12	0.7	1.99	10.5	10.1	>100	75.5
	SW-620	1.28	2.1	16.5	13.7	>100	>100
CNS Cancer	SF-268	0.71	2.17	>100	24.6	>100	>100
	SF-539	0.53	1.78	10.8	13.7	67.8	63.8
	SNB-19	0.41	0.529	>100	15.2	>100	>100
	SNB-75	1.39		9.75		>100	
	U251	0.42	0.633	7.23	4.97	82.9	29.7
Melanoma	LOX IMVI	0.5	0.64	3.28	3.36	26.3	21
	MALME-3M	0.4	1.02	2.26	3.48	>100	>100
	M14	0.68	1.38	7.16	5.37	>100	93.7
	MDA-MB-435	0.63	1.31	6.04	4.5	>100	42.7
	SK-MEL-2	0.28	0.443	0.73	1.69	5.51	8.39
	SK-MEL-28	0.68	0.865	7.05	9.28	>100	>100
	SK-MEL-5	0.26	0.345	0.88	1.26	4.61	4.39
	UACC-257	0.29	0.815	1.59	4.84	>100	>100
	UACC-62	0.28	0.319	1.14	1.22	5.59	7.21
Ovarian Cancer	IGROV1	0.55	0.909	24.3	10.7	>100	>100
	OVCAR-3	0.44	0.674	33	15.3	>100	>100
	OVCAR-4	0.86	0.841	>100	18.5	>100	>100
	OVCAR-5	4.04	5.55	>100	>100	>100	>100
	OVCAR-8	0.51	1.64	6.01	10.1	>100	>100
	NCI/ADR-RES	0.42	0.741	10.4	9.96	>100	>100
	SK-OV-3	1.29	2.68	7.3	11.8	>100	>100
Renal cancer	786-0	2.72	2.58	9.07	7.45	>100	39.7
	A498	0.24	0.263	1.52	1.93	>100	>100
	ACHN	0.82	1.73	15.5	14.4	>100	>100
	CAKI-1	0.65	0.637	>100	4.07	>100	>100
	RXF 393	1.47	2.48	5.93	6.72	>100	35.2
	SN12C	0.37	0.384	12.7	4.73	>100	>100
	TK-10	0.45	1.46	4.01	6.87	>100	82.7
	UO-31	0.41	1.14	7.18	6.95	37.4	32.4
Prostate Cancer	PC-3	0.38	1.3	3.04	5.43	>100	42.8
	DU-145	1.28	2.16	>100	23.4	>100	>100
Breast Cancer	MCF7	0.42	0.471	9.11	13.4	>100	>100
	MDA-MB231/ATCC	1.06	4.76	4.08	50.5	>100	0
	HS 578T	0.65	1.31	28.7	8.65	>100	>100
	BT-549	0.45	1.11	2.59	5.5	43.6	48.8
	T-47D	0.29	0.449	2.74	7.49	>100	>100
	MDA-MB-468	0.3	0.425	3.17	4.42	>100	>100

The GI$_{50}$ = 50% growth inhibition, TGI = total growth inhibition, LC$_{50}$ = 50% loss of cells.

Table 2. NCI synthetic compounds and standard anticancer agent sharing similar anti-cancer fingerprints and mechanistic correlation with NSC765599 and NSC765690.

Drugs	Rank	P	CCLC	Target Descriptor	MW (g/mol)	P	CCLC	Target Descriptor	Mechanism of Action
			NCI-Synthetic Compounds				**NCI-Standard Agents**		
NSC765690 Fingerprints	1	0.61	42	Antineoplastic-643812	419.3	0.74	55	Actinomycin D	Transcription inhibitor
	2	0.58	49	Combretastatin A-4	316.3	0.61	58	Mitramycin	Transcription inhibitor
	3	0.55	49	N-(3-chloro-2-methylphenyl)-2-hydroxy-3-nitrobenzamide	306.7	0.6	59	Thioguanine	Inhibit cell cycle transition
	4	0.51	46	2-Methyl-4-(phenylimino)naphth(2,3-d)oxazol-9-one	288.3	0.58	58	Cisplatin	Inhibit DNA replication
	5	0.51	46	Resibufogenin, Methacrylate De	452.6	0.58	49	Morpholino-ADR	Tubulin inhibitor
	6	0.5	43	3-Nitro-2′,4′-Salicyloxylidide	286.2	0.56	59	5-Azacytidine	Tubulin inhibior
	7	0.48	49	5,7-Dichloro-3-hydroxy-3-[2-(4-nitrophenyl)-2-oxoethyl]-1,3-dihydro-2H-indol-2-one	381.2	0.53	58	Topotecan	DNA damage inducer
	8	0.46	58	4-ipomeanol	168.1	0.48	59	Doxorubicin (Adriamycin)	DNA damage inducer
	9	0.46	48	3,3′-Diethyl-9-methylthiacarbocyanine iodide	506.5	0.39	59	5-Fluorouracil	Inhibitor of DNA replication.
	10	0.44	44	2,2-Dibutyl-3-(p-tolylsulfonyl)-1,3,2-thiazastannolidine	462.3	0.33	59	Abemaciclib	Inhibit cell cycle transition
NSC765599 Fingerprints	1	0.62	47	N-(3-chloro-2-methylphenyl)-2-hydroxy-3-nitrobenzamide	306.7	0.36	57	Trametinib	MEK Inhibitor
	2	0.57	44	Uvaretin	378.4	0.3	57	Erlotinib HCL	Growth factor receptor inhibitor
	3	0.54	44	Eunicin	334.4	0.29	55	Vandetanib	Growth factor receptor inhibitor
	4	0.54	44	Resibufogenin derivative	452.6	0.28	56	Topotecan	DNA damage inducer
	5	0.54	45	1H,3H-Thiazolo(3,4-a)benzimidazole, 1-(2-chloro-6-fluorophenyl)-	304.8	0.27	55	Ixabepilone	microtubule inhibitor
	6	0.53	44	Combretastatin A-4	316.3	0.23	57	Abemaciclib	Inhibitor of cell cycle transition
	7	0.52	44	Nagilactone C	362.4	0.25	56	Idelalisib	phosphoinositide 3-kinase
	8	0.51	56	dichloroallyl lawsone	283.1	0.23	57	Pazopanib Hydrochloride	Growth factor receptor inhibitor
	9	0.51	56	Merbarone	263.2	0.21	57	Doxorubicin (Adriamycin)	DNA damage inducer
	10	0.48	55	5-Bromo-1-[[4-methylidene-5-oxo-2-(4-phenylphenyl)oxolan-2-yl]methyl]pyrimidine-2,4-dione	453.3	0.15	57	Palbociclib	Inhibitor of cell cycle transition

P: Pearson's correlation coefficient. CCLC: Common cell lines count. MW: molecular weight.

3.4. CDK2/4/6 and STAT3 Are Potential Druggable Candidates for NSC765690 and NSC765599

Using NSC765690 and NSC765599 as query molecules on the SwissTargetPrediction algorithm, a computer-based drug target prediction tool that identifies the most probable macromolecular targets of a small molecule, on the basis of similarity with a known actives compound in the library [54], we identified a number of targetable proteins, most of which are CDKs and associated proteins. Among these predicted targets, we found that kinases, cytochrome P450, enzymes, and electrochemical transporters were the most occurring targeted classes (Table 4, Supplementary Figure S1). Specifically, STAT3, four members of CDKs (CDK1/2/4/9), and three cyclins were among the top-ranked targeted proteins, while NSC765599 was predicted to target CDK2/4/5/6. Other top-ranked proteins targetable by NSC765599 are shown in Table 4. Coherent with the SwissTarget prediction, the PASS analysis of NSC765690 and NSC765699 also predicted (all pa > pi) inhibitions of CDKs and STAT3 amongst other activities (Table 5).

Table 3. Molecular targets correlated to NSC765599 and NSC765690 activity.

P	CCLC	P	CCLC	Target ID	Gene Card Code	Target Description
NSC765599		NSC765690				
0.30	53	0.29	55	CG2399	CCNB1	Cyclin B1
0.30	56	0.32	58	CG2465	CCND1	Cyclin D1
0.29	51	0.31	52	CG2440	RARB	Retinoic Acid Receptor Beta
0.28	54	0.13	55	CG2585	CDH1	Cadherin-1
0.28	48	0.17	50	CG2558	FGFR1	Fibroblast growth factor receptor 1
0.28	55	0.28	57	CG2369	RAF1	Raf-1 Proto-Oncogene
0.23	50	-	-	CG2405	E2F4	E2F Transcription Factor 4
0.22	52	-	-	CG2555	CDKN2A	cyclin-dependent kinase inhibitor 2A
0.21	56	0.15	58	CG2357	MYCN	N-myc proto-oncogene protein
0.22	50			CG2499	CDC25A	Activator of cyclin dependent kinase 2/4
0.21	56	0.11	58	CG2531	CDK4	Cyclin dependent kinase 4
0.21	56	-	-	CG2448	TCL1A	T-cell leukemia/lymphoma protein 1A
0.20	49	-	-	CG2269	BTK	Bruton Tyrosine Kinase
0.15	56	0.16	58	CG2311	PIK3CB	Phosphatidylinositol-4,5-bisphosphate 3-kinase
0.14	55	-	-	CG2466	CCND2	Cyclin D2
0.12	56	0.1	58	CG2327	CDK6	Cyclin dependent kinase 6
-	-	0.13	57	CG2467	CDC25B	Activator of cyclin dependent kinase CDC2
-	-	0.18	58	CG2468	CDKN1A	Cyclin Dependent Kinase Inhibitor 1A

P: Pearson's correlation coefficient. CCLC: Common cell lines count. Pearson's correlation coefficient ranges from high −1 (negative correlation) to +1 (high positive correlation). The higher the positive value, the more positive correlation between gene expression and NSC765599 and NSC765690 activities.

Table 4. SwissTarget prediction of potential protein targets for NSC765690 and NSC765599.

Gene Name	Common Name	Uniprot ID	ChEMBL ID	Target Class
		NSC765690 Targets		
CDK9/cyclin T1	CDK9, CCNT1	P50750 O60563	CHEMBL2111389	Other cytosolic protein
Cyclin-dependent kinase 1	CDK1	P06493	CHEMBL308	Kinase
Cyclin-dependent kinase 1/cyclin B	CCNB3 CDK1 CCNB1 CCNB2	Q8WWL7 P06493 P14635 O95067	CHEMBL2094127	Other cytosolic protein
Cyclin-dependent kinase 2	CDK2	P24941	CHEMBL301	Kinase
Cyclin-dependent kinase 4/cyclin D1	CCND1 CDK4	P24385 P11802	CHEMBL1907601	Kinase
Epidermal growth factor receptor erbB1	EGFR	P00533	CHEMBL203	Kinase

Table 4. Cont.

Gene Name	Common Name	Uniprot ID	ChEMBL ID	Target Class
Signal transducer and activator of transcription 3	STAT3	P40763	CHEMBL4026	Transcription factor
Fibroblast growth factor receptor 1	FGFR1	P11362	CHEMBL3650	Kinase
Insulin receptor	INSR	P06213	CHEMBL1981	Kinase
MAP kinase ERK2	MAPK1	P28482	CHEMBL4040	Kinase
PI3-kinase p110-gamma subunit	PIK3CG	P48736	CHEMBL3267	Enzyme
Platelet-derived growth factor receptor	PDGFRA PDGFRB	P16234 P09619	CHEMBL2095189	Kinase
Rho-associated protein kinase 1	ROCK1	Q13464	CHEMBL3231	Kinase
Serine/threonine-protein kinase 11/16/Chk1/MST2	STK11/3/16/CHEK1	Q15831	CHEMBL5606	Kinase
Tyrosine-protein kinase ABL/ITK/JAK1/JAK2	ABL1	P00519	CHEMBL1862	Kinase
NSC765599 Targets				
Cyclin-dependent kinase 5/CDK5 activator 1	CDK5R1 CDK5	Q15078 Q00535	CHEMBL1907600	Kinase
Epidermal growth factor receptor erbB1	EGFR	P00533	CHEMBL203	Kinase
Cyclin-dependent kinase 2	CDK2	P24941	CHEMBL301	Kinase
Cyclin-dependent kinase 4/cyclin D1	CCND1, CDK4	P24385, P11802	CHEMBL1907601	Kinase
Hepatocyte growth factor receptor	MET	P08581	CHEMBL3717	Kinase
Inhibitor of NF-kappa-B kinase (IKK)	CHUK	O15111	CHEMBL3476	Kinase
Insulin-like growth factor I receptor	IGF1R	P08069	CHEMBL1957	Kinase
MAP kinase p38 alpha	MAPK14	Q16539	CHEMBL260	Kinase
CDK6/cyclin D1	CCND1, CDK6	P24385, Q00534	CHEMBL2111455	Kinase
PI3-kinase p110-alpha/p85-alpha	PIK3CA, PIK3R1	P42336, P27986	CHEMBL2111367	Enzyme
Receptor protein-tyrosine kinase erbB-2	ERBB2	P04626	CHEMBL1824	Kinase
Receptor protein-tyrosine kinase erbB-4	ERBB4	Q15303	CHEMBL3009	Kinase
Rho-associated protein kinase 1	ROCK1/2	Q13464	CHEMBL3231	Kinase
Signal transducer and activator of transcription 3	STAT3	P40763	CHEMBL4026	Transcription factor
Serine/threonine-protein kinase RIPK2	RIPK2	O43353	CHEMBL5014	Kinase
Tankyrase−1/2	TNKS, TNKS2	O95271, Q9H2K2	CHEMBL6164, 6154	Enzyme

Table 4. *Cont.*

Gene Name	Common Name	Uniprot ID	ChEMBL ID	Target Class
Tyrosine-protein kinase JAK1	JAK1	P23458	CHEMBL2835	Kinase
Tyrosine-protein kinase SRC	SRC	P12931	CHEMBL267	Kinase
Vascular endothelial growth factor receptor 1/2	FLT1, KDR	P17948, P35968	CHEMBL1868, 279	Kinase

Targets were predicted using Swiss Target Prediction, which operates on the principle of 'similarity'.

Table 5. Prediction of Biological Activity Spectra (PASS) of NSC765690 and NSC765699 Targets.

NSC765690 PASS Predicted Targets			NSC765699 PASS Predicted Targets		
Pa	Pi	Activity	Pa	Pi	Activity
0.446	0.034	CDK6/cyclin D1 inhibitor	0.505	0.012	Transcription factor inhibitor
0.430	0.037	Transcription factor STAT inhibitor	0.430	0.037	Transcription factor STAT inhibitor
0.266	0.085	Transcription factor STAT3 inhibitor	0.391	0.020	CDK6 inhibitor
0.167	0.038	CDK9/cyclin T1 inhibitor	0.255	0.072	Transcription factor STAT3 inhibitor
0.151	0.046	CDK2/cyclin A inhibitor	0.162	0.029	CDK2/cyclin A inhibitor
0.114	0.021	Transcription factor STAT6 inhibitor	0.114	0.021	Transcription factor STAT6 inhibitor
0.101	0.094	CDK1/cyclin B inhibitor	0.020	0.011	CDK4/cyclin D3 inhibitor
0.019	0.012	CDK4/cyclin D3 inhibitor	0.046	0.007	CDK5 inhibitor

Key: Pa > Pi, Pa: probability to be active, Pi: probability to be inactive.

3.5. Molecular Docking Reavealed Favoured Ligandability of NSC765690 and NSC765599 for CDK2/4/6 and STAT3

Using molecular docking studies, we found that both NSC765690 and NSC765599 exhibited strong interactions with the crystal structure of apo CDK2 (PDB; 4EK3), CDK4/cyclin D3 (PDB; 3G33), CDK6/cyclin (PDB; 1JOW), and STAT3 (PDB; 4ZIA). The observed interactions and binding affinities indicated that CDK2 is the most favored receptor for both compounds (Figures 5 and 6, Table 6, Supplementary Figures S2–S4), while NSC765690 exhibited stronger interactions with CDK2/4/6 than does NSC765599. Furthermore, we compared the docking profiles of the two compounds with a standard CDK inhibitor, palbociclib (Figure 7), and found that NSC765690 demonstrated stronger binding affinities with CDK2/4/6 compared to NSC765599 and palbociclib. Docking of all ligands (NSC765690, NSC765599, and palbociclib) exhibited short binding distances with the receptors CDK2 (2.14~3.36 Å), CDK4 (1.87~3.23 Å), and CDK6 (2.31~3.17 Å) (Table 6).

Our careful analysis of the interactions between NSC765690 and the receptors revealed a higher number of conventional H-bonding, pi interactions, and Van der Waal forces created on the ligand backbone with a higher number of amino acids residues than does NSC765599 and palbociclib, in the CDK2/4/6 binding cavities (Table 6). NSC765690-STAT3 and NSC765599-STAT3 complexes were stabilized by similar interactions. However, the overall binding affinity of STAT3 with a known inhibitor, SH-4-54, was less negative than the values observed for NSC765690-STAT3 and NSC765599-STAT3 complexes (Figure 8, Supplementary Figure S5).

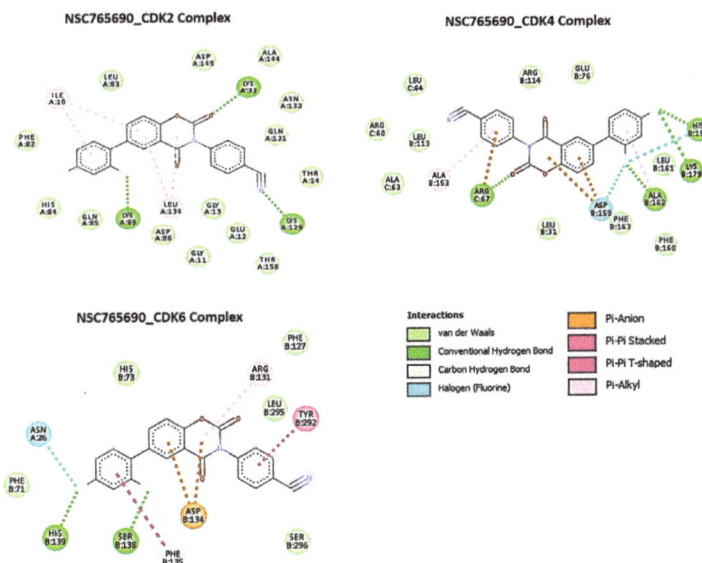

Figure 5. Docking profiles of NSC765690 with CDK2, CDK4, and CDK6. Two dimensional (2D) representations of ligand–receptor interactions occurring between NSC765690 and the target receptors (CDK2/4/6). The deep-green color indicates the strongest ligand–receptor interaction (due to conventional hydrogen bonds) of the best docking pose.

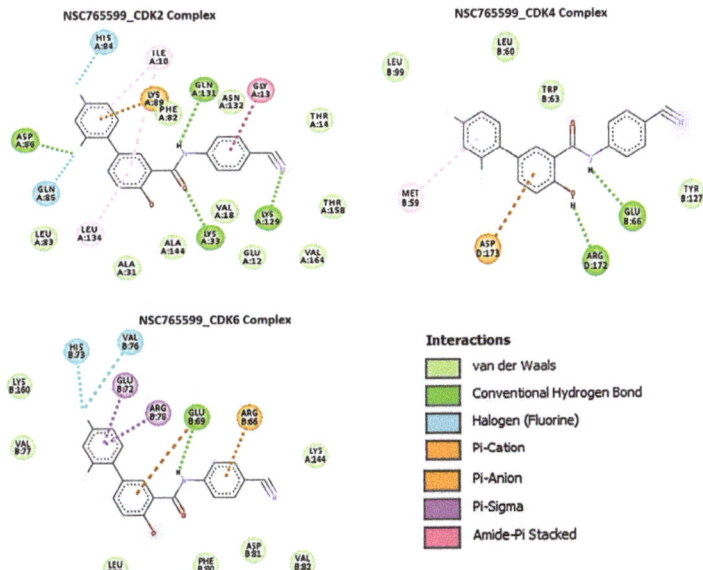

Figure 6. Docking profiles of NSC765599 with CDK2, CDK4, and CDK6. Two dimensional (2D) representations of ligand–receptor interactions occurring between NSC765599 and the target receptors (CDK2/4/6). The deep-green color indicates the strongest ligand–receptor interaction (due to conventional hydrogen bonds) of the best docking pose.

Table 6. Comparative docking profile of NSC765690, NSC765599 and standard STAT3/CDK2/4/6 inhibitors.

Docking Parameters	Cyclin Dependent Kinase 2					
	NSC765599_CDK2 Complex		NSC765690_CDK2 Complex		Palbociclib_CDK2 Complex	
ΔG = (Kcal/mol)	−11		−11.6		−9.1	
Type of Interactions	n-Bond	Interacting AA (Distance (Å))	n-Bond	Interacting AA (Distance (Å))	n-Bond	Interacting AA (Distance (Å))
Conventional H-bond	4	LYS129 (2.67), LYS33 (2.73), GLN131 (2.72) ASP86 (3.36),	3	LYS129 (2.75), LYS89 (2.15), LYS33 (2.14)	2	ARG214(2.16), ARG217 (2.65)
C-H bond					2	VAL251(3.70) LYS250 (3.70)
Halogen bond	2	HIS84 (3.69),GLN85 (3.36)				
Pi-cation	1	LYS89 (3.11)				
Pi-anion						
Pi-alkyl			2	LEU134, ILE10	2	PRO204, ARG200
Pi-pi stack						
Amide-pi stack	1	GLY13 (3.34)				
Van der waal forces	10	LEU83, PHE82, ALA144, VAL18, GLU12, VAL164, THR158, ALA31, THR14, ASN132,	14	PHE82, LEU83, ASP145, ALA144, ASN132, GLN131, THR14, THR158, GLU12, GLY13, GLY11, ASP86, GLN85, HIS84	5	GLN246, THR218, LEU202, THR198, LYS250

	Cyclin Dependent Kinase 4					
	NSC765599_CDK4 Complex		NSC765690_CDK4 Complex		Palbociclib_CDK4 Complex	
ΔG = (Kcal/mol)	−7.5		−8.5		−8.3	
Type of Interactions	n-Bond	Interacting AA (Distance (Å))	n-Bond	Interacting AA (Distance (Å))	n-Bond	Interacting AA (Distance (Å))
Conventional H-bond	2	ARG172 (2.07) GLU66 (2.06)	4	ARG67(1.84), ALA162 (2.62), LYS179 (2.90) HIS158(2.87)	4	ARG168(3.23), SER57(2.49)
Halogen bond			2	ASP159 (2.90), HIS158(3.62)		
C-H bond					1	GLY51 (3.46)
Pi-cation			1	ARG67(3.89)		
Pi-anion	1	ASP173 (4.48)	1	ASP159 (3.78)		
Pi-alkyl	1	MET59	1	ALA153, ALA162	4	TYR172, PRO55, PRO45, ILE56
Van der waal forces	3	LEU60, LEU99, TRP63	10	LEU64, ARG60, LEU113, ALA63, LEU31, PHE163, PHE160, LEU161, GLU76, ARG114	11	SER171, GLY48, GLY53, GLY52, GLY50, THR120, ILE121, LYS112, LEU108, LEU54, THR58

Table 6. Cont.

	Cyclin Dependent Kinase 6					
	NSC765599_CDK6 Complex		NSC765690_CDK6 Complex		Palbociclib_CDK6 Complex	
ΔG = (Kcal/mol)	−9.0		−9.6		−8.1	
Type of Interactions	n-Bond	Interacting AA (Distance (Å))	n-Bond	Interacting AA (Distance (Å))	n-Bond	Interacting AA (Distance (Å))
Conventional H-bond	1	GLU69 (2.22)	2	HIS139 (2.29) SER138 (2.31)	2	ARG66 (2.50) GLU69 (3.17)
C-H bond			1	PHE135(3.69)	1	PRO35(3.71)
Halogen bond	2	HIS73 (2.88) VAL76 (2.99)	1	ASN26 (3.32)		
Pi-cation	1	ARG66 (3.40)				
Pi-anion	1	GLU69 (4.90)	1	ASP134(3.99)	1	ASP146(3.59)
Pi-sigma					1	LEU34
Pi-alkyl			1	ARG131	4	ALA149, LEU33, ARG82, CYS85
Pi-pi stack	1	GLU72, ARG78	1	TYR292	1	PHE37292
Pi-pi T-shape			1	PHE135		
Van der waal forces	7	Lys160, Val77, Leu79, Phe80, Asp81, Val82, Lys144	5	Phe71, Ser296, Leu295, Phe127, His73	5	Lys36, Thr38, Thr70, Glu148, His67
	Signal Transducer and Activator of Transcription 3					
	NSC765599_STAT3 Complex		NSC765690_STAT3 Complex		SH-4-54_STAT3 Complex	
ΔG = (Kcal/mol)	−8.0		−8.3		−7.3	
Type of Interaction	n-Bond	Interacting AA (Distance (Å))	n-Bond	Interacting AA (Distance (Å))	n-Bond	Interacting AA (Distance (Å))
Conventional H-bond	2	ARG107(2.73) TRP110 (3.79)			1	SER113 (2.57)
C-H bond			1	ARG107 (3.23)	2	TRP110 (3.69) ALA106 (3.47)
Halogen	1	GLN3 (3.52)	1	ALA106 (3.67)	3	ARG107(3.65), ARG103 (3.05), ALA44 (3.26)
Pi-pi stacked	1	TRP110				
Pi-sigma			1	ALA44		
Pi-sulfur					1	TRP110 (4.49)
Pi-alkyl	3	LEU109, ALA106, ALA44	3	LEU109, ARG103, ALA44	1	ALA106
Pi-pi T-shaped			1	TRP110		
Van der waal forces	5	GLU39, GLN41, ASP42, TYR45, TRP43	4	TRP43, GLU39, GLN3, SER113	4	GLU39, GLN3, GLN117, ALA47

Interacting AA: Interacting Amino acids.

3.6. NSC765599 and NSC765690 Met the Required Criteria of Drug-Likeness and Safety

NSC765690 met the required criteria of a good drug candidate in terms of lipophilicity, polarity, flexibility, solubility, saturation, and molecular weight, while NSC765599 slightly violated the required range of solubility (Log S(ESOL) = 0~6) and lipophilicity (XlogP3 = −0.7~5) having slight outlying values of −5.71 and 5.47 respectively. Both compounds demonstrated good synthetic accessibilities, highly probable GIA absorption, and bioavailability, but poor BBB permeation (Supplementary Figures S6 and S7, Table 7). Predicted ecotoxicity and acute toxicity for different administration routes of NSC765690 and NSC765599 produce class 4 and 5 levels of acute toxicity (LD_{50}) according to OECD classification (Table 7). Collectively, NSC765599 and NSC765690 met the criteria for a drug-likeness candidate and are relatively known to be toxic.

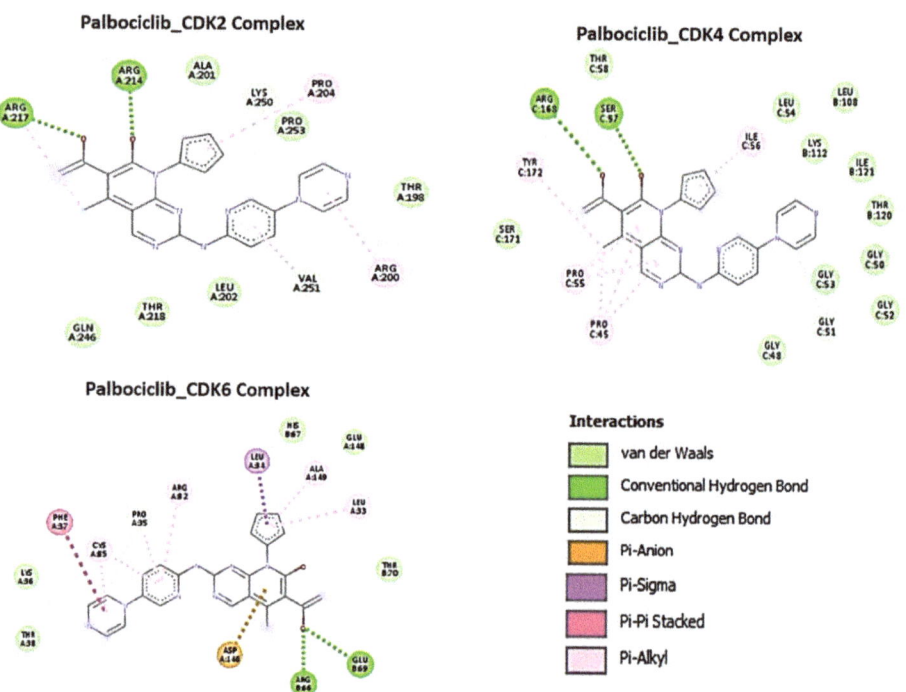

Figure 7. Docking profiles of palbociclib with CDK2, CDK4, and CDK6. Two dimensional (2D) representations of ligand–receptor interactions occurring between palbociclib and the target receptors (CDK2/4/6). The deep-green color indicates the strongest ligand–receptor interaction (due to conventional hydrogen bonds) of the best docking pose.

Table 7. Drug likeness, ADME and safety/toxicity profile of NSC765690 and NSC765599.

Properties	NSC765690	NSC765599	Reference Value
Formula	$C_{21}H_{10}F_2N_2O_3$	$C_{20}H_{12}F_2N_2O_2$	-
Molecular weight	376.31 g/mol	350.32 g/mol	150–500 g/mol
Num. rotatable bonds	2	4	0–9
Num. H-bond acceptors	6	5	0–10
Num. H-bond donors	0	2	0–5
Molar Refractivity	98.15	92.75	
TPSA	76.00 Å^2	73.12 Å^2	20–130 Å^2
Fraction Csp3	0.00	0.00	0.25~<1
Log $P_{o/w}$ (XLOGP3)	4.31	5.47	−0.7~5
Consensus Log $P_{o/w}$	4.11	4.29	
Log S (ESOL)	0.34	−5.71	0–6
Lipinski, Ghose, Veber and Egan's rule	Yes; 0 violation	Yes; 0 violation	
Bioavailability Score	0.56	0.55	>0.1 (10%)
Synthetic accessibility	3.33	2.37	1 (very easy) to 10 (very difficult).

Table 7. Cont.

Properties	NSC765690	NSC765599	Reference Value
Acute toxicity			
LD_{50} for Intraperitoneal (mg/kg)	446.100 (OECD:4)	593.200 (OECD:5)	
LD_{50} for Intravenous (mg/kg)	127.200 (OECD:4)	251.200 (OECD:4)	
LD_{50} for Oral (mg/kg)	494.000 (OECD:4)	836.900 (OECD:4)	
LD_{50} for Subcutaneous (mg/kg)	398.300 (OECD:4)	740.900 (OECD:4)	
Environmental toxicity			
Bioaccumulation factor Log10 (BCF)	1.204	1.210	
Daphnia magna LC_{50}Log10 (mol/L)	7.294	6.713	
Fathead Minnow LC_{50}Log10 (mmol/L)	−3.088	−3.099	
Tetrahymena pyriformis IGC_{50}Log10 (mol/L)	2.016	2.033	

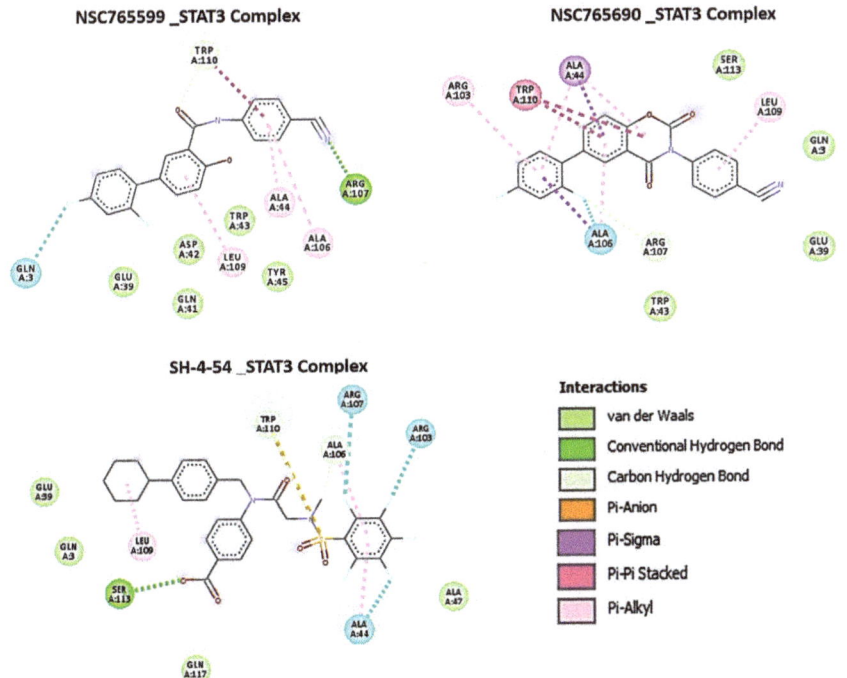

Figure 8. Comparative docking profiles of STAT3 with NSC765599, NSC765690, and SH-4-54 (a known STAT3 inhibitor). A 2D representation of ligand–receptor interactions of STAT3 with NSC765599, NSC765690, and SH-4-54 in the receptor binding pocket.

4. Discussion

Despite advances in treatment modalities, cancer survival ratios are still disappointing; thus, developing a novel chemotherapeutic strategy may improve the prognosis of the cancer patient [55]. At present, substantial attention is being focused on small molecules for targeted therapy in cancer treatments [35]. In the present study, we demonstrated the anti-proliferative and dose-dependent cytotoxic effect of NSC765690 and NSC765599 against panels of NCI human cancer cell lines, with NSC765690 demonstrating higher activities than NSC765599. However, there was the least amount of cell lethality in panels of leukemia, CNS, ovarian, and colon cancer cell lines, suggesting that NSC765690 and NSC765599 are not generally toxic to growing cell lines, but display some degree of cytotoxic preference for NSCLC, melanoma, renal, and breast cancer cell line.

The NCI60 cell lines have been well-characterized for genetic and protein expression patterns, and, a computational tool, the DTP-COMPARE algorithm, has been developed to identify the molecular targets and mechanism(s) of action for the unknown compound from known drugs as well as the known molecular targets in the NCI databases [56]. Interestingly, our analysis of correlation patterns of NSC765690 anticancer fingerprint with mechanistically known NCI-Standard Agents suggests that NSC765690 might be targeting DNA replication and cell cycle. NSC765599, on the other hand, shares similar ($p = 0.15$~0.36) antitumor mechanistic fingerprints with known inhibitors of growth factor receptor and cell cycle transition, and DNA damage inducer. However, the modest correlation with NCI-standard agents suggests that NSC765599 may have a unique mechanism of action not common to standard agent database. The strong antitumor pattern correlation ($p = 0.44$~0.6) between NSC765690 and NSC765599 fingerprint with NCI synthetic compounds suggests a mechanism of action similar to that of the seed compounds. Unfortunately, the top-ranked correlated compounds antineoplastic-643812 ($p = 0.61$) and N-(3-chloro-2-methylphenyl)-2-hydroxy-3-nitrobenzamide ($p = 0.62$) are yet to be mechanistically investigated, while combretastatin A-4 with p-value 0.58 (NSC765690) and p-value 0.53 (NSC765599) have been reported for the mechanism of action, indicating cell cycle arrest and inhibition of tubulin [57], hence providing hypothesis about the possible mechanism of actions of NSC765690 and NSC765599. The high number of cell cycle proteins and cyclin and cyclin-dependent kinases identified as molecular target fingerprints of both NSC765690 and NSC765599 strongly suggest that cyclin and cyclin-dependent kinase pathways are the core molecular targets of NSC765690 and NSC765599 predicted by COMPARE. However, the correlations ($p = 0.1$~0.3) were low, indicating the possibility of a new mechanism not captured by COMPARE.

The COMPARE prediction, together with in-silico SwissTarget and PASS prediction collectively identified STAT3/CDK2/4/6 as the most probable target for NSC765690 and NSC765599, and thus were further studied for ligand–receptor interactions. Interestingly, we found that NSC765690 and NSC765599 docked well into the receptor cavities of STAT3, CDK2, CDK4, and CDK6, with CDK2 being the most favored receptor while CDK4 appeared to be the least favored. Comparatively, the higher binding affinities and closer proximity of NSC765690 to the receptors suggested that NSC765690 is a better ligand for CDK2, CDK4, and CDK6 than is NSC765599.

NSC765690 and NSC765599 are both derivatives of NDMC101. A close look at the structure-related activities of NSC765690 and NSC765599 revealed that cyclization of salicylanilide core scaffold (Figure 1) was the structural feature associated with enhanced anticancer activity and better docking profiles of NSC765690 with STAT3/CDK2/4/6 compared to NSC765599 with an open-ring structure (Figures 7 and 8). Interestingly, when the same receptors (CDK2/4/6) were docked with palbociclib, a clinical CDK inhibitor, higher binding energies (lower binding affinities) were recorded for palbociclib compared to NSC765690, thus making the latter the more-favored ligand for CDK2/4/6.

The unique stability of NSC765690 in the binding sites of CDK2, CDK4, and CDK6 could be attributed to the larger number of H-bond and pi interactions including pi–cation, pi–anion, pi–alkyl, pi–pi stack, and pi–pi T-shaped interactions between NSC765690 and the receptors. The large numbers of pi interactions, which mostly involve charge transfer, help in intercalating the NSC765690 in the receptors' binding cavities. The higher affinity of NSC765690 was also associated with the presence of a larger number of Van der Waal forces created on its backbone with respective amino acids Phe82, Leu83, Asp145, Ala144, Asn132, Gln131, Thr14, Thr158, Glu12, Gly13, Gly11, Asp86, Gln85 and His84 of CDK2; Leu64, Arg60, Leu113, Ala63, Leu31, Phe163, Phe160, Leu161, Glu76 and Arg114 of CDK4; and Phe71, Ser296, Leu295, Phe127, and His73 of CDK6, which undoubtedly created a strong cohesive environment, thereby stabilizing the complex formed [58]. These higher numbers of interactions undoubtedly contributed to the higher affinity that NSC765690 has for CDK2, CDK4, and CDK6 than do NSC765599 and palbociclib. Palbociclib has been actively applied in multiple preclinical models and was approved for targeting CDK4/6 as anticancer therapy for breast cancer; however, acquired resistance occurs in almost all cases [20]. Although docking STAT3 with a known inhibitor, SH-4-54, revealed a higher number of conventional H-bond and halogen bond interactions with STAT3, the pi interactions were fewer, and consequently, the overall binding affinity was less negative. Therefore, higher pi interactions also contributed to the higher binding affinity that NSC765690 has for STAT3 than does SH-4-54. Our molecular simulations of ligand–receptor interactions validated the computational prediction of STAT3/CDK2/4/6 as druggable candidates for NSC765690 and NSC765599. The present study, therefore, provides useful molecular docking-based evidence of alternative small molecules that could target CDK4/6 as well as CDK2 and STAT3. They thus offer a wider targeted therapy with less probability of suffering drug resistance

The concept of drug-likeness gives useful guidelines for identifying potential drug candidates during the early stage of drug discovery and development [59]. Estimation of rodent acute toxicity (LD_{50}), an adverse effect that follows a single dose exposure to a substance, is an important task in drug design and risk assessment of chemicals [60–62]. The LD_{50} values predicted for oral, intravenous, intraperitoneal, and subcutaneous administration indicated that both NSC765690 and NSC765599 were non-toxic and will be well-tolerated by the experimental animals. In addition, NSC765690 and NSC765599 met the criteria of a good drug candidate (Table 7), suggesting that the compounds were drug-like molecules and thus possessed the potential to be considered oral drug candidates. Collectively, findings from this study have opened the door for new research direction for NSC765690 and NSC765599 as a novel and potent anti-cancer agent. We found these compounds worthy of further investigation, and both in vitro and in vivo studies in tumor-bearing mice are currently ongoing in our lab to assess the full therapeutic efficacies of these compounds.

5. Conclusions

In conclusion, this study demonstrated the anti-proliferative effect of NSC765690 and NSC765599 against the 60 panels of NCI human cancer cell lines, and dose-dependent cytotoxic preference for NSCLC, melanoma, renal, and breast cancer cell lines. STAT3/CDK2/4/6 signatures appear to be potential druggable candidates for the small molecules and interacted with high binding affinity, indicating the potential of NSC765690 and NSC765599 to dysregulate expressions of STAT3/CDK2/4/6 signature and, consequently, compromised cell survival. Further in-vitro and in-vivo confirmation studies are ongoing in our lab.

Supplementary Materials: The following are available online at https://www.mdpi.com/2227-9059/9/1/92/s1. Figure S1: Pie chart showing the repartition of protein classes of potential druggable candidates for NSC765690 and NSC765599. Figures S2–S5: Docking profiles of NSC765690, NSC765599, palbociclib with CDK2/4/6 and STAT3. Figure S6: BOILED-Egg model of brain or intestinal estimated permeation of NSC765599 and NSC765690. Figure S7: Bioavailability Radar showing suitable physicochemical spaces of the oral bioavailability of NSC765690 and NSC765599.

Author Contributions: B.L. wrote the manuscript; Y.-L.L., N.M., H.K. helped with data collection and analyses; H.-S.H. and M.R.S. synthesized and provided NSC765690 and NSC765599; H.-S.H. and A.T.H.W. designed and oversaw the study. All authors have read and agreed to the published version of the manuscript.

Funding: Hsu-Shan Huang is funded by the Ministry of Science and Technology MOST 109-2113-M-038-003. Alexander TH Wu and Yen-Lin Liu were funded by Taipei Medical University Hospital Taipei, Taiwan (Grant No. 104TMU-TMUH-11).

Institutional Review Board Statement: Not Applicable.

Informed Consent Statement: Not Applicable.

Data Availability Statement: The datasets generated and/or analyzed in this study are available on reasonable request.

Acknowledgments: The NCI Developmental Therapeutics Program (DTP) for the 60-cancer-cell-line screening of selected compounds described in this paper, funded by the National Cancer Institute National Institutes of Health (NIH-NCI).

Conflicts of Interest: The authors declare no conflict of interest.

References

1. Kim, I.; He, Y.-Y. Targeting the AMP-Activated Protein Kinase for Cancer Prevention and Therapy. *Front. Oncol.* **2013**, *3*, 15 [CrossRef] [PubMed]
2. Siegel, R.L.; Miller, K.D.; Jemal, A. Cancer statistics, 2020. *CA A Cancer J. Clin.* **2020**, *70*, 7–30. [CrossRef]
3. Lee, J.-C.; Wu, A.T.H.; Chen, J.-H.; Huang, W.-Y.; Lawal, B.; Mokgautsi, N.; Huang, H.-S.; Ho, C.-L. HNC0014, a Multi-Targeted Small-Molecule, Inhibits Head and Neck Squamous Cell Carcinoma by Suppressing c-Met/STAT3/CD44/PD-L1 Oncoimmune Signature and Eliciting Antitumor Immune Responses. *Cancers* **2020**, *12*, 3759. [CrossRef] [PubMed]
4. Kanwal, R.; Gupta, S. Epigenetic modifications in cancer. *Clin. Genet.* **2012**, *81*, 303–311. [CrossRef] [PubMed]
5. Zhang, Q.; Zheng, P.; Zhu, W. Research Progress of Small Molecule VEGFR/c-Met Inhibitors as Anticancer Agents (2016–Present) *Molecules* **2020**, *25*, 2666. [CrossRef]
6. Zhuo, L.-S.; Xu, H.-C.; Wang, M.-S.; Zhao, X.-E.; Ming, Z.-H.; Zhu, X.-L.; Huang, W.; Yang, G.-F. 2, 7-naphthyridinone-based MET kinase inhibitors: A promising novel scaffold for antitumor drug development. *Eur. J. Med. Chem.* **2019**, *178*, 705–714. [CrossRef]
7. Robinson, D.R.; Wu, Y.-M.; Lin, S.-F. The protein tyrosine kinase family of the human genome. *Oncogene* **2000**, *19*, 5548–5557. [CrossRef] [PubMed]
8. Vermeulen, K.; Van Bockstaele, D.R.; Berneman, Z.N. The cell cycle: A review of regulation, deregulation and therapeutic targets in cancer. *Cell Prolif.* **2003**, *36*, 131–149. [CrossRef] [PubMed]
9. Squires, M.S.; Feltell, R.E.; Wallis, N.G.; Lewis, E.J.; Smith, D.-M.; Cross, D.M.; Lyons, J.F.; Thompson, N.T. Biological characterization of AT7519, a small-molecule inhibitor of cyclin-dependent kinases, in human tumor cell lines. *Mol. Cancer Ther.* **2009**, *8*, 324–332. [CrossRef]
10. Brown, V.D.; Phillips, R.A.; Gallie, B.L. Cumulative effect of phosphorylation of pRB on regulation of E2F activity. *Mol. Cell. Biol.* **1999**, *19*, 3246–3256. [CrossRef]
11. Zhao, J.; Dynlacht, B.; Imai, T.; Hori, T.-A.; Harlow, E. Expression of NPAT, a novel substrate of cyclin E–CDK2, promotes S-phase entry. *Genes. Dev.* **1998**, *12*, 456–461. [CrossRef] [PubMed]
12. Goel, B.; Tripathi, N.; Bhardwaj, N.; Jain, S.K. Small Molecule CDK Inhibitors for the Therapeutic Management of Cancer. *Curr. Top. Med. Chem.* **2020**, *20*, 1535–1563. [CrossRef]
13. Kim, S.; Loo, A.; Chopra, R.; Caponigro, G.; Huang, A.; Vora, S.; Parasuraman, S.; Howard, S.; Keen, N.; Sellers, W.; et al. Abstract PR02: LEE011: An orally bioavailable, selective small molecule inhibitor of CDK4/6– Reactivating Rb in cancer. *Mol. Cancer Ther.* **2013**, *12*, PR02. [CrossRef]
14. Okada, Y.; Kato, S.; Sakamoto, Y.; Oishi, T.; Ishioka, C. Synthetic lethal interaction of CDK inhibition and autophagy inhibition in human solid cancer cell lines. *Oncol. Rep.* **2017**, *38*, 31–42. [CrossRef] [PubMed]
15. Vijayaraghavan, S.; Moulder, S.; Keyomarsi, K.; Layman, R.M. Inhibiting CDK in Cancer Therapy: Current Evidence and Future Directions. *Target. Oncol.* **2018**, *13*, 21–38. [CrossRef] [PubMed]
16. Kodym, E.; Kodym, R.; Reis, A.E.; Habib, A.A.; Story, M.D.; Saha, D. The small-molecule CDK inhibitor, SNS-032, enhances cellular radiosensitivity in quiescent and hypoxic non-small cell lung cancer cells. *Lung Cancer* **2009**, *66*, 37–47. [CrossRef] [PubMed]
17. Asghar, U.; Witkiewicz, A.K.; Turner, N.C.; Knudsen, E.S. The history and future of targeting cyclin-dependent kinases in cancer therapy. *Nat. Rev. Drug Discov.* **2015**, *14*, 130–146. [CrossRef]
18. Ramaswamy, B.; Phelps, M.A.; Baiocchi, R.; Bekaii-Saab, T.; Ni, W.; Lai, J.-P.; Wolfson, A.; Lustberg, M.E.; Wei, L.; Wilkins, D. A dose-finding, pharmacokinetic and pharmacodynamic study of a novel schedule of flavopiridol in patients with advanced solid tumors. *Investig. New Drugs* **2012**, *30*, 629–638. [CrossRef]

29. Tan, A.R.; Yang, X.; Berman, A.; Zhai, S.; Sparreboom, A.; Parr, A.L.; Chow, C.; Brahim, J.S.; Steinberg, S.M.; Figg, W.D. Phase I trial of the cyclin-dependent kinase inhibitor flavopiridol in combination with docetaxel in patients with metastatic breast cancer. *Clin. Cancer Res.* **2004**, *10*, 5038–5047. [CrossRef]
30. Pandey, K.; Park, N.; Park, K.-S.; Hur, J.; Cho, Y.B.; Kang, M.; An, H.-J.; Kim, S.; Hwang, S.; Moon, Y.W. Combined CDK2 and CDK4/6 Inhibition Overcomes Palbociclib Resistance in Breast Cancer by Enhancing Senescence. *Cancers* **2020**, *12*, 3566. [CrossRef]
31. O'Brien, N.A.; McDermott, M.S.J.; Conklin, D.; Luo, T.; Ayala, R.; Salgar, S.; Chau, K.; Di Tomaso, E.; Babbar, N.; Su, F.; et al. Targeting activated PI3K/mTOR signaling overcomes acquired resistance to CDK4/6-based therapies in preclinical models of hormone receptor-positive breast cancer. *Breast Cancer Res.* **2020**, *22*, 89. [CrossRef]
32. Pandey, K.; An, H.-J.; Kim, S.K.; Lee, S.A.; Kim, S.; Lim, S.M.; Kim, G.M.; Sohn, J.; Moon, Y.W. Molecular mechanisms of resistance to CDK4/6 inhibitors in breast cancer: A review. *Int. J. Cancer* **2019**, *145*, 1179–1188. [CrossRef] [PubMed]
33. Rawlings, J.S.; Rosler, K.M.; Harrison, D.A. The JAK/STAT signaling pathway. *J. Cell Sci.* **2004**, *117*, 1281–1283. [CrossRef] [PubMed]
34. Johnson, D.E.; O'Keefe, R.A.; Grandis, J.R. Targeting the IL-6/JAK/STAT3 signalling axis in cancer. *Nat. Rev. Clin. Oncol.* **2018**, *15*, 234. [CrossRef]
35. Ishibashi, K.; Koguchi, T.; Matsuoka, K.; Onagi, A.; Tanji, R.; Takinami-Honda, R.; Hoshi, S.; Onoda, M.; Kurimura, Y.; Hata, J. Interleukin-6 induces drug resistance in renal cell carcinoma. *Fukushima J. Med. Sci.* **2018**, *64*, 103–110. [CrossRef]
36. Priego, N.; Zhu, L.; Monteiro, C.; Mulders, M.; Wasilewski, D.; Bindeman, W.; Doglio, L.; Martínez, L.; Martínez-Saez, E.; y Cajal, S.R. STAT3 labels a subpopulation of reactive astrocytes required for brain metastasis. *Nat. Med.* **2018**, *24*, 1024–1035. [CrossRef] [PubMed]
37. Kortylewski, M.; Kujawski, M.; Wang, T.; Wei, S.; Zhang, S.; Pilon-Thomas, S.; Niu, G.; Kay, H.; Mulé, J.; Kerr, W.G. Inhibiting Stat3 signaling in the hematopoietic system elicits multicomponent antitumor immunity. *Nat. Med.* **2005**, *11*, 1314–1321. [CrossRef] [PubMed]
38. Villarino, A.V.; Kanno, Y.; O'Shea, J.J. Mechanisms and consequences of Jak-STAT signaling in the immune system. *Nat. Immunol.* **2017**, *18*, 374. [CrossRef]
39. Kettner, N.M.; Vijayaraghavan, S.; Durak, M.G.; Bui, T.; Kohansal, M.; Ha, M.J.; Liu, B.; Rao, X.; Wang, J.; Yi, M.; et al. Combined Inhibition of STAT3 and DNA Repair in Palbociclib-Resistant ER-Positive Breast Cancer. *Clin. Cancer Res.* **2019**, *25*, 3996–4013. [CrossRef] [PubMed]
40. Zou, S.; Tong, Q.; Liu, B.; Huang, W.; Tian, Y.; Fu, X. Targeting STAT3 in Cancer Immunotherapy. *Mol. Cancer* **2020**, *19*, 145. [CrossRef] [PubMed]
41. Phosrithong, N.; Ungwitayatorn, J. Molecular docking study on anticancer activity of plant-derived natural products. *Med. Chem. Res.* **2010**, *19*, 817–835. [CrossRef]
42. Ekins, S.; Mestres, J.; Testa, B. In silico pharmacology for drug discovery: Methods for virtual ligand screening and profiling. *Br. J. Pharm.* **2007**, *152*, 9–20. [CrossRef] [PubMed]
43. Ortega, S.S.; Cara, L.C.L.; Salvador, M.K. In silico pharmacology for a multidisciplinary drug discovery process. *Drug Met. Pers. Ther.* **2012**, *27*, 199–207. [CrossRef] [PubMed]
44. Kening, L.; Yuxin, D.; Lu, L.; Dong-Qing, W. Bioinformatics Approaches for Anti-cancer Drug Discovery. *Curr. Drug Target.* **2020**, *21*, 3–17. [CrossRef]
45. Coussens, N.P.; Braisted, J.C.; Peryea, T.; Sittampalam, G.S.; Simeonov, A.; Hall, M.D. Small-Molecule Screens: A Gateway to Cancer Therapeutic Agents with Case Studies of Food and Drug Administration—Approved Drugs. *Pharm. Rev.* **2017**, *69*, 479–496. [CrossRef]
46. Cheng, C.-P.; Huang, H.-S.; Hsu, Y.-C.; Sheu, M.-J.; Chang, D.-M. A Benzamide-linked Small Molecule NDMC101 Inhibits NFATc1 and NF-κB Activity: A Potential Osteoclastogenesis Inhibitor for Experimental Arthritis. *J. Clin. Immunol.* **2012**, *32*, 762–777. [CrossRef]
47. Lee, C.-C.; Liu, F.-L.; Chen, C.-L.; Chen, T.-C.; Chang, D.-M.; Huang, H.-S. Discovery of 5-(2′,4′-difluorophenyl)-salicylanilides as new inhibitors of receptor activator of NF-κB ligand (RANKL)-induced osteoclastogenesis. *Eur. J. Med. Chem.* **2015**, *98*, 115–126. [CrossRef]
48. Lee, C.-C.; Liu, F.-L.; Chen, C.-L.; Chen, T.-C.; Liu, F.-C.; Ahmed Ali, A.A.; Chang, D.-M.; Huang, H.-S. Novel inhibitors of RANKL-induced osteoclastogenesis: Design, synthesis, and biological evaluation of 6-(2,4-difluorophenyl)-3-phenyl-2H-benzo[e][1,3]oxazine-2,4(3H)-diones. *Bioorg. Med. Chem.* **2015**, *23*, 4522–4532. [CrossRef]
49. Shoemaker, R.H. The NCI60 human tumour cell line anticancer drug screen. *Nat. Rev. Cancer* **2006**, *6*, 813–823. [CrossRef]
50. Holbeck, S.L.; Collins, J.M.; Doroshow, J.H. Analysis of Food and Drug Administration-approved anticancer agents in the NCI60 panel of human tumor cell lines. *Mol. Cancer Ther.* **2010**, *9*, 1451–1460. [CrossRef]
51. Vichai, V.; Kirtikara, K. Sulforhodamine B colorimetric assay for cytotoxicity screening. *Nat. Protoc.* **2006**, *1*, 1112–1116. [CrossRef] [PubMed]
52. Boyd, M.R.; Paull, K.D. Some practical considerations and applications of the National Cancer Institute in vitro anticancer drug discovery screen. *Drug Dev. Res.* **1995**, *34*, 91–109. [CrossRef]
53. Gfeller, D.; Michielin, O.; Zoete, V. Shaping the interaction landscape of bioactive molecules. *Bioinformatics* **2013**, *29*, 3073–3079. [CrossRef] [PubMed]

44. Poroikov, V.V.; Filimonov, D.A.; Gloriozova, T.A.; Lagunin, A.A.; Druzhilovskiy, D.S.; Rudik, A.V.; Stolbov, L.A.; Dmitriev, A.V.; Tarasova, O.A.; Ivanov, S.M.; et al. Computer-aided prediction of biological activity spectra for organic compounds: The possibilities and limitations. *Russ. Chem. Bull.* **2019**, *68*, 2143–2154. [CrossRef]
45. Paull, K.; Shoemaker, R.; Hodes, L.; Monks, A.; Scudiero, D.; Rubinstein, L.; Plowman, J.; Boyd, M. Display and analysis of patterns of differential activity of drugs against human tumor cell lines: Development of mean graph and COMPARE algorithm. *JNCI J. Natl. Cancer Inst.* **1989**, *81*, 1088–1092. [CrossRef]
46. Hanwell, M.D.; Curtis, D.E.; Lonie, D.C.; Vandermeersch, T.; Zurek, E.; Hutchison, G.R. Avogadro: An advanced semantic chemical editor, visualization, and analysis platform. *J. Chem.* **2012**, *4*, 17. [CrossRef] [PubMed]
47. Trott, O.; Olson, A.J. AutoDock Vina: Improving the speed and accuracy of docking with a new scoring function, efficient optimization, and multithreading. *J. Comput. Chem.* **2010**, *31*, 455–461. [CrossRef]
48. Visualizer, D.S. *BIOVIA, Dassault Systèmes, BIOVIA Workbook, Release 2020*; BIOVIA Pipeline Pilot, Release 2020; Dassault Systèmes: San Diego, CA, USA, 2020.
49. Daina, A.; Michielin, O.; Zoete, V. SwissADME: A free web tool to evaluate pharmacokinetics, drug-likeness and medicinal chemistry friendliness of small molecules. *Sci. Rep.* **2017**, *7*, 42717. [CrossRef]
50. Lipinski, C.A. Lead-and drug-like compounds: The rule-of-five revolution. *Drug Discov. Today Technol.* **2004**, *1*, 337–341. [CrossRef] [PubMed]
51. Martin, Y.C. A bioavailability score. *J. Med. Chem.* **2005**, *48*, 3164–3170. [CrossRef]
52. Daina, A.; Zoete, V. A BOILED-Egg To Predict Gastrointestinal Absorption and Brain Penetration of Small Molecules. *ChemMedChem* **2016**, *11*, 1117–1121. [CrossRef]
53. Lagunin, A.A.; Zakharov, A.V.; Filimonov, D.A.; Poroikov, V.V. A new approach to QSAR modelling of acute toxicity. *SAR QSAR Environ. Res.* **2007**, *18*, 285–298. [CrossRef]
54. Daina, A.; Michielin, O.; Zoete, V. SwissTargetPrediction: Updated data and new features for efficient prediction of protein targets of small molecules. *Nucleic Acids Res.* **2019**, *47*, W357–W364. [CrossRef]
55. Rathnagiriswaran, S.; Wan, Y.-W.; Abraham, J.; Castranova, V.; Qian, Y.; Guo, N.L. A population-based gene signature is predictive of breast cancer survival and chemoresponse. *Int. J. Oncol.* **2010**, *36*, 607–616. [CrossRef]
56. Bates, S.E.; Fojo, A.T.; Weinstein, J.N.; Myers, T.G.; Alvarez, M.; Pauli, K.D.; Chabner, B.A. Molecular targets in the National Cancer Institute drug screen. *J. Cancer Res. Clin. Oncol.* **1995**, *121*, 495–500. [CrossRef] [PubMed]
57. Hamze, A.; Rasolofonjatovo, E.; Provot, O.; Mousset, C.; Veau, D.; Rodrigo, J.; Bignon, J.; Liu, J.-M.; Wdzieczak-Bakala, J.; Thoret, S. B-ring-modified isocombretastatin A-4 analogues endowed with interesting anticancer activities. *ChemMedChem* **2011**, *6*, 179–191. [CrossRef] [PubMed]
58. Arthur, D.E.; Uzairu, A. Molecular docking studies on the interaction of NCI anticancer analogues with human Phosphatidylinositol 4,5-bisphosphate 3-kinase catalytic subunit. *J. King Saud Univ. Sci.* **2019**, *31*, 1151–1166. [CrossRef]
59. Keller, T.H.; Pichota, A.; Yin, Z. A practical view of 'druggability'. *Curr. Opin. Chem. Biol.* **2006**, *10*, 357–361. [CrossRef] [PubMed]
60. Lawal, B.; Shittu, O.K.; Oibiokpa, F.I.; Mohammed, H.; Umar, S.I.; Haruna, G.M. Antimicrobial evaluation, acute and sub-acute toxicity studies of Allium sativum. *J. Acute Dis.* **2016**, *5*, 296–301. [CrossRef]
61. Shittu, O.K.; Lawal, B.; Alozieuwa, B.U.; Haruna, G.M.; Abubakar, A.N.; Berinyuy, E.B. Alteration in biochemical indices following chronic administration of methanolic extract of Nigeria bee propolis in Wistar rats. *Asian Pac. J. Trop. Dis.* **2015**, *5*, 654–657. [CrossRef]
62. Lagunin, A.; Zakharov, A.; Filimonov, D.; Poroikov, V. QSAR Modelling of Rat Acute Toxicity on the Basis of PASS Prediction. *Mol. Inf.* **2011**, *30*, 241–250. [CrossRef] [PubMed]

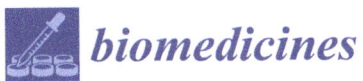

Article

Efficaciousness of Low Affinity Compared to High Affinity TSPO Ligands in the Inhibition of Hypoxic Mitochondrial Cellular Damage Induced by Cobalt Chloride in Human Lung H1299 Cells

Nidal Zeineh [1,†], Nunzio Denora [2,3,†], Valentino Laquintana [2], Massimo Franco [2], Abraham Weizman [4,5] and Moshe Gavish [1,*]

1. The Ruth and Bruce Rappaport Faculty of Medicine, Technion Institute of Technology, Haifa 31096, Israel; nidalz1988@gmail.com
2. Department of Pharmacy–Pharmaceutical Sciences, University of Bari "Aldo Moro", 70125 Bari, Italy; nunzio.denora@uniba.it (N.D.); valentino.laquintana@uniba.it (V.L.); massimo.franco@uniba.it (M.F.)
3. Institute for Chemical and Physical Processes (IPCF)-CNR SS Bari, Via Orabona 4, 70126 Bari, Italy
4. Research Unit at Geha Mental Health Center and Laboratory of Biological Psychiatry at Felsenstein Medical Research Center, Petah Tikva 4910002, Israel; weizmana@gmail.com
5. Sackler Faculty of Medicine, Tel Aviv University, Tel Aviv 6997801, Israel
* Correspondence: mgavish@technion.ac.il; Tel.: +972-4829-5275; Fax: +972-4829-5330
† These authors contributed equally to this work.

Received: 5 April 2020; Accepted: 30 April 2020; Published: 2 May 2020

Abstract: The 18 kDa translocator protein (TSPO) plays an important role in apoptotic cell death, including apoptosis induced by the hypoxia mimicking agent cobalt chloride ($CoCl_2$). In this study, the protective effects of a high (CB86; Ki = 1.6 nM) and a low (CB204; Ki = 117.7 nM) affinity TSPO ligands were investigated in H1299 lung cancer cell line exposed to $CoCl_2$. The lung cell line H1299 was chosen in the present study since they express TSPO and able to undergo programmed cell death. The examined cell death markers included: ATP synthase reversal, reactive oxygen species (ROS) generation, mitochondrial membrane potential ($\Delta\psi m$) depolarization, cellular toxicity, and cellular viability. Pretreatment of the cells with the low affinity ligand CB204 at a concentration of 100 µM suppressed significantly ($p < 0.05$ for all) $CoCl_2$-induced cellular cytotoxicity (100%), ATP synthase reversal (67%), ROS generation (82%), $\Delta\psi m$ depolarization (100%), reduction in cellular density (97%), and also increased cell viability (85%). Furthermore, the low affinity TSPO ligand CB204, was harmless when given by itself at 100 µM. In contrast, the high affinity ligand (CB86) was significantly effective only in the prevention of $CoCl_2$–induced ROS generation (39%, $p < 0.001$), and showed significant cytotoxic effects when given alone at 100 µM, as reflected in alterations in ADP/ATP ratio, oxidative stress, mitochondrial membrane potential depolarization and cell death. It appears that similar to previous studies on brain-derived cells, the relatively low affinity for the TSPO target enhances the potency of TSPO ligands in the protection from hypoxic cell death. Moreover, the high affinity TSPO ligand CB86, but not the low affinity ligand CB204, was lethal to the lung cells at high concentration (100 µM). The low affinity TSPO ligand CB204 may be a candidate for the treatment of pulmonary diseases related to hypoxia, such as pulmonary ischemia and chronic obstructive pulmonary disease COPD.

Keywords: translocator protein (TSPO); $CoCl_2$; mitochondrial membrane potential; reactive oxygen species (ROS); cell viability; cell death; lung cancer cell line

1. Introduction

In this study the hypoxic toxic agent cobalt chloride ($CoCl_2$) was used to induce hypoxic death in H1299 lung cancer cells. Hypoxia is a state in which the oxygen supply to a tissue within an organ is compromised [1]. Decreased oxygen levels or tension in a tissue results in hypoxic damage due to altered cellular signaling networks. Hypoxia may occur both in physiological conditions such as climbing to high altitudes, as well as in pathological conditions such as myocardial ischemia, chronic obstructive pulmonary disease (COPD), and obstructive sleep apnea [2]. Hypoxia affects cellular homeostasis, which may lead to reactive oxygen species (ROS) production, elevated vasoconstrictive substances, increased expression of pro-inflammatory cytokines, and increased intercellular and vascular cell adhesion molecules [3–9]. Impaired protein homeostasis in the muscle system is a well-known condition in COPD patients [10–12].

$CoCl_2$ mimics hypoxic state when applied to cell cultures [13–19]. Previous studies in neural-derived PC12 cells, demonstrated that $CoCl_2$ might induce apoptotic cell death via the P38-MAPK-caspase 3 pathway [20]. $CoCl_2$ interferes with heme production from protoporphyrin IX (PPIX) [19,21]. PPIX acts as an endogenous ligand for the mitochondrial 18 kDa translocator protein (TSPO) [22]. It was shown that decreased ROS levels due to TSPO knockdown lead to accumulation of PPIX and consequently increased heme production [23]. The hypoxia mimicking effect of $CoCl_2$ is related to its stabilizing effect on the α-subunit of HIF (hypoxia inducible transcription factor), in addition to inhibition of cytochrome-C oxidase subunit 4 (COX4) precursor processing and enhancement of its degradation [16].

Mitochondria are involved in some of the hypoxia-induced cellular injury mechanisms, and it acts as an energy source, as well as a source for metabolic signals, cellular proliferation, inflammation, and intrinsic cell death [24]. The TSPO located in the outer mitochondrial membrane plays an important role in the mitochondrial apoptotic processes [25–29], along with other cellular roles [30–32]. A previous study has indicated the role of TSPO in $CoCl_2$-induced apoptotic cell death. TSPO knockdown in U118MG glioblastoma cells, demonstrated the important role of TSPO in apoptosis induced by $CoCl_2$, including processes such as: Δψm depolarization, cardiolipin peroxidation, and ROS generation. Administration of the TSPO ligand PK 11195 inhibited partially a sequence of TSPO-related processes relevant to $CoCl_2$-induced cell death reminiscent of the effects of TSPO knockdown determined in the same study [22]. In the present study, TSPO ligands characterized by a 2-phenyl-imidazo [1–a] pyridine nucleus (Scheme 1) that express various affinities were investigated (Table 1). The goal of the current study was to examine, for the first time, the protective effect of two novel TSPO ligands (CB86 and CB204), in the attenuation of the hypoxic effect of $CoCl_2$ in H1299 lung cancer cell line. The two ligands differ in their affinity to TSPO: CB204 has low affinity (K_i = 117.7 nM) and CB86 has high affinity (K_i = 1.6 nM) [33]. Among the few examples known of TSPO ligands containing hydrophilic groups, there is the 8-amino imidazopyridine CB86 ligand. In a previous study it was evaluated whether further polar substituents or ionizable functional groups could be introduced on the amino group of CB86 [33]. Data indicated that introduction of a -COOH group led to a significant decrease in affinity to TSPO, as observed for the compound CB204. Furthermore, in addition to the structure-activity relationship studies, reported by some of us, highlighting the main physicochemical factors eliciting the binding of imidazopyridines to TSPO, the pharmacological profile of these compounds by measuring their modulatory effects on the $GABA_A$ receptors was also explored [33].

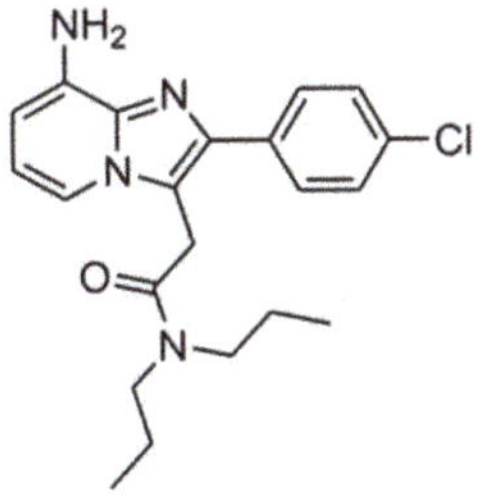

CB86

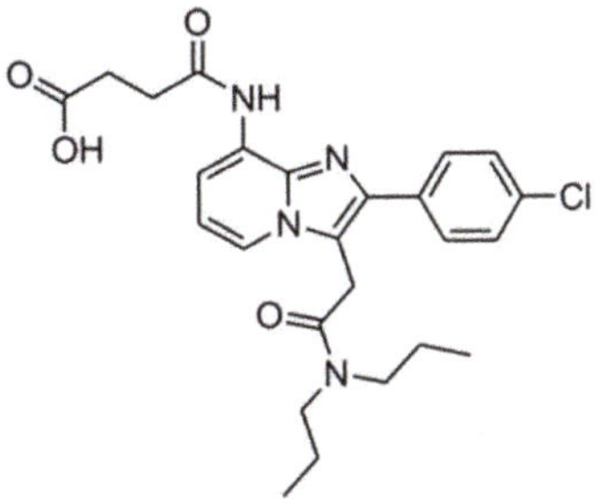

CB194

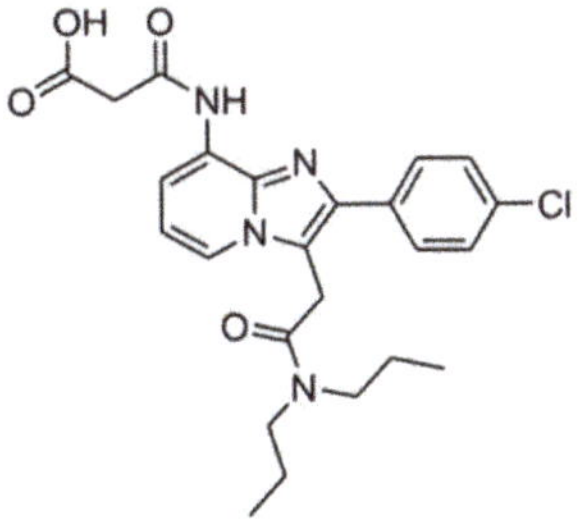

CB199

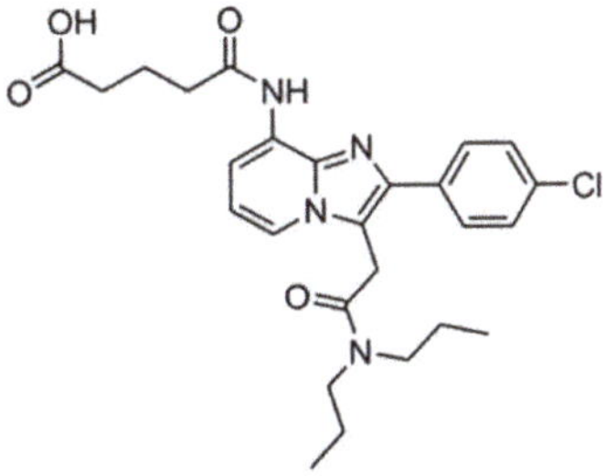

CB204

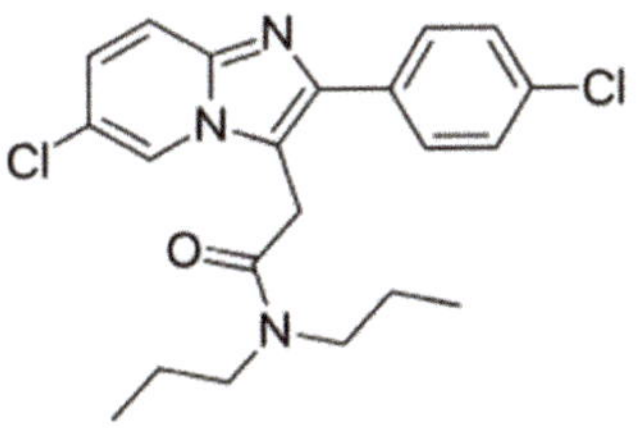

Alpidem

Scheme 1. Molecular structure of CB86, CB194, CB199, CB204, and Alpidem assayed in the present study.

Table 1. The affinity data of translocator protein (TSPO) ligands used in the current study.

Ligand Name	CB86	CB194	CB199	CB204	Alpidem
Molecular weight	384	484	470	498	404
TSPO *Ki* (nM)	1.6	285.3	193.1	117.7	0.6

CB86 and CB204 were chosen in the present study for their diverging affinities to the TSPO. This choice was prompted by previous findings with other TSPO ligands, presenting low to moderate affinity, that showed efficacy regarding cellular protective effects and without cellular toxic activity. In contrast, high affinity TSPO ligands can induce cellular toxic effects and conspicuous lethal effects at relatively high concentrations [34–36]. These previous studies were conducted on microglia, astrocytic, neuronal, and cancer cells and in animal models [35,37,38]. A previous review of numerous cell types reported that classical high affinity TSPO ligands show lethal effects at high concentrations (typically > 50 μM), but protective effects at low concentrations [39]. A subsequent experimental research reported that indeed in a paradigm of astrocytic cells challenged with ammonia, the classical high affinity TSPO ligands (PK 11195, Ro5 4864 and FGIN-1-27) induced cell death at concentrations above 50 µM, but were protective at the nM range [40]. Thus, the hypothesis of the present study was that the high affinity TSPO ligand (CB86 in Scheme 1) would show cytotoxic effects at a concentration of 100 µM, while the low affinity TSPO ligand with a comparable structure (CB204 in Scheme 1) would show cellular protective effects at the same concentration of 100 µM. We applied this to a paradigm of cells vastly different from the cells regularly used by us (lung cancer cells vs. brain cells). We attempted to confirm or disprove previous findings on the relationship between the affinity of ligands to TSPO and their cytotoxic or protective effects. Furthermore, the question was whether these cellular effects are specific for brain cells, or valid also for other types of cells as well, in our case lung cells. The present report provides new data since: (1) The TSPO ligands in the current study were not used in the previous studies; (2) low affinity and high affinity TSPO ligands based on a common structural framework are compared in one paradigm, so they can reliably represent their unique pharmacological properties; and (3) another type of cells (lung cells) are used, while in the previous similar studies brain derived cells were used. The present study was designed to provide indication whether the previous findings on the effects of TSPO ligands on brain derived cells can also be discerned with novel TSPO ligands when applied to other types of cells, and thus are not restricted to the cells of brain origin (microglia, astrocytes, and neuronal cells). Thus, the present attempted to verify and unify the image suggested by the scattered information of previous studies. We chose H1299 lung cells because they represent peripheral respiratory mitochondrial-relevant system, express TSPO and can undergo programmed cell death when exposed to cytotoxic agents [41].

Thus, the correlation between TSPO ligand affinity and their protective effects in a putative TSPO-associated hypoxic cellular model was evaluated in the present study.

2. Materials and Methods

2.1. Study Design

In this study, the H1299 lung cancer cells from human origin were used. The maintenance of the cells was performed according to the American Type Culture Collection (ATCC) instructions, as follows: Culture medium consisted of RPMI (high glucose, without L-glutamine and sodium pyruvate), supplemented with 10% Fetal Bovine Serum (FBS), 2% glutamine, and gentamycin (50 mg/mL). The serum-deprived medium contained similar components, just with 2.5 mL FCS (0.5%), instead of 50 mL (10%). According to a previous study, hypoxic damage due to exposure to toxic agent (e.g., cigarette smoke) demonstrated an association between TSPO and apoptotic cell death. Since the conditions needed were the existence of TSPO and the possibility to induce apoptosis via TSPO, H1299 fulfilled these criteria, and were chosen in the current study [41].

The cells were incubated at 37 °C in 5% CO_2 until 80–90% confluency was reached. Initially, pretreatment of the cells with the TSPO ligands: CB86, CB194, CB199, CB204, and Alpidem, at increasing concentrations was performed 24 h prior to incubation with $CoCl_2$ for another 24 h. According to the collected results, the high affinity CB86 and the low affinity CB204 TSPO ligands were chosen for the proceeding experiments.

2.2. $CoCl_2$ Exposure and Its Treatment with TSPO Ligands

According to previous studies, the $CoCl_2$ at a concentration of 0.5 mM was used in our experiments [22,42,43].

Treatment consisted of 24 h of TSPO ligand pretreatment prior to the subsequent 24 h simultaneous exposure to $CoCl_2$ and TSPO ligands/or vehicle. In more detail, pretreatment of the cells was conducted using DMSO (1%) (vehicle) in serum-deprived medium for the control groups, and ligand-containing serum-deprived medium for the experimental groups. After 24 h of pretreatment, the medium of the control groups and the ligand-containing groups was replaced by the same medium, but in the "experimental groups" it contained also 0.5 mM CoCl$_2$. Then, the groups of cells were incubated for another 24 h (the treatment), as previously described [43–45]. The pretreatment groups included: vehicle and vehicle plus ligand groups. For treatment, the groups included: Vehicle, vehicle plus ligand, vehicle plus CoCl$_2$, and vehicle plus ligand plus CoCl$_2$ groups. Following this subsequent exposure to CoCl$_2$ for 24 h, the cells were collected and processed. According to a previous study using U118MG cells [22], dose response analysis with increasing CoCl$_2$ concentrations was performed. It was shown that at concentrations of 0.3–0.5 mM cell death levels increased by 10–25%, while at concentrations above 0.6 mM cell death elevated by 40% to 90% [22]. In accord with the previous study [22], the 0.5 mM concentration of CoCl$_2$ was selected for the current experiments, in order obtain reversible and treatable cellular toxic effects. The dose response curve for H1299 cells exposed to CoCl$_2$ was very similar to the one described by us previously on U118MG cells [22].

2.3. ADP/ATP Ratio

White 96-well plates were used to measure the levels of ADP and ATP. After pretreatment of cells in medium with and without CB86 and CB204, followed by CoCl$_2$ exposure, the ADP/ATP ratio was measured and calculated, according to the manufacturer's protocol (MAK135; Sigma-Aldrich, St. Louis, MO, USA), as previously described [46]. Luminescence levels of the ratio between ADP and ATP were measured by ELISA using Infinite M200 Pro plate reader (Tecan, Männedorf, Switzerland), according to the instructions of the manufacturer.

2.4. Reactive Oxygen Species (ROS) Levels

ROS/superoxide detection assay kit (Abcam, Cambridge, UK) was used to measure ROS and superoxide levels according to the manufacturer's instructions. Following treatment of the cells as described above, they were washed using 1X wash buffer followed by application of 100 µL/well of ROS/superoxide detection solution and then incubated in dark for 60 min. ELISA with Infinite M200 Pro plate reader (Tecan, Männedorf, Switzerland) was used with standard fluorescein (excitation 488 nm and emission 520 nm) and rhodamine (excitation 550 nm and emission 610 nm) filter sets, and fluorescence levels were measured, according to the instructions of the manufacturer.

2.5. Depolarization of the Mitochondrial Membrane Potential ($\Delta\Psi m$)

Mitochondrial membrane potential ($\Delta\Psi m$) depolarization was assayed using the dye JC-1(5,5′,6,6′-tetrachloro-1,1′,3,3′-tetraethylbenzimidazolylcarbocyanine-chloride), as described previously [22]. JC-1 is a marker for mitochondrial function and cell health. Intact cells characterized by high $\Delta\psi_M$, the cationic lipophilic JC-1 dye selectively enters the mitochondria, forms aggregates and thus reversibly changes color from green to red inside the mitochondria (orange-red fluorescence emitting at 590 nm wavelength). In case of $\Delta\psi_M$ depolarization, monomers of JC-1 remain in the cytoplasm, and these monomers emit at 527 nm (green fluorescence). Thus, $\Delta\psi_M$ depolarization is expressed by decreased red/green ratio.

The cells were trypsinized and collected by centrifugation (660× g, 5 min, 4 °C). The proton ionophore carbonyl cyanide was used as a positive control, as previously described [22]. The samples were incubated in 400 µL of diluted JC-1 dye (1/500) for 30 min. Then, the cells were centrifuged (660× g, 5 min, 4 °C), the pellets then resuspended in 500 µL of PBS and transferred into FACS tubes. The mean fluorescence intensity (MFI) was measured using FACS device, and the results were analyzed using FlowJo (10th version, FlowJo LLC, Ashland, OR, USA). In the calculation of the mitochondrial depolarization the basal 590/527 ratio was subtracted. This is an assay demonstrating cell number-wise, namely, the percentage of the measured cell population presents mitochondrial depolarization sufficient to prevent JC-1 entry and conversion to red emitting aggregates.

2.6. Cellular Cytotoxicity Assay (LDH)

Cellular cytotoxicity levels were measured by the Cytotoxicity Detection Kit (Roche Pharmaceuticals, Basel, Switzerland), which measures the LDH enzyme levels in the medium. LDH enzyme is released from the cells when the cell membrane is disrupted in case of necrosis and late apoptosis [47].

Cytotoxicity levels were measured by an absorbance at 492 nm wavelength and a reference wavelength of 620 nm, according to the manufacturer's protocol. ELISA with spectrophotometer Zenyth 200 (Anthos, Eugendorf, Austria) was used for measurements and the results were calculated and normalized (calibrated) according to the formula given by the manufacturer.

2.7. XTT Based Colorimetric Assay

Cell viability was measured using XTT cell viability assay kit (Abcam, Cambridge, UK), according to the manufacturer's protocol. In this assay, in viable cells the 2,3-bis [2-methoxy-4-nitro-5-sulphophenyl]-2H-tetrazolium-5-carboxylanilide inner salt (XTT) is reduced by mitochondrial dehydrogenases, and this reaction leads to an orange formazan product. This assay measures cell metabolism as an indication of cell viability. The spectrophotometer Zenyth 200 (Anthos, Eugendorf, Austria) was used to assess optical density (OD) as reflected by absorbance at 492 nm wavelength and a reference wavelength of 620 nm (ELISA technology).

2.8. Cell Density

Photographs from wells of a 96-well plate with the various experimental groups were taken using a Basler scA1400–30gm camera, a CCD camera with Sony ICX285 CCD sensor (Essen Bioscience, Ann Arbor, MI, USA). The confluency of the cells was measured using the high throughput, continuous live cell imager Incucyte Zoom HD/2CLR System (Essen Bioscience, Ann Arbor, MI, USA) to assess the effects of $CoCl_2$ exposure on the density of the cells. The same number of cells were used in each assay for all wells. To ensure this, plating was done from one tube with cell suspension by collecting equal amounts from the tube for each well. In numbers, 40,000 cells per cm^2 were seeded and then the cells were cultured till they reached 80–90% confluency.

2.9. Statistical Analysis and Data Presentation

Relative changes (%) were used for comparisons among assays. GraphPad prism (GraphPad Software, San Diego, CA, USA) was used for statistical analysis. The results were expressed as mean ± SEM. One-way analysis of variance (ANOVA) was performed followed by Bonferroni's post hoc test for multiple comparisons as appropriate. $p < 0.05$ was considered as statistically significant.

3. Results

3.1. Screening of TSPO Ligand Efficacy in the Protection of Cellular Viability

Assessment of the efficacy of the TSPO ligands in the prevention of $CoCl_2$ cytotoxicity was determined using a cellular viability assay (XTT) with different TSPO ligands CB86, CB194, CB199, CB204, and alpidem, at concentrations of 1 µM, 10 µM, 25 µM, 50 µM, and 100 µM for each of them (Figure 1A–E). It was demonstrated that the high affinity CB86 ligand and the high affinity alpidem, did not protect against the cytotoxicity caused by $CoCl_2$ (0.5 mM), while the low affinity CB204 achieved significant protective capacity by 76% at a concentration of 25 µM (Figure 1C) and by 85% at 100 µM (Figure 1E). In addition, the low affinity CB194 and CB199 ligands displayed significant protection by 61% and by 59%, respectively, against $CoCl_2$ cytotoxicity only at a concentration of 100 µM (Figure 1E). According to these data (Figure 1), the high affinity ligand CB86 and the low affinity ligand CB204 at a concentration of 100 µM were chosen for further investigation of the potential effects of the affinity of the TSPO ligands in the protection from $CoCl_2$-induced cellular damage.

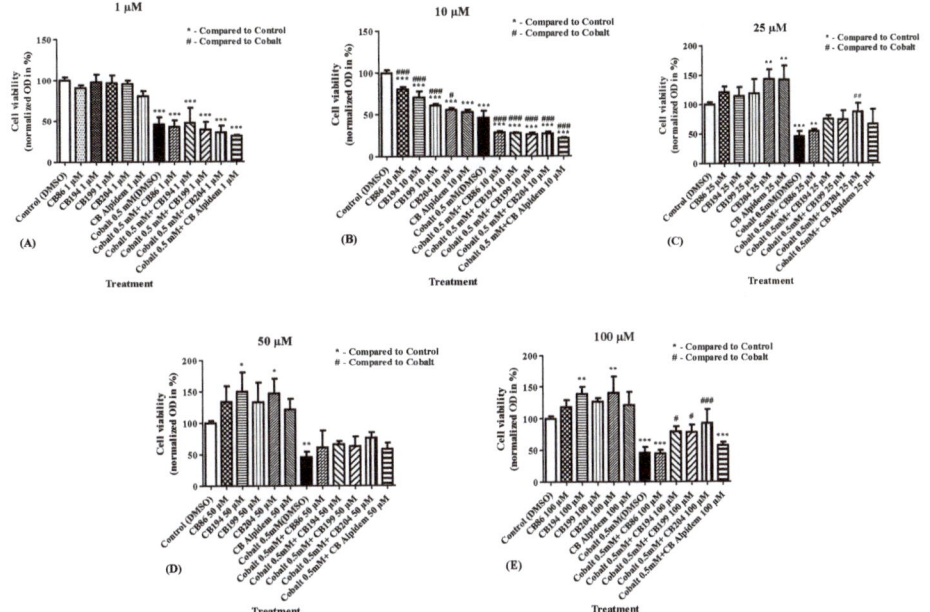

Figure 1. Determination of the ligand efficacy in inhibition of CoCl$_2$-induced decrease in cellular viability (XTT assay). Cell viability was assessed following pretreatment with TSPO ligands at various concentrations of 1 µM, 10 µM, 25 µM, 50 µM, and 100 µM (**A–E**). Results are expressed as mean ± SEM (n = 5 replicates in each group). # and * $p < 0.05$, ## and ** $p < 0.01$, ### and *** $p < 0.001$.

In general, going from high affinity to low affinity TSPO ligands (Table 1) was associated with larger protective effect (Figure 1).

3.2. Dose–Response Analyses for the Efficacy of CB86 and CB204 Ligands in the Prevention of CoCl$_2$-Induced Decrease in Cellular Viability

To verify the indications described in Figure 1, the modulatory effect of CB86 and CB204 on cell viability following exposure to CoCl$_2$ was assessed. The range of concentrations of these two ligands was expanded, from 1 µM to 100 µM (Figure 1), and from 5 nM to 100 µM (Figure 2), to ensure that no major concentration-dependent effects were overlooked. Dose–response assessment was performed for CB86 and CB204 using cellular viability assay (XTT). Pretreatment with increasing concentrations of CB86 did not inhibit the cytotoxic effect of 0.5 mM CoCl$_2$ at any tested concentration (Figure 2A). In contrast, the low affinity TSPO ligand CB204 at concentrations of 25 µM and 100 µM prevented 50% and 81% of the cellular damage, respectively (Figure 2B). At 100 µM, CB204 caused maintenance at control levels, i.e., cell viability was not significantly different from vehicle-exposed cells. Figures 1 and 2 show that 100 µM is the optimal concentration for CB204 capacity to provide protection from CoCl$_2$-induced cell death.

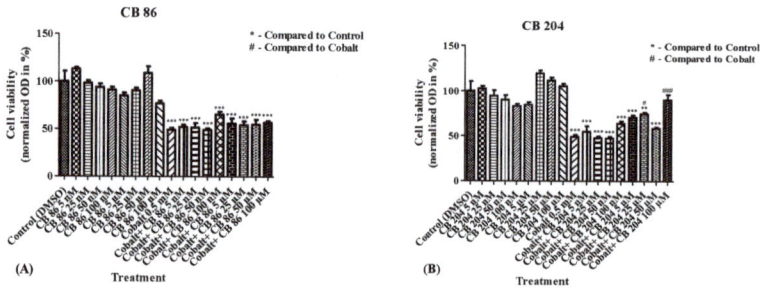

Figure 2. Dose response analysis of CB86 and CB204 ligands in inhibition of cellular viability decrease induced by $CoCl_2$. XTT assay was performed to measure the levels of cellular viability following exposure to $CoCl_2$ after pretreatment with (**A**) CB86 and (**B**) CB204 at increasing concentrations. Results are expressed as mean ± SEM (n = 5 replicates in each group). # $p < 0.05$, ## and ** $p < 0.01$, ### and *** $p < 0.001$.

3.3. ADP/ATP Ratio

Following $CoCl_2$ exposure for 24 h, the ADP/ATP ratio significantly increased by 84% ($p < 0.001$) as compared to the control group (absolute level of ADP/ATP luminescence ratio was 0.1). This increase was not attenuated significantly by pretreatment with CB86 at a concentration of 100 μM (49%; $p > 0.05$), while pretreatment with CB204 at a concentration of 100 μM significantly attenuated (67%; $p < 0.01$) the increase in ADP/ATP ratio, as compared to the $CoCl_2$-exposed group (Figure 3).

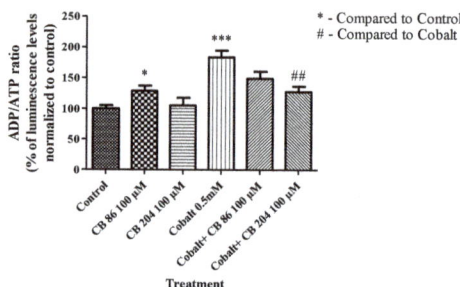

Figure 3. The ability of TSPO ligands to attenuate $CoCl_2$-induced ATP synthase reversal. ELISA was performed to measure the alterations in ADP/ATP ratio with and without pretreatment with the TSPO ligands. Results are expressed as mean ± SEM (n = 5 replicates in each group). * $p < 0.05$, ## $p < 0.01$, and *** $p < 0.001$.

Regarding ADP/ATP ratio, CB86 appears to have a dual effect: slightly cytotoxic by itself, but protective from the cytotoxic effects of $CoCl_2$. Reminiscent of the effects on ROS levels described in Section 3.4 (Figure 4).

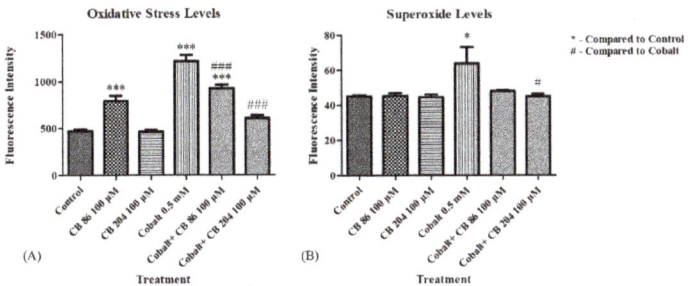

Figure 4. The protective effect of the TSPO ligands in prevention of reactive oxygen species (ROS) elevation. ELISA was performed to evaluate the levels of oxidative stress and superoxide levels. (**A**) Represents the oxidative stress levels, and (**B**) Represents the superoxide levels, with and without pretreatment with TSPO ligands. Results are expressed as mean ± SEM (n = 6 replicates in each group). $^{\#}$ and * $p < 0.05$, $^{\#\#\#}$ and *** $p < 0.001$.

3.4. Oxidative Stress and Superoxide Levels

ROS levels were measured following $CoCl_2$ exposure of CB86 and CB204 pretreated cells. Significant elevation in ROS levels was detected following pretreatment of the cells with CB86 ligand alone, while no elevation occurred following pretreatment with the TSPO ligand CB204 alone. $CoCl_2$ induced a significant elevation in oxidative stress levels by (158%; $p < 0.001$) as compared to the control group. Pretreatment with CB86 at a concentration of 100 μM significantly prevented (39%; $p < 0.001$) of the $CoCl_2$-induced increase in ROS generation, however remained significantly higher than the control ($p < 0.001$). In contrast, pretreatment with CB204 at a concentration of 100 μM significantly prevented 82% of the $CoCl_2$-induced elevation (at the control range; $p < 0.001$; Figure 4A). In a second assay, superoxide levels were not elevated in response to the incubation with both ligands alone. $CoCl_2$ exposure for 24 h induced a significant elevation (41%; $p < 0.05$) as compared to the control group, while pretreatment with CB86 did not prevent significantly the elevation in superoxide levels ($p > 0.05$; Figure 4B). CB204 was more effective in preventing this elevation (actually to control range; $p < 0.05$; Figure 4B).

3.5. Depolarization of the Mitochondrial Membrane Potential ($\Delta\Psi m$)

$\Delta\Psi m$ depolarization was measured by JC-1 fluorescence changes as described in the methods. Significant depolarization of the $\Delta\Psi m$ (18%; $p < 0.001$) occurred after exposure to $CoCl_2$, as compared to the control group. Pre-treatment with CB86 at a concentration of 100 μM did not show any protective effect and $\Delta\Psi m$ remained significantly different from the control group ($p < 0.001$). Pretreatment with CB204 prevented completely the depolarization of the $\Delta\Psi m$ ($p < 0.001$) induced by $CoCl_2$ (Figure 5A–G). Carbonyl cyanide chlorophenylhydrazone (CCCP) was used as a positive control and its administration resulted in a significant increase in depolarization of $\Delta\Psi m$ (by 48% vs. control raw level; $p < 0.001$) (Figure 5H).

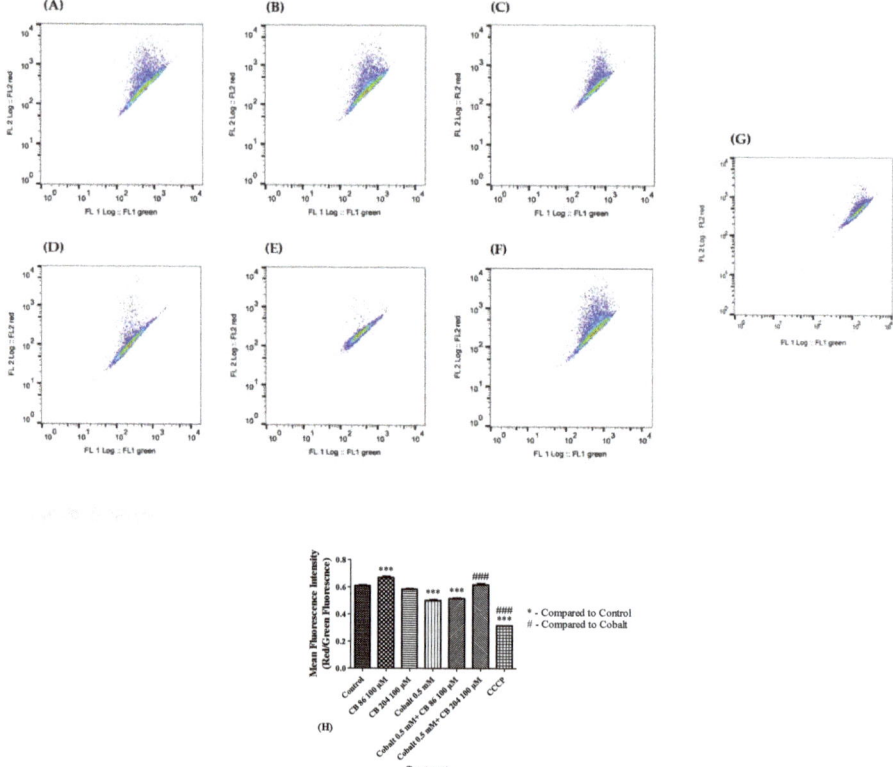

Figure 5. Comparison of the protective capacities of CB86 and CB204 in prevention of mitochondrial membrane potential depolarization. FACS was used to evaluate the Δψm depolarization in (**A**) Control group, (**B**) cells pretreated with CB86 alone, (**C**) cells pretreated with CB204 alone, (**D**) cells exposed to 0.5 mM of CoCl$_2$, (**E**) cells pretreated with CB86 and exposed to CoCl$_2$, (**F**) cells pretreated with CB204 and exposed to CoCl$_2$, (**G**) positive control group exposed to CCCP, and (**H**) representative bar graph of the raw data. Results are expressed as mean ± SEM (n = 7 replicates in each group). ### and *** $p < 0.001$.

3.6. LDH Assay of Cell Death

Cytotoxicity levels were measured by release of LDH enzyme into the media. CoCl$_2$ exposure resulted in a significant elevation in cytotoxicity levels by 52% ($p < 0.001$) as compared to the control group (absolute LDH level measured by OD was 0.5). Pretreatment with the TSPO ligand CB86 at a concentration of 100 μM did not attenuate significantly the LDH elevation, while CB204 at a concentration of 100 μM completely prevented the LDH elevation (100%; $p < 0.001$) as compared to the CoCl$_2$-exposed group. Both CB86 and CB204 had no effect when applied alone (Figure 6).

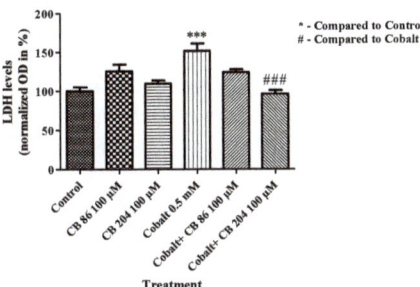

Figure 6. Prevention of CoCl$_2$-induced cellular cytotoxicity by TSPO ligands. LDH cytotoxicity assay was performed to measure cytotoxicity levels following exposure to CoCl$_2$ with or without TSPO ligands pretreatment. Results are expressed as mean ± SEM ($n = 5$ replicates in each group). ### and *** $p < 0.001$.

3.7. XTT Assay of Cell Viability

Following CoCl$_2$ exposure, cellular viability significantly decreased by 54% ($p < 0.001$) as compared to the control group. Pretreatment with CB86 at a concentration of 100 μM did not prevent the decrease in cell viability, while CB204 at a concentration of 100 μM significantly prevented the decrease in cell viability as compared to the CoCl$_2$-exposed group (85%; $p < 0.001$; Figure 7).

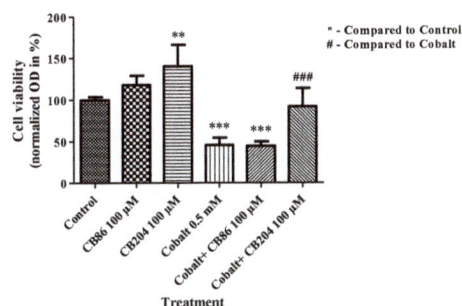

Figure 7. The protective effect of TSPO ligands in preventing the decrease in cellular viability. XTT assay was performed to measure the levels of cellular viability following CoCl$_2$ exposure with or without TSPO ligands pretreatment. Results are expressed as mean ± SEM ($n = 5$ replicates in each group). ** $p < 0.01$, ### and *** $p < 0.001$.

3.8. Cellular Density

Representative illustration of the alterations in cell density are depicted in Figure 8A–F. The density of the cells significantly decreased by 32% (Figure 8G) following exposure to 0.5 mM CoCl$_2$ for 24 h, relative to the control group (set as 100%) (Figure 8G). The application of the high affinity ligand CB86 alone at a concentration of 100 μM induced a robust reduction in cell density (by 79%; $p < 0.001$; Figure 8G). No further decrease in cell density occurred when CB86 (100 μM) was applied as a pretreatment to CoCl$_2$ exposure (by 82%; $p < 0.001$; Figure 8G). In the case of pretreatment with the low affinity ligand CB204 at a concentration of 100 μM, the density of the cells remained within the control range (Figure 8C). Also, when exposed to CoCl$_2$, the pretreatment with CB204 prevented 97% of the CoCl$_2$-induced decrease in cell density (Figure 8G). The collected data are summarized in Figure 8G.

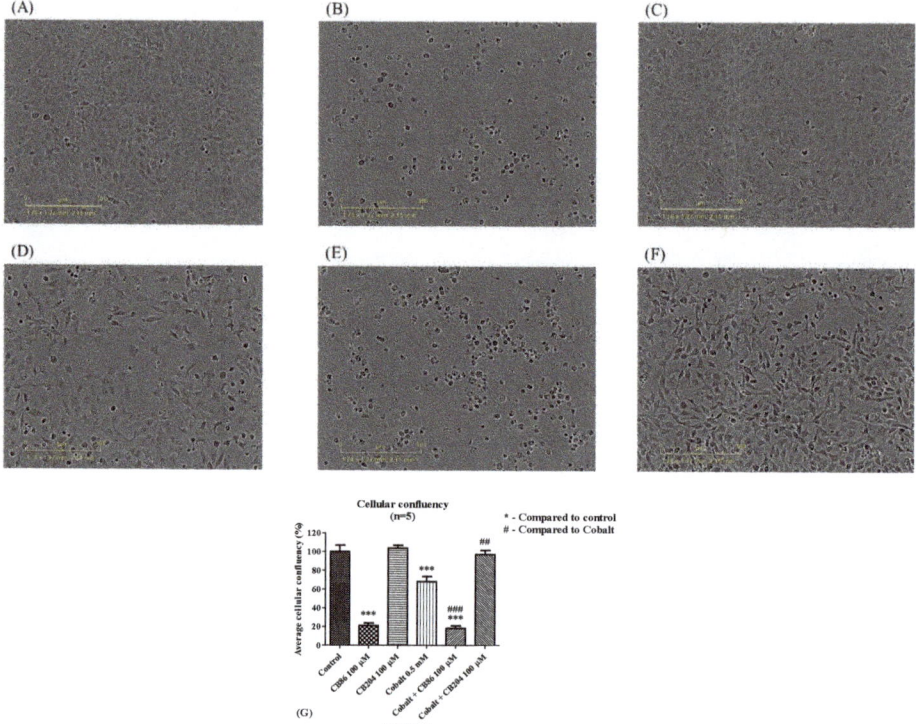

Figure 8. The effects of CB86 and CB204 on reductions of cell density caused by $CoCl_2$. Photographs showing the density of H1299 cells in (**A**) control group, (**B**) following pretreatment with the high affinity CB86 ligand alone (100 µM), (**C**) following pretreatment with the low affinity CB204 ligand alone (100 µM), (**D**) following exposure to 0.5 mM of $CoCl_2$, (**E**) following pretreatment with the high affinity CB86 at a concentration of 100 µM and exposure to 0.5 mM $CoCl_2$, (**F**) following pretreatment with the low affinity CB204 at a concentration of 100 µM and exposure to 0.5 mM $CoCl_2$, and (**G**) a bar graph summarizing the results. Results in Figure 8G are presented as mean ± SEM (n = 5 replicates in each group). ## $p < 0.01$, ### and *** $p < 0.001$.

In summary, CB86 (with and without $CoCl_2$) caused robust reductions in cell density, while CB204 alone has no harmful effect on cell density and prevented completely reductions in cell density induced by exposure $CoCl_2$.

3.9. Summary of the Collected Data

As the results show (Figures 3–8), application of the high affinity TSPO ligand CB86 applied alone at a concentration of 100 µM caused: (1) Increase in the ADP/ATP ratio (Figure 3); (2) increase in ROS generation, but without effect on superoxide levels (Figure 4); (3) increase in the occurrence of ΔΨm depolarization (Figure 5); (4) increase of cell membrane disruption as assessed by LDH levels in the supernatant (Figure 6). In contrast, the low affinity TSPO ligand CB204 at the same concentration (100 µM) did not induce any cytotoxic effects (Figures 3–8). The overall efficient protective effects indicate a favorable profile of the low affinity TSPO ligand CB204 (Figures 1–8) with regard to efficacy and safety in hypoxic cellular conditions.

4. Discussion

In this study, we focused on the capacity of two TSPO ligands, the high affinity CB86 and the low affinity CB204 (affinity and structure presented in Table 1 and Scheme 1) to prevent cellular damage induced by $CoCl_2$ (Figures 3–8 and Scheme 2). Based on ligand efficacy in prevention of $CoCl_2$-induced cytotoxicity (Figure 1) and dose–response analysis (Figure 2), the high affinity CB86 ligand and the low affinity CB204 ligand at a concentration of 100 µM were chosen for this study. A previous study demonstrated the protective effects of the high affinity TSPO ligand PK 11195 (25 µM), in $CoCl_2$-induced cell death, which was reminiscent to the protective effect of TSPO gene knockdown [22]. The protective effect of the TSPO ligands was established in several $CoCl_2$-induced cytotoxic assays, including ADP/ATP ratio, ROS generation, superoxide levels, LDH cytotoxicity assay, cellular viability assay (XTT), and viable cell density. The low affinity ligand CB204 significantly inhibited the cytotoxic effect of $CoCl_2$ on H1299 lung cells in all the tested assays (Figures 3–8), furthermore, it was harmless when given alone. In contrast, the high affinity ligand CB86 was ineffective in the prevention of the cytotoxicity in most of the assays, except ROS generation. Moreover, CB86 was harmful when given alone in the assay of density of viable cells (Figure 8). Our results show that the effects of TSPO ligands reported in brain cells, are not restricted to cells of the central nervous system [35,37,38], but also applicable to lung cancer cells. It would be interesting to test whether this could be true for other types of cells as well.

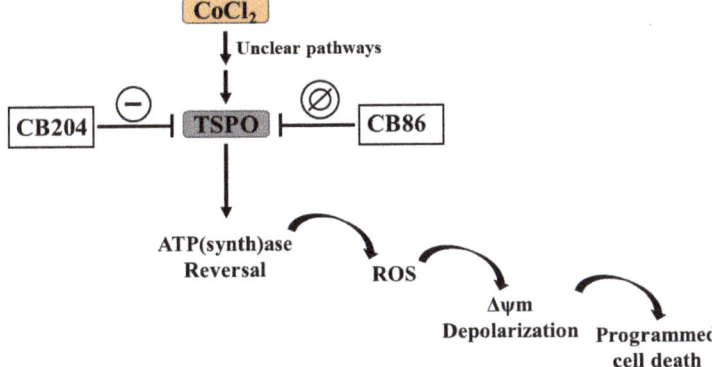

Scheme 2. The capacity of TSPO ligand to inhibit the initiation of the $CoCl_2$ cytotoxic effect and its propagation towards mitochondrial apoptosis cascade. The progression was inhibited by the low affinity CB204, but not by the high affinity CB86, TSPO ligands.

The difference in the protective capacity of the two ligands could be related to differences in their affinity to TSPO or could be related to their putative agonistic or antagonistic activities at the TSPO. Several studies attempted to identify the agonistic or antagonistic properties of TSPO ligands and to sort them as agonists and antagonists. Unfortunately, such classification of TSPO ligands was abandoned, since the same ligand may exert an agonistic activity or an antagonistic activity, depending on the investigated TSPO function [48,49]. The present study confirms the observation that high affinity TSPO ligands can exert harmful, and even lethal, cellular effects, as was described in other paradigms [34–36]. On the other hand, most importantly, the present study supports the notion that low affinity TSPO ligands, may possess protective cellular effects and are devoid of cytotoxic effects, as was demonstrated in previous studies [35,37,38].

Different ligands have varying cellular impact in nanomolar or micromolar range concentrations depending on the TSPO complex composition and the varying affinities to the TSPO complex present in a specific cell [49]. For example, the TSPO2 isoform, the main isoform at the red blood cells membrane requires micromolar concentrations for modulation of cellular functions, while the TSPO1 isoform requires nanomolar concentrations for modulation of cellular functions [49–52]. Such difference in specific ligand-interacting structural domains, within the TSPO protein or the protein complex, could explain the variability in the impact of TSPO ligands at different concentrations in different cell types. The presence of a high affinity and a low affinity binding sites can explain the dose-dependent dual effects of some TSPO ligands [39,40,53,54]. For example, the high affinity TSPO ligands PK 11195, Ro5-4864, and FGIN-1-27 at nanomolar concentrations protect U118MG human glioma cells from ammonia-induced cytotoxicity, while at micromolar concentrations the same ligands induce cytotoxic effects [36]. We suggest that this association between affinity of the ligands to TSPO and their protective potency regarding cell viability may be the rule rather than a coincidence. Yet, this notion should be investigated further in other cell types. The two ligands CB194 and CB199 with the lowest affinity (Table 1) did not show lethal cellular effect, but they may influence other TSPO functions. It is unclear whether these ligands act at the same ligand binding site, or at different ones. At present, only a restricted number of ligand binding sites were identified [36]. Previous studies showed that binding of the ligands might be influenced by the interaction between TSPO and the TSPO-associated proteins, such as mitochondrial voltage-dependent anion channels (or mitochondrial porins; VDAC) [55,56]. For example, the anticancer drugs ErPC and ErPC3, do not bind directly to TSPO, but they exert their anti-proliferative effect indirectly through TSPO [29], while TRO 19622 binds to both the TSPO and its associated protein VDAC [57].

TSPO is associated with regulation of various intracellular and mitochondrial processes. In the current study, the cytotoxic impact of CB86 on viable cellular density was accompanied by inability to protect most of the vital cellular metabolic processes. Modulation of TSPO protein expression leads to a cascade of events, including reversal of ATP synthase activity, followed by elevated ROS generation causing oxidative stress [23,29,58,59], which is associated with $\Delta\psi M$ depolarization, and eventually cell death (Scheme 2) [60]. Such a correlation between TSPO and cell death, mainly apoptotic cell death, was investigated previously. Exposure of U118MG glioblastoma cells to $CoCl_2$ resulted in increased apoptotic cell death, while TSPO knockdown prevented this cytotoxic effect of $CoCl_2$. Moreover, exposure of the cells to the proapoptotic agent $CoCl_2$ resulted in parallel increases in TSPO expression levels, as determined by Western blot and binding capacity. The same study demonstrated the role of TSPO in cellular processes leading to apoptosis [22]. Regarding another function, apart from $\Delta\Psi m$ collapse initiating the mitochondrial apoptosis cascade, TSPO via the mitochondria-to-cell-nucleus-pathway may also affect apoptosis induction due to modulation of cell nuclear gene expression for proteins that play a role in functional pathways regulating apoptosis [61]. Thus, the present observations on lung cells are similar to previous observations in brain cells, i.e., indicative of a common property, rather than a cell, tissue, or organ specific effect. However, research on different cell types, from different tissues and organs are required to further substantiate notion.

It was shown previously that 0.1–1 mM of $CoCl_2$ can mimic hypoxia in urinary bladder smooth muscle cells as well as cardiomyocytes [62,63]. In the current study in H1299 lung cancer cell line, it was shown that the $CoCl_2$-induced cascade of apoptotic events demonstrated in Scheme 2, may be prevented by TSPO ligands. The results emphasize the superiority of the low affinity TSPO ligand (CB204) in preventing cell death as well the preceding cascade of events leading to cell death as compared to the high affinity ligand (CB86). Previous studies have shown that TSPO ligands affect also cell proliferation, hence, it would also be interesting to test this for CB86 and CB204. It may be assumed that different binding domains modulate different TSPO functions.

In conclusion, our study demonstrated the robust efficacy of the low affinity TSPO ligand (CB204) in the prevention of $CoCl_2$-induced cellular damages in lung cells. The protective effect of the low affinity ligand was reflected in the inhibition of the appearance of classical makers of cytotoxicity assessed in this study. In contrast, the high affinity ligand (CB86) was effective only in the prevention of oxidative stress (ROS generation). These results may have clinical implications, namely, the potential use of the low affinity TSPO ligand CB204, but not the high affinity ligand CB86, for the treatment of lung cell pathologies related to hypoxia, such as pulmonary ischemia and COPD.

Future studies should address the following issues: the impact of TSPO knockdown and other TSPO ligands, to clarify further the role of TSPO in the $CoCl_2$-related cellular damage as well as the role of the TSPO ligands, preferably low affinity ligands, in the protection from non-$CoCl_2$-related hypoxic damage. Noteworthy, the current study, as well as a similar previous study on U118MG glioblastoma cells, were conducted on cells from human origin. Thus, it would be of interest to investigate the effects of TSPO ligands on cells of other species. The mechanism underpinning the impact of $CoCl_2$ on TSPO remains unclear (Scheme 2), further gene expression studies must be performed to identify the cellular pathways that are involved in the inhibitory effect of TSPO on in vitro and in vivo hypoxic states.

Author Contributions: Conceptualization, investigation, formal analysis, and writing—original draft preparation, N.Z.; methodology and data curation, N.Z., A.W. and M.G.; writing—review and editing, M.G., A.W., N.D., V.L. and M.F.; supervision, M.G. and A.W.; funding acquisition, M.G. and N.D. All authors have read and agreed to the published version of the manuscript.

Funding: The Israel Science Foundation is acknowledged for their support for this research (Moshe Gavish 1931/14).

Conflicts of Interest: The authors declare no conflict of interest.

References

1. Tuder, R.M.; Yun, J.H.; Bhunia, A.; Fijalkowska, I. Hypoxia and chronic lung disease. *J. Mol. Med.* **2007**, *85*, 1317–1324. [CrossRef]
2. Bensaid, S.; Fabre, C.; Fourneau, J.; Cieniewski-Bernard, C. Impact of different methods of induction of cellular hypoxia: Focus on protein homeostasis signaling pathways and morphology of C2C12 skeletal muscle cells differentiated into myotubes. *J. Physiol. Biochem.* **2019**, *75*, 367–377. [CrossRef] [PubMed]
3. Chen, D.; Fang, F.; Yang, Y.; Chen, J.; Xu, G.; Xu, Y.; Gao, Y. Brahma-related gene 1 (Brg1) epigenetically regulates CAM activation during hypoxic pulmonary hypertension. *Cardiovasc. Res.* **2013**, *100*, 363–373. [CrossRef] [PubMed]
4. Chen, D.; Yang, Y.; Cheng, X.; Fang, F.; Xu, G.; Yuan, Z.; Fang, M. Megakaryocytic leukemia 1 directs a histone H3 lysine 4 methyltransferase complex to regulate hypoxic pulmonary hypertension. *Hypertension* **2015**, *65*, 821–833. [CrossRef] [PubMed]
5. Janaszak-Jasiecka, A.; Siekierzycka, A.; Bartoszewska, S.; Serocki, M.; Dobrucki, L.W.; Collawn, J.F.; Bartoszewski, R. eNOS expression and NO release during hypoxia is inhibited by miR-200b in human endothelial cells. *Angiogenesis* **2018**, *21*, 711–724. [CrossRef] [PubMed]
6. Omura, J.; Satoh, K.; Kikuchi, N.; Satoh, T.; Kurosawa, R.; Nogi, M.; Sunamura, S. Protective Roles of Endothelial AMP-Activated Protein Kinase Against Hypoxia-Induced Pulmonary Hypertension in Mice. *Circ. Res.* **2016**, *119*, 197–209. [CrossRef] [PubMed]
7. Stenmark, K.R.; Fagan, K.A.; Frid, M.G. Hypoxia-induced pulmonary vascular remodeling: Cellular and molecular mechanisms. *Circ. Res.* **2006**, *99*, 675–691. [CrossRef]
8. Xu, W.; Erzurum, S.C. Endothelial cell energy metabolism, proliferation, and apoptosis in pulmonary hypertension. *Compr. Physiol.* **2011**, *1*, 357–372.
9. Ferrero, E.; Fulgenzi, A.; Belloni, D.; Foglieni, C.; Ferrero, M.E. Cellfood improves respiratory metabolism of endothelial cells and inhibits hypoxia-induced reactive oxygen species (ros) generation. *J. Physiol. Pharmacol.* **2011**, *62*, 287–293.
10. Debigaré, R.; Marquis, K.; Côté, C.H.; Tremblay, R.R.; Michaud, A.; LeBlanc, P.; Maltais, F. Catabolic/anabolic balance and muscle wasting in patients with COPD. *Chest* **2003**, *124*, 83–89. [CrossRef]
11. Egerman, M.A.; Glass, D.J. Signaling pathways controlling skeletal muscle mass. *Crit. Rev. Biochem. Mol. Biol.* **2014**, *49*, 59–68. [CrossRef] [PubMed]
12. Langen, R.C.J.; Gosker, H.R.; Remels, A.H.V.; Schols, A.M.W.J. Triggers and mechanisms of skeletal muscle wasting in chronic obstructive pulmonary disease. *Int. J. Biochem. Cell Biol.* **2013**, *45*, 2245–2256. [CrossRef] [PubMed]
13. Goldberg, M.A.; Schneider, T.J. Similarities between the Oxygen-Sensing Mechanisms Regulating the Expression of Vascular Endothelial Growth-Factor and Erythropoietin. *J. Biol. Chem.* **1994**, *269*, 4355–4359. [PubMed]

14. Griguer, C.E.; Oliva, C.R.; Kelley, E.E.; Giles, G.I.; Lancaster, J.R.; Gillespie, G.Y. Xanthine oxidase-dependent regulation of hypoxia-inducible factor in cancer cells. *Cancer Res.* **2006**, *66*, 2257–2263. [CrossRef] [PubMed]
15. Harris, G.K.; Shi, X. Signaling by carcinogenic metals and metal-induced reactive oxygen species. *Mutat. Res.* **2003**, *533*, 183–200. [CrossRef]
16. Hervouet, E.; Pecina, P.; Demont, J.; Vojtíšková, A.; Simonnet, H.; Houštěk, J.; Godinot, C. Inhibition of cytochrome c oxidase subunit 4 precursor processing by the hypoxia mimic cobalt chloride. *Biochem. Biophys. Res. Commun.* **2006**, *344*, 1086–1093. [CrossRef]
17. Leonard, S.S.; Harris, G.K.; Shi, X. Metal-induced oxidative stress and signal transduction. *Free Radic. Biol. Med.* **2004**, *37*, 1921–1942. [CrossRef]
18. Santore, M.T.; McClintock, D.S.; Lee, V.Y.; Budinger, G.S.; Chandel, N.S. Anoxia-induced apoptosis occurs through a mitochondria-dependent pathway in lung epithelial cells. *Am. J. Physiol. Lung Cell. Mol. Physiol.* **2002**, *282*, L727–L734. [CrossRef]
19. Vijayasarathy, C.; Damle, S.; Lenka, N.; Avadhani, N.G. Tissue variant effects of heme inhibitors on the mouse cytochrome c oxidase gene expression and catalytic activity of the enzyme complex. *Eur. J. Biochem.* **1999**, *266*, 191–200. [CrossRef]
20. Liu, J.; Zhu, Y.; Chen, S.; Shen, B.; Yu, F.; Zhang, Y.; Shen, R. Apocynin Attenuates Cobalt Chloride-Induced Pheochromocytoma Cell Apoptosis by Inhibiting P38-MAPK/Caspase-3 Pathway. *Cell. Physiol. Biochem.* **2018**, *48*, 208–214. [CrossRef]
21. Padmanaban, G.; Sarma, P.S. Cobalt toxicity and iron metabolism in Neurospora crassa. *Biochem. J.* **1966**, *98*, 330–334. [CrossRef] [PubMed]
22. Zeno, S.; Zaaroor, M.; Leschiner, S.; Veenman, L.; Gavish, M. CoCl(2) induces apoptosis via the 18 kDa translocator protein in U118MG human glioblastoma cells. *Biochemistry* **2009**, *48*, 4652–4661. [CrossRef] [PubMed]
23. Zeno, S.; Veenman, L.; Katz, Y.; Bode, J.; Gavish, M.; Zaaroor, M. The 18 kDa mitochondrial translocator protein (TSPO) prevents accumulation of protoporphyrin IX. Involvement of reactive oxygen species (ROS). *Curr. Mol. Med.* **2012**, *12*, 494–501. [PubMed]
24. Tang, X.; Luo, Y.X.; Chen, H.Z.; Liu, D.P. Mitochondria, endothelial cell function, and vascular diseases. *Front. Physiol.* **2014**, *5*, 175. [CrossRef] [PubMed]
25. Kugler, W.; Veenman, L.; Shandalov, Y.; Leschiner, S.; Spanier, I.; Lakomek, M.; Gavish, M. Ligands of the mitochondrial 18 kDa translocator protein attenuate apoptosis of human glioblastoma cells exposed to erucylphosphohomocholine. *Cell. Oncol.* **2008**, *30*, 435–450. [PubMed]
26. Levin, E.; Premkumar, A.; Veenman, L.; Kugler, W.; Leschiner, S.; Spanier, I.; Pasternak, G.W. The peripheral-type benzodiazepine receptor and tumorigenicity: Isoquinoline binding protein (IBP) antisense knockdown in the C6 glioma cell line. *Biochemistry* **2005**, *44*, 9924–9935. [CrossRef]
27. Shoukrun, R.; Veenman, L.; Shandalov, Y.; Leschiner, S.; Spanier, I.; Karry, R.; Gavish, M. The 18-kDa translocator protein, formerly known as the peripheral-type benzodiazepine receptor, confers proapoptotic and antineoplastic effects in a human colorectal cancer cell line. *Pharm. Genom.* **2008**, *18*, 977–988. [CrossRef]
28. Veenman, L.; Levin, E.; Weisinger, G.; Leschiner, S.; Spanier, I.; Snyder, S.H.; Gavish, M. Peripheral-type benzodiazepine receptor density and in vitro tumorigenicity of glioma cell lines. *Biochem. Pharmacol.* **2004**, *68*, 689–698. [CrossRef]
29. Veenman, L.; Shandalov, Y.; Gavish, M. VDAC activation by the 18 kDa translocator protein (TSPO), implications for apoptosis. *J. Bioenerg. Biomembr.* **2008**, *40*, 199–205. [CrossRef]
30. Gavish, M.; Bachman, I.; Shoukrun, R.; Katz, Y.; Veenman, L.; Weisinger, G.; Weizman, A. Enigma of the peripheral benzodiazepine receptor. *Pharmacol. Rev.* **1999**, *51*, 629–650.
31. Papadopoulos, V.; Baraldi, M.; Guilarte, T.R.; Knudsen, T.B.; Lacapère, J.J.; Lindemann, P.; Gavish, M. Translocator protein (18kDa): New nomenclature for the peripheral-type benzodiazepine receptor based on its structure and molecular function. *Trends Pharmacol. Sci.* **2006**, *27*, 402–409. [CrossRef] [PubMed]
32. Veenman, L.; Gavish, M. The peripheral-type benzodiazepine receptor and the cardiovascular system. Implications for drug development. *Pharmacol. Ther.* **2006**, *110*, 503–524. [CrossRef] [PubMed]
33. Denora, N.; Laquintana, V.; Pisu, M.G.; Dore, R.; Murru, L.; Latrofa, A.; Sanna, E. 2-Phenyl-imidazo[1,2-a]pyridine Compounds Containing Hydrophilic Groups as Potent and Selective Ligands for Peripheral Benzodiazepine Receptors: Synthesis, Binding Affinity and Electrophysiological Studies. *J. Med. Chem.* **2008**, *51*, 6876–6888. [CrossRef] [PubMed]

34. Azrad, M.; Zeineh, N.; Weizman, A.; Veenman, L.; Gavish, M. The TSPO Ligands 2-Cl-MGV-1, MGV-1, and PK11195 Differentially Suppress the Inflammatory Response of BV-2 Microglial Cell to LPS. *Int. J. Mol. Sci.* **2019**, *20*, 594. [CrossRef]
35. Vainshtein, A.; Veenman, L.; Shterenberg, A.; Singh, S.; Masarwa, A.; Dutta, B.; Maniv, I. Quinazoline-based tricyclic compounds that regulate programmed cell death, induce neuronal differentiation, and are curative in animal models for excitotoxicity and hereditary brain disease. *Cell Death Discov.* **2015**, *1*, 1–17. [CrossRef]
36. Veenman, L.; Vainshtein, A.; Yasin, N.; Azrad, M.; Gavish, M. Tetrapyrroles as Endogenous TSPO Ligands in Eukaryotes and Prokaryotes: Comparisons with Synthetic Ligands. *Int. J. Mol. Sci.* **2016**, *17*, 880. [CrossRef]
37. Chen, Y.; Veenman, L.; Singh, S.; Ouyang, F.; Liang, J.; Huang, W.; Gavish, M. 2-Cl-MGV-1 Ameliorates Apoptosis in the Thalamus and Hippocampus and Cognitive Deficits After Cortical Infarct in Rats. *Stroke* **2017**, *48*, 3366–3374. [CrossRef]
38. Shehadeh, M.; Palzur, E.; Apel, L.; Soustiel, J.F. Reduction of Traumatic Brain Damage by Tspo Ligand Etifoxine. *Int. J. Mol. Sci.* **2019**, *20*, 2639. [CrossRef]
39. Veenman, L.; Papadopoulos, V.; Gavish, M. Channel-like functions of the 18-kDa translocator protein (TSPO): Regulation of apoptosis and steroidogenesis as part of the host-defense response. *Curr. Pharm. Des.* **2007**, *13*, 2385–2405. [CrossRef]
40. Caballero, B.; Veenman, L.; Bode, J.; Leschiner, S.; Gavish, M. Concentration-dependent bimodal effect of specific 18 kDa translocator protein (TSPO) ligands on cell death processes induced by ammonium chloride: Potential implications for neuropathological effects due to hyperammonemia. *CNS Neurol. Disord. Drug Targets* **2014**, *13*, 574–592. [CrossRef]
41. Zeineh, N.; Nagler, R.; Gabay, M.; Weizman, A.; Gavish, M. Effects of Cigarette Smoke on TSPO-related Mitochondrial Processes. *Cells* **2019**, *8*, 694. [CrossRef] [PubMed]
42. Borcar, A.; Menze, M.A.; Toner, M.; Hand, S.C. Metabolic preconditioning of mammalian cells: Mimetic agents for hypoxia lack fidelity in promoting phosphorylation of pyruvate dehydrogenase. *Cell Tissue Res.* **2013**, *351*, 99–106. [CrossRef]
43. Kim, K.S.; Rajagopal, V.; Gonsalves, C.; Johnson, C.; Kalra, V.K. A novel role of hypoxia-inducible factor in cobalt chloride- and hypoxia-mediated expression of IL-8 chemokine in human endothelial cells. *J. Immunol.* **2006**, *177*, 7211–7224. [CrossRef] [PubMed]
44. Jones, N.M.; Kardashyan, L.; Callaway, J.K.; Lee, E.M.; Beart, P.M. Long-term functional and protective actions of preconditioning with hypoxia, cobalt chloride, and desferrioxamine against hypoxic-ischemic injury in neonatal rats. *Pediatr. Res.* **2008**, *63*, 620–624. [CrossRef] [PubMed]
45. Jung, J.Y.; Roh, K.H.; Jeong, Y.J.; Kim, S.H.; Lee, E.J.; Kim, M.S.; Kim, W.J. Estradiol protects PC12 cells against CoCl2-induced apoptosis. *Brain Res. Bull.* **2008**, *76*, 579–585. [CrossRef]
46. Wu, K.C.; Cheng, K.S.; Wang, Y.W.; Chen, Y.F.; Wong, K.L.; Su, T.H.; Leung, Y.M. Perturbation of Akt Signaling, Mitochondrial Potential, and ADP/ATP Ratio in Acidosis-Challenged Rat Cortical Astrocytes. *J. Cell Biochem.* **2017**, *118*, 1108–1117. [CrossRef]
47. Weiner, D.; Levy, Y.; Khankin, E.V.; Reznick, A.Z. Inhibition of salivary amylase activity by cigarette smoke aldehydes. *J. Physiol. Pharmacol.* **2008**, *59* (Suppl. S6), 727–737.
48. Le Fur, G.; Vaucher, N.; Perrier, M.L.; Flamier, A.; Benavides, J.; Renault, C.; Uzan, A. Differentiation between two ligands for peripheral benzodiazepine binding sites, [3H]RO5-4864 and [3H]PK 11195, by thermodynamic studies. *Life Sci.* **1983**, *33*, 449–457. [CrossRef]
49. Marginedas-Freixa, I.; Alvarez, C.L.; Moras, M.; Hattab, C.; Bouyer, G.; Chene, A.; Ostuni, M.A. Induction of ATP Release, PPIX Transport, and Cholesterol Uptake by Human Red Blood Cells Using a New Family of TSPO Ligands. *Int. J. Mol. Sci.* **2018**, *19*, 3098. [CrossRef]
50. Canat, X.; Carayon, P.; Bouaboula, M.; Cahard, D.; Shire, D.; Roque, C.; Casellas, P. Distribution profile and properties of peripheral-type benzodiazepine receptors on human hemopoietic cells. *Life Sci.* **1993**, *52*, 107–118. [CrossRef]
51. Olson, J.M.; Ciliax, B.J.; Mancini, W.R.; Young, A.B. Presence of peripheral-type benzodiazepine binding sites on human erythrocyte membranes. *Eur. J. Pharmacol.* **1988**, *152*, 47–53. [CrossRef]
52. Ostuni, M.A.; Ducroc, R.; Peranzi, G.; Tonon, M.C.; Papadopoulos, V.; Lacapere, J.J. Translocator protein (18 kDa) ligand PK 11195 induces transient mitochondrial Ca2+ release leading to transepithelial Cl- secretion in HT-29 human colon cancer cells. *Biol. Cell* **2007**, *99*, 639–647. [CrossRef] [PubMed]

53. Awad, M.; Gavish, M. Species differences and heterogeneity of solubilized peripheral-type benzodiazepine binding sites. *Biochem. Pharmacol.* **1989**, *38*, 3843–3849. [CrossRef]
54. Kanegawa, N.; Collste, K.; Forsberg, A.; Schain, M.; Arakawa, R.; Jucaite, A.; Halldin, C. In vivo evidence of a functional association between immune cells in blood and brain in healthy human subjects. *Brain Behav. Immun.* **2016**, *54*, 149–157. [CrossRef] [PubMed]
55. Garnier, M.A.R.T.I.N.E.; Dimchev, A.B.; Boujrad, N.O.U.R.E.D.D.I.N.E.; Price, J.M.; Musto, N.A.; Papadopoulos, V.A.S.S.I.L.I.O.S. In vitro reconstitution of a functional peripheral-type benzodiazepine receptor from mouse Leydig tumor cells. *Mol. Pharmacol.* **1994**, *45*, 201–211.
56. Veenman, L.; Leschiner, S.; Spanier, I.; Weisinger, G.; Weizman, A.; Gavish, M. PK 11195 attenuates kainic acid-induced seizures and alterations in peripheral-type benzodiazepine receptor (PBR) protein components in the rat brain. *J. Neurochem.* **2002**, *80*, 917–927. [CrossRef]
57. Bordet, T.; Buisson, B.; Michaud, M.; Drouot, C.; Galea, P.; Delaage, P.; Lacapere, J.J. Identification and characterization of cholest-4-en-3-one, oxime (TRO19622), a novel drug candidate for amyotrophic lateral sclerosis. *J. Pharmacol. Exp. Ther.* **2007**, *322*, 709–720. [CrossRef]
58. Caballero, B.; Veenman, L.; Gavish, M. Role of mitochondrial translocator protein (18 kDa) on mitochondrial-related cell death processes. *Recent Pat. Endocr. Metab. Immune Drug Discov.* **2013**, *7*, 86–101. [CrossRef]
59. Veenman, L.; Alten, J.; Linnemannstöns, K.; Shandalov, Y.; Zeno, S.; Lakomek, M.; Kugler, W. Potential involvement of F0F1-ATP(synth)ase and reactive oxygen species in apoptosis induction by the antineoplastic agent erucylphosphohomocholine in glioblastoma cell lines: A mechanism for induction of apoptosis via the 18 kDa mitochondrial translocator protein. *Apoptosis* **2010**, *15*, 753–768.
60. Veenman, L.; Gavish, M.; Kugler, W. Apoptosis induction by erucylphosphohomocholine via the 18 kDa mitochondrial translocator protein: Implications for cancer treatment. *Anticancer Agents Med. Chem.* **2014**, *14*, 559–577. [CrossRef]
61. Yasin, N.; Veenman, L.; Singh, S.; Azrad, M.; Bode, J.; Vainshtein, A.; Gavish, M. Classical and Novel TSPO Ligands for the Mitochondrial TSPO Can Modulate Nuclear Gene Expression: Implications for Mitochondrial Retrograde Signaling. *Int. J. Mol. Sci.* **2017**, *18*, 786. [CrossRef]
62. Sawada, N.; Yao, J.; Hiramatsu, N.; Hayakawa, K.; Araki, I.; Takeda, M.; Kitamura, M. Involvement of hypoxia-triggered endoplasmic reticulum stress in outlet obstruction-induced apoptosis in the urinary bladder. *Lab. Invest.* **2008**, *88*, 553–563. [CrossRef] [PubMed]
63. Shu, B.; Yang, W.W.; Yang, H.T. Expression pattern of E2F6 in physical and chemical hypoxia-induced apoptosis. *Sheng Li Xue Bao* **2008**, *60*, 1–10. [PubMed]

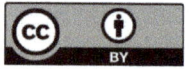

© 2020 by the authors. Licensee MDPI, Basel, Switzerland. This article is an open access article distributed under the terms and conditions of the Creative Commons Attribution (CC BY) license (http://creativecommons.org/licenses/by/4.0/).

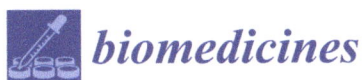

Article

Detailed Characterization of the Cooperative Binding of Piperine with Heat Shock Protein 70 by Molecular Biophysical Approaches

Gabriel Zazeri [1], Ana Paula Ribeiro Povinelli [1], Marcelo de Freitas Lima [2] and Marinônio Lopes Cornélio [1],*

[1] Departamento de Física, Instituto de Biociências, Letras e Ciências Exatas (IBILCE), UNESP, Rua Cristovão Colombo 2265, CEP 15054-000 São José do Rio Preto, SP, Brazil; gabriel.zazeri@unesp.br (G.Z.); ana.povinelli@unesp.br (A.P.R.P.)
[2] Departamento de Química, Instituto de Biociências, Letras e Ciências Exatas (IBILCE), UNESP, Rua Cristovão Colombo 2265, CEP 15054-000 São José do Rio Preto, SP, Brazil; marcelo.f.lima@unesp.br
* Correspondence: m.cornelio@unesp.br

Received: 30 November 2020; Accepted: 16 December 2020; Published: 18 December 2020

Abstract: In this work, for the first time, details of the complex formed by heat shock protein 70 (HSP70) independent nucleotide binding domain (NBD) and piperine were characterized through experimental and computational molecular biophysical methods. Fluorescence spectroscopy results revealed positive cooperativity between the two binding sites. Circular dichroism identified secondary conformational changes. Molecular dynamics along with molecular mechanics Poisson Boltzmann surface area (MM/PBSA) reinforced the positive cooperativity, showing that the affinity of piperine for NBD increased when piperine occupied both binding sites instead of one. The spontaneity of the complexation was demonstrated through the Gibbs free energy ($\Delta G < 0$ kJ/mol) for different temperatures obtained experimentally by van't Hoff analysis and computationally by umbrella sampling with the potential of mean force profile. Furthermore, the mean forces which drove the complexation were disclosed by van't Hoff and MM/PBSA as being the non-specific interactions. In conclusion, the work revealed characteristics of NBD and piperine interaction, which may support further drug discover studies.

Keywords: heat shock protein 70; Hsp70; piperine; fluorescence spectroscopy; molecular docking; molecular dynamics; molecular biophysics

1. Introduction

Heat shock proteins (HSPs) constitute the first line of protection for cells exposed to stressful conditions [1]. HSPs belong to the family of intracellular molecular chaperones, which are involved in many cellular processes including protein folding, prevention of protein aggregation, modulation of protein complexes and protein transport between cellular compartments [2].

The comprehension of HSPs functions was very accepted by the scientific community until Asea et al. [3] initiated a paradigm in the understanding of the function of one of the heat shock proteins (HSP70), revealing that this protein may be found in the extracellular medium acting as an inflammatory cytokine that stimulates innate immune response through the activation of Nuclear Factor-κB (NF-κB) [4–6], which in turn is responsible for the transcription of more than 150 inflammatory cytokines genes including TNF-α, IL-1β and IL6 [6].

HSP70 is a 70 kDa protein that consists of an independent conserved N-terminal nucleotide binding domain (NBD ≈ 40 kDa) with ATPase activity, a substrate binding domain (SBD ≈ 25 kDa) and a weakly conserved C-terminal domain [2]. The NBD and SBD are linked by a short inter-domain linker [7]. The NBD consists of two subdomains, I and II, which are further divided into regions a and b. The Ia and IIa regions interact with ATP [7]. The interaction with ATP leads the NBD structure to conformational changes that affect the affinity of HSP70 for its receptors (TLRs), revealing the plasticity of this protein [8]. Cheeseman et al. [9] and Jones et al. [2] identified some ligands that caused conformational changes in NBD, reinforcing the plasticity of the domain. Moreover, the authors highlighted the need to find small ligands with the potential to inhibit HSP70. Considering the NBD structural flexibility, the key to inhibit the cytokine function of HSP70 may be the search for small molecules able to induce conformational changes that reduce the affinity for the receptors.

Studies reported in the literature showed by means of biological assays that piperine, a bioactive natural product (inset of Figure 1) [10], inhibited IL-1β-mediated activation of NF-κB, leading to the downregulation of pro-inflammatory proteins in human osteoarthritis chondrocyte [11], in human interleukin 1β-stimulated fibroblast-like synoviocytes and in rat arthritis models [12]. Further, it was reported that piperine also inhibited the LPS-mediated activation of NF-κB in RAW 264.7, not allowing the expression of inflammatory mediators [13]. Although it was recently reported in the literature that HSP70 also triggers the NF-κB activation pathway playing a similar role to IL-1β and LPS, there are no studies either at a cellular level or at a molecular level regarding the interaction of the anti-inflammatory molecule piperine and HSP70.

From this perspective, the present work comes to describe a detailed biophysical characterization of the interaction between NDB and piperine to point out the main features of the interaction, supporting drug discovery teams in order to give them an insight into the possible inhibitory role of piperine. Fluorescence spectroscopy and circular dichroism spectroscopic methods were employed to disclose the number of binding sites, the cooperativity, the binding affinity, the thermodynamic parameters of interaction and the protein conformational changes due to the interactions. To have a complete description of the complex, molecular docking and dynamics were employed to predict and confirm the binding sites, to disclose the molecular interactions involved and to calculate the binding free energy.

2. Materials and Methods

2.1. Reagents

Piperine (>97%) was purchased from Sigma-Aldrich Chemical Co. (Schnelldorf, Bavaria, Germany), as dibasic sodium phosphate (>99%) reagents, anhydrous citric acid (>99%) and sodium chloride (>99%). Lyophilised NBD (>97%) was purchased from GenScript. Methanol alcohol was purchased from Dynamics Química Contemporânea LTDA (Indaiatuba, SP, Brazil). Ultrapure water was prepared by a Millipore water purification system—Direct-Q UV-3 (Merck KGaA, Darmstadt, Germany). Lyophilized NBD was reconstituted in 50 mM phosphate buffer containing 150 mM of sodium chloride, and the pH was adjusted to 7.4 with anhydrous citric acid. Stock solutions of piperine were prepared in pure methanol. The concentrations of piperine and NBD solutions were determined by UV-VIS experiments performed on a Biospectro spectrophotometer (Biospectro, Curitiba, PR, Brazil), using the extinction coefficient at 16,500 $M^{-1}cm^{-1}$ at 345 nm for piperine and 20,525 $M^{-1}cm^{-1}$ at 280 nm for NBD.

2.2. Steady-State Fluorescence Spectroscopy

Fluorescence experiments were performed on the Lumina (Thermo Fisher Scientific, Waltham, MA, USA) stationary state spectrofluorimeter equipped with a thermal bath and Xenon lamp. A 100 µL quartz cuvette with a 10 × 2 mm optical path was used in the experiments. The widths of the excitation and the emission slits were adjusted to 10 nm. A wavelength of 295 nm was used to excite the single tryptophan residue of NBD (Trp90). The emission spectra were obtained in the range of 305 to 570 nm with a resolution of 1.0 ± 5.0 nm. Each emission point collected was the average of 15 accumulations. The software ScanWave was used to collect the measured data.

In the binding equilibrium experiments, aliquots of piperine (increment of 0.5 µM) were added in NBD solution at 4 µM. Measurements were performed at 288, 298 and 308 K. In the interaction density function analysis, small aliquots of piperine (increments of 1 µM) were added to NBD solutions at 4 µM, 6 µM and 8 µM at a fixed temperature (288 K). In all experiments, the final volume of methanol in the buffer was less than 1.0%.

The correction of the inner filter effects was performed with Equation (1), where F_{corr} and F_{obs} are corrected and observed fluorescence intensities, and A_{ex} and A_{em} are the absorbance at the excitation and the emission wavelengths, respectively, considering a cuvette of 10 × 10 mm of optical path [14].

$$F_{corr} = F_{obs} \cdot 10^{\frac{(5 \cdot A_{ex} + A_{em})}{10}} \qquad (1)$$

2.3. Time-Resolved Fluorescence

Fluorescence lifetime measurements were performed using a mini-tau filter-based fluorescence lifetime spectrometer coupled to a time-correlated single-photon counting (TCSPC) system (Edinburgh Instruments, Livingston, UK). Aliquots of piperine were added in the NBD solution at 4 µM. The piperine concentration varied from 0 to 20 µM. Experiments were carried out at 298 K.

The sample was excited at 295 nm using a picosecond pulsed light emitting diode (LED), and fluorescence decay was collected using a 340 nm filter. The fluorescence decay profile (Figure S1) was fitted using multiexponential decay (Equation (2)), where τ_i is the lifetime of each component, and α_i is the contribution of each component to total fluorescence decay. The average lifetime $<\tau_{avg}>$ was calculated using Equation (3) (Table S1).

$$I_T = \sum_{i=1}^{n} \alpha_i \cdot e^{\frac{-T}{\tau_i}} \qquad (2)$$

$$\tau_{avg} = \frac{\alpha_1 \tau_1^2 + \alpha_2 \tau_2^2}{\alpha_1 \tau_1 + \alpha_2 \tau_2} \qquad (3)$$

2.4. Circular Dichroism

Circular dichroism spectra were recorded at 288, 298 and 308 K on a Jasco J-815 spectropolarimeter model DRC-H (Jasco, Easton, MD, USA) equipped with a demountable quartz cell with a 0.01 cm optical path length. The CD spectra were recorded from the 200 to 260 nm range with a scan rate of 20 nm/min and a spectral resolution of 0.1 nm. For each spectrum, 15 accumulations were performed. The molar ratios of NBD and piperine were 1:0, 1:2.5, 1:5, 1:7.5, 1:10 and 1:12.5, and the buffer spectrum was subtracted. The ellipticity θ collected in millidegrees was converted to mean residue ellipticity [θ] (deg.cm^2.dmol^{-1}) using Equation (4).

$$[\theta] = \frac{\theta(\text{mdeg})}{10 \cdot [P] \cdot l \cdot n} \qquad (4)$$

The secondary structures' percentages were calculated with CDPro, applying the CONTIN method with the SP43 protein library [15].

2.5. Molecular Docking

The piperine structures used in the molecular docking were obtained from ab initio calculations from our previous work [16]. The NBD structure used in the molecular docking was extracted from PDB (1S3X). AutoDockTools [17] software of the MGL program Tools 1.5.4 was used to prepare the NBD by adding polar hydrogen atoms and Gasteiger charges. The maps were generated by the AutoGrid 4.2 program [18] with a spacing of 0.541 Å, a dimension of 126 × 126 × 126 points and grid center coordinates of 51.315, 43.754 and 48.905 for x, y and z coordinates, respectively. The AutoDock 4.2 program [17] was used to investigate the NBD binding sites using the Lamarckian genetic algorithm (LGA) with a population size of 150, a maximum number of generations of 27,000 and energy evaluations equal to 2.5×10^6. The other parameters were selected as software defaults. To generate different conformations, the total number of runs was set to 100. The final conformations were chosen among the most negative energies and belonging to the most representative cluster (Figure S2). The final conformations were visualized on VMD [19]. The binding microenvironment was generated by LigPlot [20].

2.6. Molecular Dynamics

The simulations of the complex NBD/piperine were performed with the GROMOS54a6 force field [21] by Gromacs v.5.1.4 [22]. The complex was placed in a rectangular box, solvated with simple point charge water (SPC) [23] and neutralized with NaCl in a concentration of 150 mM. The energy minimization was performed with the steepest descent. The first step of equilibration was performed in an NVT ensemble for 100 ps. The system was coupled to a V-rescale thermostat [24] at 298 K. All bonds were constrained with the LINCS algorithm [25], the cut-off for short-range non-bonded interactions was set at 1.4 nm and long-range electrostatics were calculated using the particle mesh ewald (PME) algorithm [26]. The second step of equilibration was performed in the NPT ensemble coupled to a Parrinello-Rahman barostat [27] to isotropically regulate the pressure for 100 ps. The pulling of piperine from the NBD pocket was performed without restraints to allow the protein conformational changes. The reaction coordinate ξ, was chosen as being the distance between the Thr14 oxygen atom (O index 97) and piperine carbon atom (CAA 3802) for piperine into binding site 1 (Figure S3a) and between the Leu309 carbon atom (CA index 3073) and piperine carbon atom (CAL index 3800) for piperine into binding site 2 (Figure S3b). Piperine was pulled away from the NBD binding site in a Z direction until the reaction coordinate reached 7 nm for binding site 1 and 6 nm for binding site 2, using a spring constant of 1000 kJ/mol^{-1}nm^{-2} and a pull rate of 0.01 nm/ns (Figure S4). A sampling of the pullings was analyzed to guarantee a good sampling (Figure S5). The potential of mean force (PMF) profile [28] along the reaction coordinate was calculated with the WHAM method [29]. Statistical errors were estimated with a bootstrap analysis, with 1000 bootstraps properly autocorrelated.

The free energy of the binding process of piperine toward NBD was calculated by a G_mmpbsa tool [30], using the molecular mechanics Poisson Boltzmann surface area (MM/PBSA) method applied to the snapshots obtained from the molecular dynamics simulations. The snapshots were extracted from the trajectory after the system reached equilibrium, which was verified by the root mean square deviation (RMSD) obtained by the program *gmx rms* from Gromacs (Figure S6). The snapshots were extracted in intervals of 250 ps. The coarse grid-box (cfac) was set as 2 and the finner grid-box (fadd) was set as 20. The concentration of positive and negative ions was set as 0.150, being the positive and negative radii set as 0.95 and 1.81 Å, which correspond to sodium and chloride atoms, respectively. The values for the vacuum (vdie) and solvent (sdie) dielectric constants were set as 1 and 80, respectively. The solute dielectric constant (pdie) was set as 4.

3. Results and Discussions

3.1. Fluorescence Spectroscopy

Figure 1 shows the effect in the NBD Trp90 fluorescence caused by the addition of piperine in the solution. According to the spectra, there are two fluorescent bands centered at 330 nm and at 485 nm. The first one refers to protein Trp90 fluorescence emission while the second one refers to piperine fluorescence emission. The full-width half maximum (FWHM) for the band at 330 is ±30 nm and for the band at 480 is ±46 nm, which guarantees that the bands do not overlap and allows the fluorescence intensity at 330 nm to be handled accurately. Figure 1 also shows the fluorescence intensity of tryptophan decreased while piperine was added to the solution, which evidenced that Trp90 was quenched. Another characteristic observed is that the Trp90 fluorescence band remained centered at 330 nm during the piperine titration, which showed the fluorophore was not exposed to an environment with a different polarity [31].

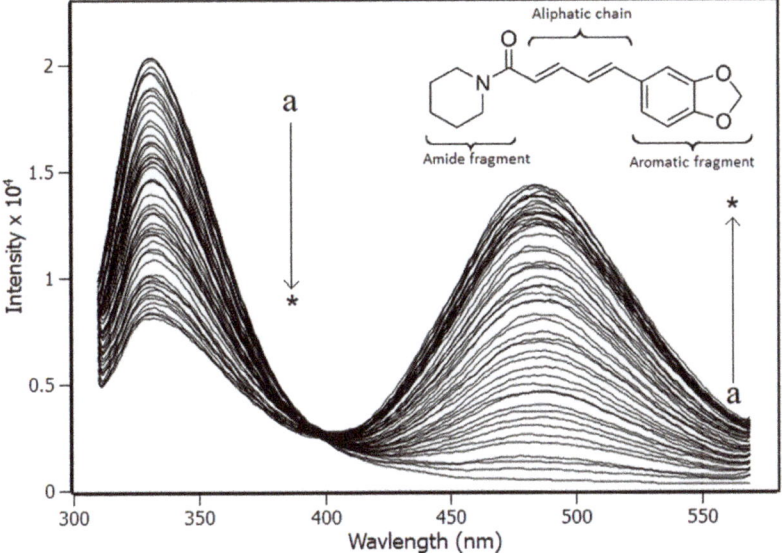

Figure 1. Spectra of fluorescence emission of nucleotide binding domain (NBD) obtained from titration experiments with increments in the concentration of piperine (pH 7.4, T = 288 K, λ_{exc} = 295 nm). (NBD) = 4.0 µM; piperine titrations with increment of 0.5 µM (a → * = 0 µM → 20 µM).

There are two possible different quenching mechanisms. One is dynamic quenching, when the ligand deactivates the excited form of the protein fluorophore by collisions. Another is static quenching, when there is a complex formation between the protein and the ligand. A simple way to distinguish the quenching mechanisms is by analyzing the Stern-Volmer constants (K_{SV}) at different temperatures [14] obtained by Equation (5). If the K_{SV} decreases with the rise in temperature, it is evidence of static quenching. On the other hand, if the K_{SV} increases with the rise in temperature, the quenching mechanism is not directly determined because the increase of K_{SV} may be an effect of either a complex formation drove by entropic factors or an effect of collisions.

A complementary method to determine the quenching mechanism is the association of the steady-state and time-resolved fluorescence data [32]. If the fluorophore is quenched by collisions, the ratio of fluorescence intensities F_0/F is equivalent to the ratio of fluorophore lifetime τ_0/τ, e.g.,: $F_0/F = \tau_0/\tau$. On the other hand, if such equivalence is not verified, static quenching is occurring. In addition, the combination of steady-state and time-resolved fluorescence data can result in a constant known as bimolecular quenching rate constant (k_q), which can be obtained through Equation (5). This constant is related to processes of diffusion, and in the case that the system is under collisions between the fluorophore and the ligand, the constant cannot exceed the order of 10^{10} M$^{-1} \cdot$s^{-1} [32]; otherwise the quenching is static.

$$\frac{F_0}{F} = 1 + K_{SV} \cdot [\text{piperine}] = 1 + k_q \cdot \tau_0 \cdot [\text{piperine}] \tag{5}$$

The Stern-Volmer plots (Figure 2) exhibited a linear response under piperine titration, indicating a single class of fluorophore in the protein and therefore the presence of one quenching mechanism process [33]. According to the results obtained for the K_{SV} constants presented in Table 1, the increase in temperature also caused the values of the constants to follow it. Figure 2 also shows that piperine poorly affected the Trp90 lifetime, once τ_0/τ remained close to the unity. Further, according to the plots, no equivalence is found between the ratios of fluorescence intensities and the lifetime values ($F_0/F \neq \tau_0/\tau$). The set of these results indicated that the system is under static quenching. To reinforce this indication, an analysis of the bimolecular constant at different temperatures was carried out (Table 1). It was found that for the three temperatures, k_q magnitude was of the order of 10^{12} M$^{-1}\cdot$s^{-1}, which is two orders of magnitude greater than that observed for collisional quenching (10^{10} M$^{-1}\cdot$s^{-1}). In conclusion, all these results revealed that the quenching mechanism is undoubtedly static and therefore a complex is formed by NBD and piperine.

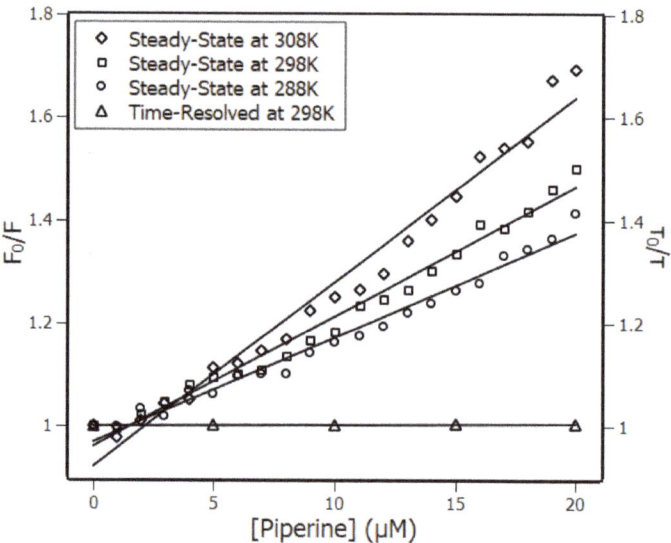

Figure 2. Left ordinate Stern–Volmer plots at three temperatures, 288 K, 298 K and 308 K, and right ordinate time-resolved fluorescence lifetime plot at 298 K; (NBD) = 4 µM, (piperine) = 0–20 µM. $R^2 > 0.98$.

Table 1. Stern-Volmer constant (K_{SV}), bimolecular constants (k_q) and binding constant (K_a) for the complex NBD and piperine at 288, 298 and 308 K.

Temperature (K)	Stern-Volmer (K_{SV}) ×10^4 M^{-1}	Bimolecular (K_q) ×10^{12} M$^{-1}\cdot$s^{-1}	Binding (K_a) ×10^5 M^{-1}
288	2.02 ± 0.07	9.18 ± 0.01	8.82 ± 0.07
298	2.52 ± 0.08	11.45 ± 0.01	44.60 ± 0.10
308	3.58 ± 0.1	16.27 ± 0.01	301.37 ± 1.1

Once the complex formation is proven, the next step was to obtain the binding constant (K_a), applying the binding equilibrium model. The K_a was obtained from the plot of Figure 3 using the double-logarithm equation (Equation (6)), which relates the quenching fluorescence intensities with the total concentration of piperine.

$$\log\left(\frac{F_0 - F}{F}\right) = \log K_a - n\cdot \log[\text{piperine}] \quad (6)$$

The results of K_a at different temperatures for the first order model ($n \approx 1$) are presented in Table 1. The binding constants found at different temperatures have a magnitude order of 10^5 M^{-1}, however their values differ at each temperature, meaning that it is under the direct influence of the available thermal energy.

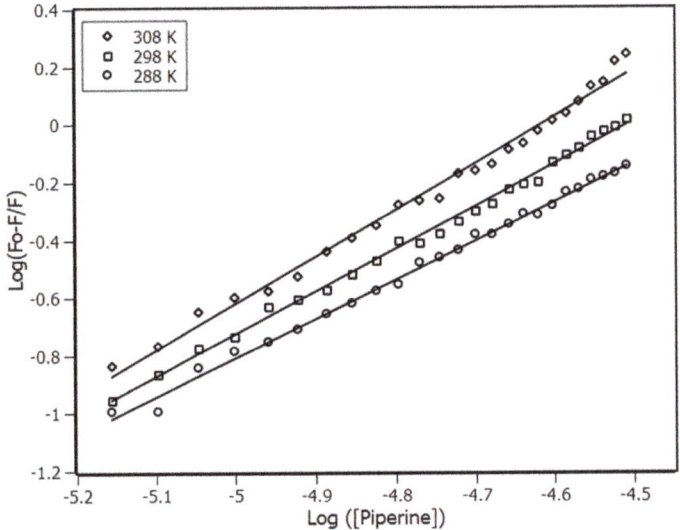

Figure 3. Double-log plots for the fluorescence quenching of NBD (4 µM) in the presence of piperine at 288 K, 298 K and 308 K. $R^2 > 0.99$.

3.2. Thermodynamic Parameters

Based on thermodynamic parameters such as ΔS (entropy variation), ΔH (enthalpy variation) and ΔG (Gibbs free variation) it is possible to gain more information about the complex formation and the forces that drive the process [34]. The parameters ΔS and ΔH are obtained from the van't Hoff plot (Figure 4) according to Equation (7) and ΔG is calculated from Equation (8).

$$\ln K_a = -\frac{\Delta H}{R \cdot T} + \frac{\Delta S}{R} \qquad (7)$$

$$\Delta G = \Delta H - T\Delta S \qquad (8)$$

The results of ΔS, ΔH and ΔG are shown in Table 2. Regarding the results, ΔG values were negative at the range of the applied temperatures, indicating that the complexation was a spontaneous process. Furthermore, the values of ΔG moved to more negative values with the rise in temperature due to the influence of the entropic factor, which favored the complex formation. Moreover, both terms T.ΔS and ΔH are positive, which indicated the non-specific interactions as the main contributor for the complexation. In addition, the entropic term is higher than the enthalpic, which reinforced the non-specific characteristic of the interactions.

Table 2. Thermodynamic parameters of the complex NBD-piperine at temperatures of 288 K, 298 K and 308 K.

T (K)	ΔG (kJ/mol)	ΔH (kJ/mol)	T.ΔS (kJ/mol)
288	−32.65 ± 1.31	130.13 ± 8.69	162.78 ± 8.4
298	−38.3 ± 1.94	130.13 ± 8.69	168.43 ± 8.69
308	−43.95 ± 2.06	130.13 ± 8.69	174.01 ± 8.98

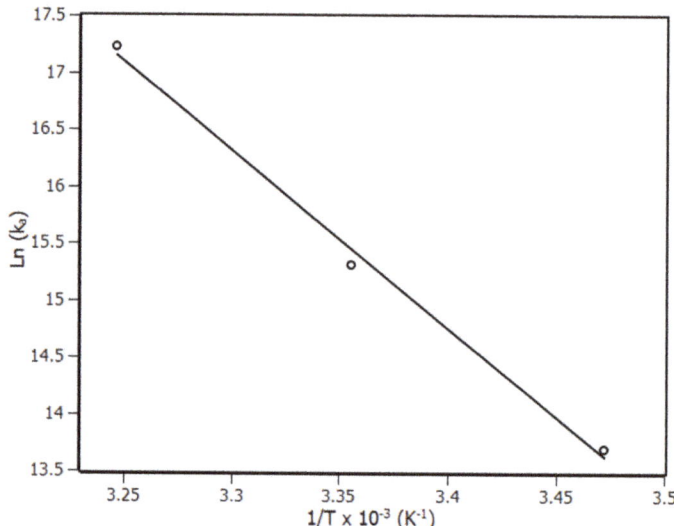

Figure 4. van't Hoff plot for the complex NBD-piperine at 288 K, 298 K and 308 K. $R^2 > 0.99$.

3.3. Interaction Density Function (IDF)

Considering the need to understand the way in which an NBD domain accommodates piperine in its sites, the IDF method was applied to the system as an alternative method in comparison to the binding equilibrium model in order to obtain a more complete description of the system. Interaction density function is a methodology used to treat experimental data, but it is different from the binding equilibrium model, as IDF does not make use of any model a priori and it is based on mass conservation law [35]. The advantage of applying IDF is the possibility of determining the real number of binding sites and identifying any matching factor between the sites. IDF considers that, if the free ligand concentration ((piperine)$_{free}$) is the same for two or more solutions at different concentrations of total protein ((NBD)), the average interaction density (Σv_i) will also be the same and consequently the system will have the same variation on the percentage of quenching (ΔF). The percentage of fluorescence quenching is given by Equation (9), where F and F_0 are the observed fluorescence signal with and without piperine, respectively. Figure 5 shows the plot of ΔF against the log [piperine] for three concentrations of NBD adjusted by a sigmoidal function.

$$\Delta F = \frac{|F - F_0|}{F_0} \cdot 100\% \tag{9}$$

Free ligand concentration and the average interaction density are related to each other through the expression of mass conservation (Equation (10)).

$$[piperine] = [piperine]_{free} + \left(\sum v_i\right) \cdot [NBD] \tag{10}$$

By means of the plot shown in Figure 5, the values of (NBD) and (piperine) for each ΔF was obtained. The inset of Figure 5 shows an example of 3 datasets of the plot of (piperine) versus (NBD) for each ΔF, in which Σv_i is obtained from the slope, and (piperine)$_{free}$ is obtained from the y-intercept of the linear function.

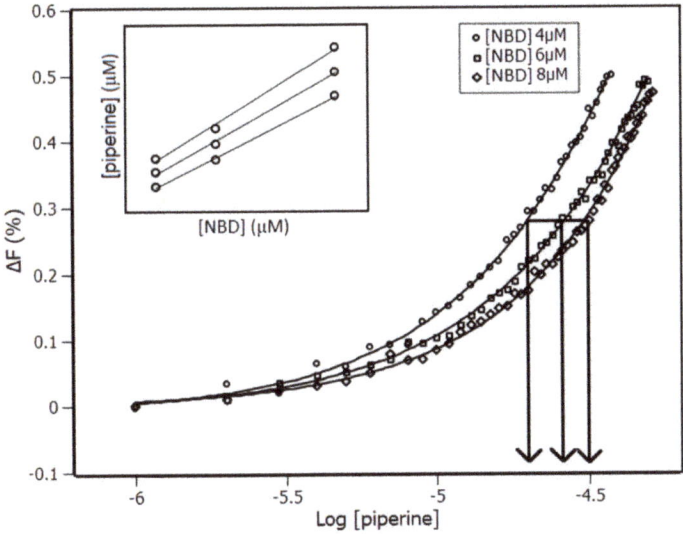

Figure 5. Plot of ΔF versus the log (piperine) obtained from piperine titration experiments with NBD concentrations of 4 µM, 6 µM and 8 µM at 288 K. The inset contains 3 datasets of (piperine) and (NBD) as an example of using Equation (5) to obtain the values of Σv_i and (piperine)$_{free}$.

With the parameters Σv_i and (piperine)$_{free}$ obtained from IDF, a Scatchard plot was built (Figure 6a), an important source of information about cooperativity. It may reveal if the binding sites of the protein are equivalents or non-equivalents, if there is cooperativity among them as well as if the cooperativity is positive or negative [36,37]. Figure 6a shows a line profile with negative concavity, pointing out positive cooperativity. Although Scatchard's plot reveals the occurrence of cooperativity, it does not identify the number of sites that NBD has. To complement this information, it is necessary to use the Hill's plot to disclose additional features such as the number of binding sites (n) and the binding constants (K_b) [38,39]. The Hill's plot is shown in Figure 6b, whose parameters n and K_b were obtained by Equation (11). The parameter h is called the Hill coefficient, which indicates the type of cooperativity. The Hill coefficient can assume values of >1, <1 and =1 indicating positive cooperativity, negative cooperativity and non-cooperativity, respectively.

$$\sum_i v_i = \sum_j \frac{n.(k_b \cdot [\text{piperine}]_{free})^h}{1 + (k_b \cdot [\text{piperine}]_{free})^h} \quad (11)$$

Regarding the results obtained by the Hill equation, the protein has two equivalent binding sites with $K_b = (2.67 \pm 0.12) \times 10^5 \text{ M}^{-1}$ and positive cooperativity (h = 2.4). The results show that both methods (Scatchard and Hill) are in full agreement, revealing a positive cooperativity system. Further, the binding constant found with Hill's method is in the magnitude order of 10^5 M^{-1}, which is in agreement with that found by the binding equilibrium method. Both methods (the binding equilibrium and Hill methods) differed somewhat in terms of the absolute value of the binding constant. This difference found is due to the fact that the binding equilibrium method uses a first order chemical reaction model while the Hill method does not, as discussed previously in the literature [16,31,40].

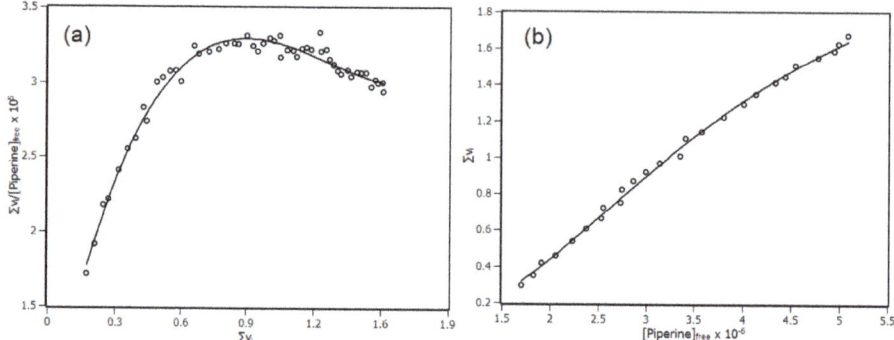

Figure 6. (a) Scatchard plot for the interaction of NBD and piperine obtained at 288 K based on interaction density function (IDF) data. (b) Hill plot for the interaction of NBD and piperine obtained at 288 K based on IDF data. $R^2 > 0.99$.

3.4. Circular Dichroism

A protein that presents cooperativity when interacting with a ligand may be susceptible to conformational changes, adjusting its structure. To have a complete description about the influence of piperine in NBD structure, circular dichroism experiments were performed (Figure 7).

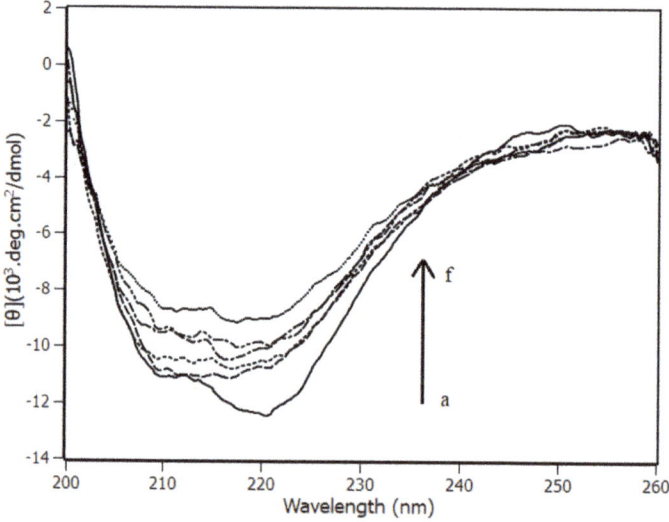

Figure 7. NBD circular dichroism experiments at 298 K in the presence and absence of piperine. Aliquots of piperine were added to the solution from a → f = 1:0 → 1:12.5.

The circular dichroism spectrum of NBD in solution has well-defined bands at 208 nm and 222 nm, which is characteristic of an alpha-helices secondary structure. In order to obtain more details about the secondary structures, the protein spectra were deconvolved by CDPro software aided by the CONTINNL algorithm with 43 soluble proteins spectra deposited in its library. According to the analyses, NBD has 34% of alpha-helices, 16% of beta sheet, 20% of turns and 30% of coil. These results are in good agreement with the data reported in the literature for the same protein using CDNN software [41].

According to the results presented in Figure 7, the protein underwent structural changes during the titration. At the highest concentration of piperine and NDB (1:12.5), its secondary structure was composed 25% of alpha-helices, 21% of beta-sheet, 22% of turn and 32% of coil. Turn and coil content results did not undergo significant secondary structural changes (≈2%). In the meantime, alpha-helices dropped from 34% to 26% and beta sheet content rose from 16% to 31%. These results revealed that the positive cooperativity found by the Scatchard and Hill methods are followed by the NBD structural changes.

3.5. Molecular Modeling

3.5.1. Molecular Docking

Molecular docking was applied to predict the two binding sites found experimentally. The binding environment of the two sites is shown in Figure 8 and according to the results, the predominant molecular interactions are non-specific, with just one hydrogen bond with 2.79 Å of length performed by piperine and His89. This result is in agreement with the experimental van't Hoff analysis that indicated the non-specific interactions were predominant. The binding site 1 is composed of the non-polar amino acids Pro91, Phe68, Phe92, Phe150 and Trp90, by the polar amino acids Gln154, Asn151, Tyr149, Thr13 and His89, by amino acids charged positively, Arg76, Lys71, Arg72 and His89, and a negative Asp69.

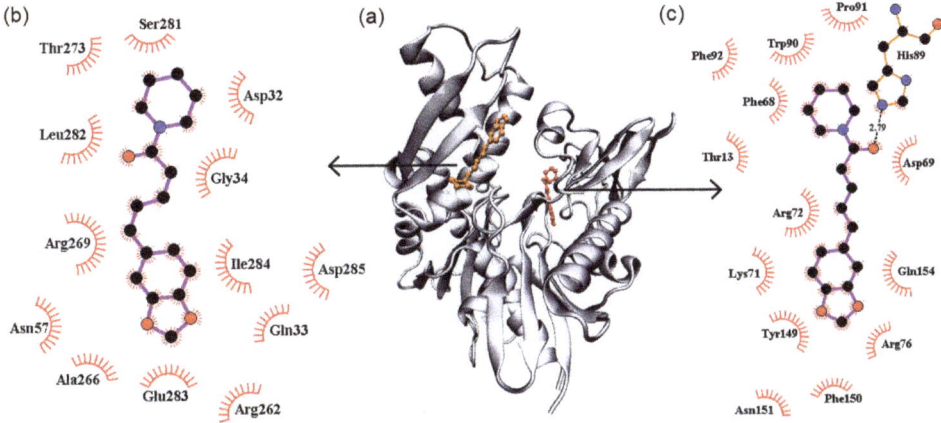

Figure 8. The central picture represents the molecular docking (**a**) in a general view. In red is piperine in binding site 1, in orange in site 2. Pose (**b**) binding environment of site 2, and (**c**) site 1 with a dotted line indicating the hydrogen bonds.

Binding site 2 is composed of the non-polar amino acids Gly34, Ile284, Ala266 and Leu282, by the polar amino acids Ser281, Gln33, Asn57 and Thr273, by amino acids charged positively, Arg262 and Arg269, and by amino acids charged negatively, Asp32, Asp285 and Glu283.

3.5.2. Molecular Dynamics

The two most promising binding sites predicted by molecular docking were explored by the umbrella sampling method. Figure 9 shows the potential of mean force profiles resulting from the complex dissociation obtained for the two binding sites. According to the results, both binding site profiles presented the minimum of energy at the configuration predicted by molecular docking, which indicated that the two configurations are stable. Potential of mean force (PMF) profiles also revealed that the energetic barrier to unbind piperine from the binding sites is higher in site 1 than in site 2. The standard free energy for the binding sites (ΔG$_{pred}$) was determined from WHAM analyses, with (−45 ± 5) kJ/mol for binding site 1 and (−41.8 ± 4) kJ/mol for binding site 2. Although the PMF profiles revealed that the binding sites are distinct in terms of the energetic barrier profile to dissociate piperine, the binding free energy values determined with WHAM analyses are very close considering the statistical errors, corroborating the results obtained from Hill's plot that showed equivalence between the binding affinities of both sites.

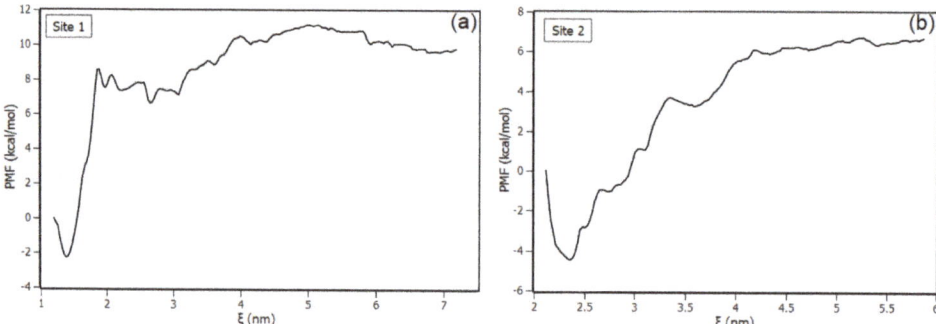

Figure 9. Potential of mean force (PMF) for the dissociation of piperine from NBD, (**a**) for binding site 1 and for (**b**) binding site 2.

The lower computational time consuming method MM/PBSA was employed to highlight the effect on binding free energy caused by piperine into the two binding sites (Table 3). It is an advantageous method to compare binding energies and comprehend which interaction has the highest binding affinity. The binding free energy calculations were performed in two steps. The first step consisted of calculating the binding free energy of the complex with one binding site occupied. The second step consisted of calculating the binding free energy of the complex with both binding sites occupied. According to the results summarized in Table 3, the binding free energy when both binding sites were accessed (columns 4 and 5) is more negative than when just one site is accessed by piperine (columns 2 and 3), with approximately 10 kJ/mol of difference. These results showed a higher binding affinity of piperine for NBD accessing both sites than a single site, which is evidence of cooperativity, in agreement with the experimental fluorescence analyses of the interaction.

Table 3. Energies obtained from molecular mechanics Poisson Boltzmann surface area (MM/PBSA) for piperine occupying both sites and for piperine occupying just one site. Van der Waals, Electrostatic, polar solvation and SASA were obtained from a PBSA calculation.

Energies (kJ/mol)	Site 1	Site 2	Both Sites Occupied	
			Site 1	Site 2
Binding free energy ΔG	−35.22 ± 2.45	−34.59 ± 2.60	−49.92 ± 3.01	−46.15 ± 2.03
van der Waals	−97.63 ± 1.86	−119.61 ± 2.25	−73.74 ± 1.98	−96.12 ± 1.45
Electrostatic	−11.76 ± 0.85	−25.23 ± 0.95	−2.80 ± 1.73	−12.31 ± 1.17
Polar solvation	86.80 ± 2.89	124.32 ± 3.52	36.25 ± 3.34	73.88 ± 2.1
SASA	−12.64 ± 0.24	−14.07 ± 0.23	−9.64 ± 0.25	−11.59 ± 0.12

The root mean square fluctuation (RMSF) of NBD simulated in the absence of ligand disclosed the dynamic of the protein residues, indicating that NBD presented some specific regions with high fluctuation (>0.25 nm). The RMSF of NBD simulated with site 1 and 2 occupied by piperine showed that the interaction with ligand induced a decrease in the fluctuation of some regions that was previously high; such regions where marked with blue dots in Figure S7a. According to the results, most of the amino acids that exhibited expressive changes in RMSF surround piperine in binding site 2 (blue new cartoon regions of Figure S7b,c), while it was noted that there were few fluctuation changes for residues surrounding piperine in binding site 1.

4. Conclusions

In the present work, the interaction between piperine and NBD was investigated by means of experimental and computational molecular biophysical tools. Steady-state and time-resolved fluorescence showed that NBD in the presence of piperine presented a static-quenching process, which means that a complex was formed. Fluorescence spectroscopy revealed with a Scatchard plot and Hill's method an important feature about the interaction of NBD and piperine, which was the presence of positive cooperativity between the two binding sites. In addition, the thermodynamic parameters were disclosed, showing the spontaneity of a complex formation ($\Delta G < 0$ kJ/mol) for the three temperatures. Circular dichroism revealed that the protein underwent conformational changes due to the interaction with piperine. The binding sites were unveiled by molecular docking and molecular dynamics, which reinforced the binding free energy found experimentally. Molecular dynamics along with MM/PBSA reinforced the positive cooperativity found experimentally, showing that the binding free energy was more negative when both binding sites were occupied by piperine. In other words, the affinity was higher under this condition than when just one binding site was occupied. A multispectroscopic evaluation aided by molecular docking and dynamics elucidated in detail the NBD/piperine molecular interaction, which may support further drug discovery studies.

Supplementary Materials: The following are available online at http://www.mdpi.com/2227-9059/8/12/629/s1. Figure S1: Time-resolved fluorescence decay of (a) NBD with Piperine (→e) from 0 to 20 µM. [IL-1β] = 10 µM, T = 298 K and λex = 295 nm, Figure S2: Molecular docking clusters with their respectives energy scores, Figure S3: The atoms picked to define the reaction coordinate (ξ) for (a) binding site 1 and (b) binding site 2, Figure S4: Pulling profile during the pulling simulation. Y-axis is the value of reaction coordinate (ξ) and x-axis is the time of simulation, Figure S5: Configuration histograms of the pulling in z-axis with the windows distance as being 0.1 nm for (a) binding site 1 and (b) binding site 2, Figure S6: Root mean square deviation (RMSD) of (a) NBD in the presence of piperine and (b) piperine occupying the binding sites, Figure S7: (a) Root mean square fluctuation (RMSF) of NBD residues in the absence and presence of piperine in both binding sites (red and black, respectively), blue dots represent the residues that altered the fluctuation from high to low when the ligands were inserted in the binding sites. (b) and (c) Blue cartoon represents the regions that altered the fluctuation from high to low when the ligands were inserted in the binding sites. Red and Orange represent piperine in site 1 and in site 2, respectively, Table S1: Tryptophan lifetime in different stoichiometries NBD: Piperine.

Author Contributions: Experimental data acquisition: G.Z. and A.P.R.P. Theoretical models: G.Z., A.P.R.P. and M.d.F.L. Data analysis: G.Z., A.P.R.P., M.d.F.L. and M.L.C. Manuscript writing: G.Z., A.P.R.P. and M.L.C. Project Administration and Supervision: M.L.C. All authors have read and agreed to the published version of the manuscript.

Funding: The authors A.P.R.P and G.Z are recipients of scholarships from Coordenação de Aperfeiçoamento de Pessoal de Nível Superior—(CAPES), Brazil-Finance Code 001, and Conselho Nacional de Desenvolvimento Científico e Tecnológico (CNPq), Brazil—(Grant 141953/2017-9), respectively. The author M.L.C acknowledges the financial support from Fundação de Amparo à Pesquisa do Estado de São Paulo-FAPESP (Grant 2017/08834-9), Brazil. The APC was funded by Conselho Nacional de Desenvolvimento Científico e Tecnológico (CNPq, Grant 141953/2017-9).

Acknowledgments: Molecular Dynamics simulations were performed at the Center for Scientific Computing (NCC/GridUNESP) of São Paulo State University (UNESP), Brazil. The authors thank João Ruggiero Neto for availability of spectropolarimeter and Valdecir Ximenes for availability of fluorescence lifetime spectrometer.

Conflicts of Interest: The authors declare no conflict of interest.

References

1. Dubrez, L.; Causse, S.; Bonan, N.B.; Dumetier, B.; Garrido, C. Heat-shock proteins: Chaperoning DNA repair. *Oncogene* **2019**, *39*, 1–14. [CrossRef] [PubMed]
2. Jones, A.M.; Westwood, I.M.; Osborne, J.D.; Matthews, T.P.; Cheeseman, M.D.; Rowlands, M.G.; Jeganathan, F.; Burke, R.; Lee, D.; Kadi, N. A fragment-based approach applied to a highly flexible target: Insights and challenges towards the inhibition of HSP70 isoforms. *Sci. Rep.* **2016**, *6*, 34701. [CrossRef] [PubMed]

3. Asea, A.; Kraeft, S.-K.; Kurt-Jones, E.A.; Stevenson, M.A.; Chen, L.B.; Finberg, R.W.; Koo, G.C.; Calderwood, S.K. HSP70 stimulates cytokine production through a CD14-dependant pathway, demonstrating its dual role as a chaperone and cytokine. *Nat. Med.* **2000**, *6*, 435–442. [CrossRef] [PubMed]
4. Asea, A.; Rehli, M.; Kabingu, E.; Boch, J.A.; Baré, O.; Auron, P.E.; Stevenson, M.A.; Calderwood, S.K. Novel signal transduction pathway utilized by extracellular HSP70 role of Toll-like receptor (TLR) 2 and TLR4. *J. Biol. Chem.* **2002**, *277*, 15028–15034. [CrossRef] [PubMed]
5. Somensi, N.; Brum, P.O.; de Miranda Ramos, V.; Gasparotto, J.; Zanotto-Filho, A.; Rostirolla, D.C.; da Silva Morrone, M.; Moreira, J.C.F.; Gelain, D.P. Extracellular HSP70 activates ERK1/2, NF-kB and pro-inflammatory gene transcription through binding with RAGE in A549 human lung cancer cells. *Cell. Physiol. Biochem.* **2017**, *42*, 2507–2522. [CrossRef]
6. Pahl, H.L. Activators and target genes of Rel/NF-κB transcription factors. *Oncogene* **1999**, *18*, 6853–6866. [CrossRef]
7. Evans, C.G.; Chang, L.; Gestwicki, J.E. Heat shock protein 70 (hsp70) as an emerging drug target. *J. Med. Chem.* **2010**, *53*, 4585–4602. [CrossRef]
8. de Oliveira, A.A.; Faustino, J.; de Lima, M.E.; Menezes, R.; Nunes, K.P. Unveiling the interplay between the TLR4/MD2 complex and HSP70 in the human cardiovascular system: A computational approach. *Int. J. Mol. Sci.* **2019**, *20*, 3121. [CrossRef]
9. Cheeseman, M.D.; Westwood, I.M.; Barbeau, O.; Rowlands, M.; Dobson, S.; Jones, A.M.; Jeganathan, F.; Burke, R.; Kadi, N.; Workman, P. Exploiting protein conformational change to optimize adenosine-derived inhibitors of HSP70. *J. Med. Chem.* **2016**, *59*, 4625–4636. [CrossRef]
10. Zazeri, G.; Povinelli, A.P.R.; Le Duff, C.S.; Tang, B.; Cornelio, M.L.; Jones, A.M. Synthesis and Spectroscopic Analysis of Piperine-and Piperlongumine-Inspired Natural Product Scaffolds and Their Molecular Docking with IL-1β and NF-κB Proteins. *Molecules* **2020**, *25*, 2841. [CrossRef]
11. Ying, X.; Chen, X.; Cheng, S.; Shen, Y.; Peng, L.; Xu, H. Piperine inhibits IL-β induced expression of inflammatory mediators in human osteoarthritis chondrocyte. *Int. Immunopharmacol.* **2013**, *17*, 293–299. [CrossRef] [PubMed]
12. Bang, J.S.; Choi, H.M.; Sur, B.-J.; Lim, S.-J.; Kim, J.Y.; Yang, H.-I.; Yoo, M.C.; Hahm, D.-H.; Kim, K.S. Anti-inflammatory and antiarthritic effects of piperine in human interleukin 1β-stimulated fibroblast-like synoviocytes and in rat arthritis models. *Arthritis Res. Ther.* **2009**, *11*, R49. [CrossRef] [PubMed]
13. Ying, X.; Yu, K.; Chen, X.; Chen, H.; Hong, J.; Cheng, S.; Peng, L. Piperine inhibits LPS induced expression of inflammatory mediators in RAW 264.7 cells. *Cell. Immunol.* **2013**, *285*, 49–54. [CrossRef] [PubMed]
14. Lakowicz, J.R. *Principles of Fluorescence Spectroscopy*; Springer Science & Business Media: Berlin/Heidelberg, Germany, 2004.
15. Sreerama, N.; Woody, R.W. Estimation of protein secondary structure from circular dichroism spectra: Comparison of CONTIN, SELCON, and CDSSTR methods with an expanded reference set. *Anal. Biochem.* **2000**, *287*, 252–260. [CrossRef]
16. Zazeri, G.; Povinelli, A.P.R.; de Lima, M.F.; Cornélio, M.L. Experimental Approaches and Computational Modeling of Rat Serum Albumin and Its Interaction with Piperine. *Int. J. Mol. Sci.* **2019**, *20*, 2856. [CrossRef]
17. Morris, G.M.; Huey, R.; Lindstrom, W.; Sanner, M.F.; Belew, R.K.; Goodsell, D.S.; Olson, A.J. AutoDock4 and AutoDockTools4: Automated docking with selective receptor flexibility. *J. Comput. Chem.* **2009**, *30*, 2785–2791. [CrossRef]
18. Morris, G.M.; Goodsell, D.S.; Pique, M.E.; Lindstrom, W.; Huey, R.; Forli, S.; Hart, W.E.; Halliday, S.; Belew, R.; Olson, A.J. *User Guide AutoDock Version 4.2. Automated Docking of Flexible Ligands to Flexible Receptors*; AutoGrid: Redwood City, CA, USA, 2010.
19. Humphrey, W.; Dalke, A.; Schulten, K. VMD: Visual molecular dynamics. *J. Mol. Graph.* **1996**, *14*, 33–38. [CrossRef]
20. Wallace, A.C.; Laskowski, R.A.; Thornton, J.M. LIGPLOT: A program to generate schematic diagrams of protein-ligand interactions. *Protein Eng. Des. Sel.* **1995**, *8*, 127–134. [CrossRef]
21. Oostenbrink, C.; Villa, A.; Mark, A.E.; Van Gunsteren, W.F. A biomolecular force field based on the free enthalpy of hydration and solvation: The GROMOS force-field parameter sets 53A5 and 53A6. *J. Comput. Chem.* **2004**, *25*, 1656–1676. [CrossRef]
22. Van Der Spoel, D.; Lindahl, E.; Hess, B.; Groenhof, G.; Mark, A.E.; Berendsen, H.J.C. GROMACS: Fast, flexible, and free. *J. Comput. Chem.* **2005**, *26*, 1701–1718. [CrossRef]

23. Wu, Y.; Tepper, H.L.; Voth, G.A. Flexible simple point-charge water model with improved liquid-state properties. *J. Chem. Phys.* **2006**, *124*, 24503. [CrossRef] [PubMed]
24. Bussi, G.; Donadio, D.; Parrinello, M. Canonical sampling through velocity rescaling. *J. Chem. Phys.* **2007**, *126*, 14101. [CrossRef] [PubMed]
25. Hess, B.; Bekker, H.; Berendsen, H.J.C.; Fraaije, J.G.E.M. LINCS: A linear constraint solver for molecular simulations. *J. Comput. Chem.* **1997**, *18*, 1463–1472. [CrossRef]
26. Batcho, P.F.; Case, D.A.; Schlick, T. Optimized particle-mesh Ewald/multiple-time step integration for molecular dynamics simulations. *J. Chem. Phys.* **2001**, *115*, 4003–4018. [CrossRef]
27. Parrinello, M.; Rahman, A. Polymorphic transitions in single crystals: A new molecular dynamics method. *J. Appl. Phys.* **1981**, *52*, 7182–7190. [CrossRef]
28. Roux, B. The calculation of the potential of mean force using computer simulations. *Comput. Phys. Commun.* **1995**, *91*, 275–282. [CrossRef]
29. Kumar, S.; Rosenberg, J.M.; Bouzida, D.; Swendsen, R.H.; Kollman, P.A. The weighted histogram analysis method for free-energy calculations on biomolecules. I. The method. *J. Comput. Chem.* **1992**, *13*, 1011–1021. [CrossRef]
30. Kumari, R.; Kumar, R.; Consortium, O.S.D.D.; Lynn, A. g_mmpbsa A GROMACS tool for high-throughput MM-PBSA calculations. *J. Chem. Inf. Model.* **2014**, *54*, 1951–1962. [CrossRef]
31. Povinelli, A.P.R.; Zazeri, G.; de Freitas Lima, M.; Cornélio, M.L. Details of the cooperative binding of piperlongumine with rat serum albumin obtained by spectroscopic and computational analyses. *Sci. Rep.* **2019**, *9*, 1–11. [CrossRef]
32. Lakowicz, J.R.; Weber, G. Quenching of fluorescence by oxygen. Probe for structural fluctuations in macromolecules. *Biochemistry* **1973**, *12*, 4161–4170. [CrossRef]
33. Soares, S.; Mateus, N.; De Freitas, V. Interaction of different polyphenols with bovine serum albumin (BSA) and human salivary α-amylase (HSA) by fluorescence quenching. *J. Agric. Food Chem.* **2007**, *55*, 6726–6735. [CrossRef] [PubMed]
34. Ross, P.D.; Subramanian, S. Thermodynamics of protein association reactions: Forces contributing to stability. *Biochemistry* **1981**, *20*, 3096–3102. [CrossRef] [PubMed]
35. Lohman, T.M.; Bujalowski, W. Thermodynamic methods for model-independent determination of equilibrium binding isotherms for protein-DNA interactions: Spectroscopic approaches to monitor binding. *Methods Enzymol.* **1991**, *208*, 258–290. [PubMed]
36. Scatchard, G. The attractions of proteins for small molecules and ions. *Ann. N. Y. Acad. Sci.* **1949**, *51*, 660–672. [CrossRef]
37. Povinelli, A.P.R.; Zazeri, G.; Cornélio, M.L. Molecular Mechanism of Flavonoids Using Fluorescence Spectroscopy and Computational Tools. In *Flavonoids-A Coloring Model For Cheering Up Life*; IntechOpen: Rijeka, Croatia, 2019.
38. Bordbar, A.K.; Saboury, A.A.; Moosavi-Movahedi, A.A. The shapes of Scatchard plots for systems with two sets of binding sites. *Biochem. Educ.* **1996**, *24*, 172–175. [CrossRef]
39. Barcroft, J.; Hill, A.V. The nature of oxyhaemoglobin, with a note on its molecular weight. *J. Physiol.* **1910**, *39*, 411. [CrossRef]
40. Zazeri, G.; Povinelli, A.P.R.; de Freitas Lima, M.; Cornélio, M.L. The Cytokine IL-1β and Piperine Complex Surveyed by Experimental and Computational Molecular Biophysics. *Biomolecules* **2020**, *10*, 1337. [CrossRef]
41. Borges, J.C.; Ramos, C.H.I. Spectroscopic and thermodynamic measurements of nucleotide-induced changes in the human 70-kDa heat shock cognate protein. *Arch. Biochem. Biophys.* **2006**, *452*, 46–54. [CrossRef]

Publisher's Note: MDPI stays neutral with regard to jurisdictional claims in published maps and institutional affiliations.

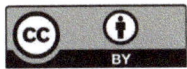

© 2020 by the authors. Licensee MDPI, Basel, Switzerland. This article is an open access article distributed under the terms and conditions of the Creative Commons Attribution (CC BY) license (http://creativecommons.org/licenses/by/4.0/).

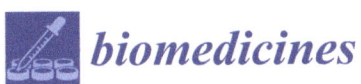

Article

Brassicasterol with Dual Anti-Infective Properties against HSV-1 and *Mycobacterium tuberculosis*, and Cardiovascular Protective Effect: Nonclinical In Vitro and In Silico Assessments

Sherif T. S. Hassan

Department of Applied Ecology, Faculty of Environmental Sciences, Czech University of Life Sciences Prague, Kamýcká 129, 6-Suchdol, 16521 Prague, Czech Republic; sherif.hassan@seznam.cz; Tel.: +420-774-630-604

Received: 8 April 2020; Accepted: 19 May 2020; Published: 24 May 2020

Abstract: While few studies have revealed the biological properties of brassicasterol, a phytosterol, against some biological and molecular targets, it is believed that there are still many activities yet to be studied. In this work, brassicasterol exerts a therapeutic utility in an in vitro setting against herpes simplex virus type 1 (HSV-1) and *Mycobacterium tuberculosis* (Mtb) as well as a considerable inhibitory property against human angiotensin-converting enzyme (ACE) that plays a dynamic role in regulating blood pressure. The antireplicative effect of brassicasterol against HSV-1 is remarkably detected (50% inhibitory concentration (IC_{50}): 1.2 µM; selectivity index (SI): 41.7), while the potency of its effect is ameliorated through the combination with standard acyclovir with proper SI (IC_{50}: 0.7 µM; SI: 71.4). Moreover, the capacity of this compound to induce an adequate level of antituberculosis activity against all Mtb strains examined (minimum inhibitory concentration values ranging from 1.9 to 2.4 µM) is revealed. The anti-ACE effect (12.3 µg/mL; 91.2% inhibition) is also ascertained. Molecular docking analyses propose that the mechanisms by which brassicasterol induces anti-HSV-1 and anti-Mtb might be related to inhibiting vital enzymes involved in HSV-1 replication and Mtb cell wall biosynthesis. In summary, the obtained results suggest that brassicasterol might be promising for future anti-HSV-1, antituberculosis, and anti-ACE drug design.

Keywords: brassicasterol; phytosterols; HSV; *Mycobacterium tuberculosis*; HSV-1 DNA polymerase; HSV-1 TK; human CDK2; ACE; UDP-galactopyranose mutase

1. Introduction

Herpesviruses are one of the major causes of human viral diseases with highly infectious properties. Herpes simplex virus type 1 (HSV-1) is a type of alpha-herpesviruses with double-stranded DNA placed in an icosahedral capsid and a lipidic envelope made by various glycoproteins [1,2]. This pathogen is known to be a thoroughly contagious infection, which is frequent and endemic globally. Most HSV-1 infections are acquired during childhood, and infection is lifelong. Infections with HSV-1 are typically oral herpes but HSV-1 can also be transmitted to the genitals and causes genital herpes [3–5]. Oral herpes infection is commonly asymptomatic, however, in immunocompromised patients with advanced HIV infection, HSV-1 could generate obvious and severe symptoms with regular recurrences [6]. In some cases, complications such as encephalitis or keratitis were observed to be associated with HSV-1 infection [7]. Antiviral drugs, such as acyclovir, famciclovir, and valacyclovir are the best effective medicines to decrease the severity and frequency of HSV symptoms. These medications act as inhibitors of viral replication with reported undesirable effects. With the extensive use of these drugs in therapy, the problem of drug resistance has been established, leading to treatment failure [1,8].

Tuberculosis (TB) is an infectious disease induced by the Gram-negative bacterium *Mycobacterium tuberculosis* (Mtb) that most often infects the lungs and can also affect the brain, kidneys, or spine [9]. Patients infected with HIV, people with a weak immune system, and people with undernutrition are more likely to acquire active TB infection than healthy people [10]. TB infection is typically symptomatic, where the most frequent symptoms of active lung TB are cough with sputum and blood, at times, and fever, chest pains, weight loss, and overall weakness [11]. Although TB is a treatable disease, the extensive and or inappropriate use of anti-TB medications led to developing multidrug-resistant tuberculosis (MDR-TB), where drugs such as isoniazid and rifampicin, the two most potent first-line anti-TB medicines failed to treat the disease [12,13]. In 2018, the World Health Organization declared that MDR-TB continues to be a public health crisis and a health security threat with an increased level of resistance to first-line drugs [14].

Angiotensin-converting enzyme (ACE) is a key enzyme in the regulation of the renin-angiotensin system, with the ability to cleave angiotensin-I to angiotensin-II and hydrolyze several peptides [15]. It is known that angiotensin-II mainly circulates in the blood and triggers the muscles surrounding blood vessels to contract, thus narrowing the vessels, leading to an increase in blood pressure (hypertension) [16]. Therefore, ACE inhibition is an essential therapeutic approach in controlling acute and chronic hypertension, treating left ventricular dysfunction and heart failure, preventing strokes, and preventing and treating kidney disease (nephropathy), especially with patients suffering from hypertension or diabetes [17,18].

Brassicasterol is a natural product that belongs to phytosterols (called plant sterol/stanol esters) and is biosynthesized by various unicellular algae and few terrestrial plants (Figure 1). This compound is a major sterol in rapeseed and canola oil and known to have nutritional value as a food additive [19]. Generally, cholesterol-lowering properties are the major beneficial effects of phytosterols on human health. However, the health benefits of phytosterols on humans have been a subject of debate for years [20]. Recently, a health claim on phytosterols has been clarified and verified by the U.S. Food and Drug Administration (FDA) with a statement: "Foods containing at least 0.65 g per serving of vegetable oil plant sterol esters, eaten twice a day with meals for a daily total intake of at least 1.3 g, as part of a diet low in saturated fat and cholesterol, may reduce the risk of heart disease." [21].

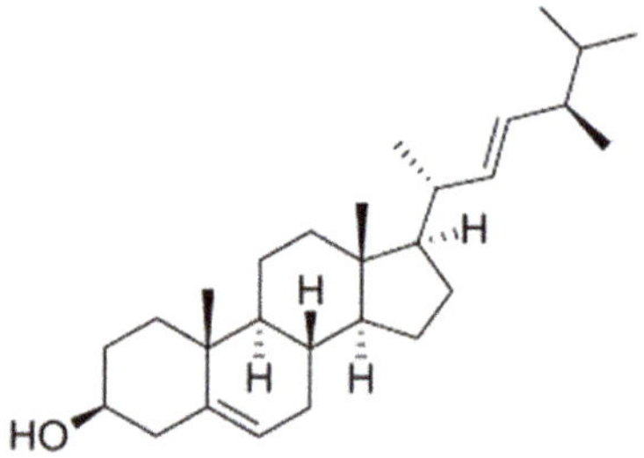

Figure 1. Chemical structure of brassicasterol.

So far, brassicasterol remains a little investigated phytosterol-type molecule with reported few biological activities [19,22,23]. Therefore, in this study, brassicasterol is examined using properly in vitro assay systems for its anti-infective properties against HSV-1 and Mtb along with its cardiovascular protective effect via inhibiting the activity of ACE. Additionally, molecular docking analyses are achieved to predict the mechanisms of action against the molecular targets as well as confirm the results obtained by the in vitro biological assay (for ACE). The investigated molecular targets for HSV-1 are HSV-1 DNA polymerase, HSV-1 thymidine kinase, and human cyclin-dependent kinase 2, while for Mtb it is UDP-galactopyranose mutase.

2. Materials and Methods

Compounds under investigation: Brassicasterol (purity ≥ 98%), standard acyclovir (ACV), and standard rifampicin (European Pharmacopoeia (EP) Reference Standard) were purchased from

Sigma-Aldrich, Berlin, Germany, while standard captopril (EP reference standard) was acquired from Sigma Aldrich, Prague, Czech Republic. The combination of brassicasterol with ACV was prepared as a form of combinatory treatment.

2.1. Antiherpetic Activity

2.1.1. Preparation of Vero Cells and the Virus

Vero cells (ATCC: CCL 81™; UK) and an ACV- susceptible strain of HSV-1 (KOS) were collected from Motol University Hospital (MUH; Prague, Czech Republic). Vero cells were prepared and grown following the previously reported protocol [2,6]. HSV-1 stocks were obtained after propagation of the virus in Vero cells. A plaque assay was further used to titrate the HSV-1 stocks on the basis of the plaque-forming unit (PFU) and the HSV-1 stocks were then kept at –80 °C, as previously specified [2,6].

2.1.2. Cell Viability Assay for Determination of Cytotoxicity

The viability of Vero cells was assessed by the neutral red dye-uptake assay, as previously detailed [8]. Briefly, the experiment was initiated by treating Vero cell monolayers grown in 96-well microtiter plates with two-fold serial dilutions of the test compounds (100 µM as a starting concentration) and then exposed to incubation for 48 h at 37 °C in 5% CO_2. After incubation, the treated cells were examined for the morphological changes by an inverted optical microscope (Leitz, Wetzlar, Germany) and the maximum non-toxic concentrations (MNTC) were ascertained. The 50% cytotoxic concentrations (CC_{50}; expressed in µM) of test compounds were calculated as the concentrations that decreased the cell viability by 50% when compared to the untreated control cells.

2.1.3. Plaque Reduction Assay for Determination of Antiherpetic Activity

To evaluate the antiviral activity against the replication of HSV-1, a plaque reduction assay was performed using ACV as a standard antiherpetic drug as earlier detailed [2,6]. The assay was initiated by infecting Vero cell monolayers with the virus (100 PFU) for 1 h at 37 °C. The infected cells were further overlapped with Eagle's minimum essential medium containing carboxymethyl cellulose (1.5%; Sigma-Aldrich, Berlin, Germany) and treated with test compounds at different concentrations. The untreated cells were considered as controls. To determine the plaque reduction, cells were incubated for 72 h at 37 °C and then dyed with naphthol blue-black (Sigma-Aldrich, Berlin, Germany). The concentrations of test molecules that diminished 50% of the number of HSV-1 plaques were assessed in comparison with the untreated control cells and expressed as 50% inhibitory concentration (IC_{50} in µM) values. The ratio CC_{50}/IC_{50} was assigned for each compound to calculate the selectivity index (SI).

2.2. Antimycobacterial Assay

2.2.1. Bacterial Strains, Identification protocols, and Culturing Procedures

The anti-Mtb activity was processed using an in vitro microdilution assay with ten Mtb strains (CI1–CI10; bacterial isolates acquired from MUH, Prague, Czech Republic), along with a reference strain (H37Rv; CNCTC My 331-88: ATCC 27294; Czech National Collection of Type Cultures (CNCTC), National Institute of Public Health, Prague, Czech Republic. For identification, all Mtb isolates were subjected to various microbiological, biochemical, and molecular protocols following the accredited guideline of Clinical and Laboratory Standards Institute (CLSI) [24]. All bacterial strains used in this study were identified as rifampicin-susceptible and were cultured and grown as previously described by CLSI guideline [25].

2.2.2. Drug Susceptibility Assay

Minimum inhibitory concentrations (MICs) of test substances (brassicasterol and rifampicin) against mycobacterial strains were investigated by employing a 96-well plate microdilution broth method under optimal assay conditions according to the specified procedure of the CLSI guideline with slight modification [25]. Briefly, the broth Middlebrook OADC (Oleic Albumin Dextrose Catalase) growth supplement was used as a supplement in 7H9 liquid medium to culture Mtb (Sigma-Aldrich, Berlin, Germany) at pH (6.6). Rifampicin was applied as a positive control, while Dimethyl sulfoxide (DMSO; 1%) and the broth were utilized as the negative controls. The test drugs were prepared in DMSO with broth (25 µL of DMSO solution in 4 mL of broth) and an aliquot of 100 µL was placed into microplate wells. An isotonic saline solution was used to suspend Mtb inocula with an adjusted density of 0.5–1.0 McFarland. Further, the suspensions (diluted by 10^{-1}) were employed to inoculate the testing wells with a mixture of suspension (100 µL) and the test drugs (100 µL). After five days of incubation, an aliquot of 30 µL of Alamar Blue solution containing a mixture (1:1) of an aqueous solution of resazurin sodium salt (0.1%) and Tween 80 (10%) was supplemented. Further, the results were finalized after 24 h of incubation and expressed as MIC values that hindered the blue to pink color change.

2.3. Anti-Angiotensin-Converting Enzyme (ACE) Assay

Brassicasterol and standard captopril were investigated for their anti-ACE properties. ACE inhibition activities of test compounds were determined by a spectrophotometric method based on the production of hippuric acid from hippuryl-$_L$-histidyl-$_L$-leucine (HHL; substrate) [15]. Concisely, the assay was performed by incubating the test substances at a fixed concentration of 12.3 µg/mL with 120 mU/mL of human ACE (Sigma-Aldrich, Prague, Czech Republic) prepared in Tris Buffer (50 mM, pH = 8.3) for 80 min at 37 °C. After incubation, ACE activity was initiated by adding 110 µL of HHL (10 mM; Sigma-Aldrich, Prague, Czech Republic) to the mixture. A spectrophotometer (UV–VIS; SPECTROstar^{Nano} BMG Labtech, Ortenberg, Germany) was utilized to detect the hippuric acid from the reaction at λ 228 nm and, subsequently, the degree of inhibition (%) was calculated.

2.4. In Silico Molecular Docking Analyses

The molecular docking studies were performed following the previously described protocol [26] and processed with a PyRx virtual screening tool merged with Autodock VINA software (version 0.8, The Scripps Research Institute, La Jolla, CA, USA). Discovery studio visualizer version v19.1.0.18287 (BIOVIA, San Diego, CA, USA) was further employed to graphically illustrate the docking results.

The three-dimensional (3D) crystal structure of HSV-1 DNA polymerase (PDB ID: 2GV9), the 3D-crystal structure of thymidine kinase from HSV-1 complexed with 5-iododeoxyuridine (HSV-1 TK; PDB ID: 1KI7), the 3D-crystal structure of human cyclin-dependent kinase 2 in complex with roscovitine (CDK2; PDB ID: 2A4L), the 3D-crystal structure of UDP-galactopyranose mutase from Mtb docked with UDP (UGM; PDB ID: 4RPJ), and the 3D-crystal structure of human angiotensin-converting enzyme complexed with captopril (ACE; PDB ID: 1UZF) were obtained from the RCSB Protein Data Bank (www.rcsb.org), while the SDF file of the 3D-structure of brassicasterol (CID: 5281327) was retrieved from PubChem database.

To validate the molecular docking outcomes, 5-iododeoxyuridine, roscovitine, UDP, and captopril were removed from (PDB ID: 1KI7), (PDB ID: 2A4L), (PDB ID: 4RPJ), and (PDB ID: 1UZF), respectively and re-docked back into their receptors. The docking results were expressed as binding energy values (kcal/mol) of ligand-receptor complexes; these are based on hydrogen bond, hydrophobic, and electrostatic interactions. All required docking settings including the preparation of PDBQT files for the receptors and ligands, determination of binding sites, the protonation state, calculations, and the overall charges were established as hitherto described [26].

3. Results and Discussion

3.1. Assessment of Cytotoxicity and Antiherpetic Properties

As shown in Table 1, the cytotoxicity (evaluated by the neutral red dye-uptake assay using Vero cells and expressed as 50% cytotoxic concentration (CC_{50}) value) for brassicasterol, brassicasterol combined with acyclovir (ACV), along with standard ACV was detected to be greater than 50 µM. After the determination of cytotoxicity, Vero cells were infected with HSV-1. Further, the infected cells were treated with the test compounds using an in vitro plaque reduction assay.

Table 1. Antireplicative actions of brassicasterol and brassicasterol in combination with acyclovir against herpes simplex virus type 1 compared to standard acyclovir along with cytotoxicity properties.

Molecules	CC_{50} (µM)	IC_{50} (µM)	SI (CC_{50}/IC_{50})
Brassicasterol	>50	1.2 ± 0.12	>41.7
Brassicasterol combined with ACV	>50	0.7 ± 0.24	>71.4
ACV (standard)	>50	2.1 ± 0.13	>23.8

The acquired values are means ± standard deviation (SD) of three independent measurements assayed in duplicate. CC_{50}: 50% cytotoxic concentration, IC_{50}: 50% inhibitory concentration. CC_{50} and IC_{50} values were determined by nonlinear regressions of concentration-response curves. The differences between treatments with test molecules and the controls were analyzed using a one-way ANOVA test tracked by post-hoc comparison tests (Dunnett and Student–Newman–Kuels), where statistical significance was $p < 0.05$, SI: Selectivity index defined as the ratio CC_{50}/IC_{50}, ACV: Acyclovir. For performing the statistical analyses, PRISM software version 8.0 (GraphPad Software, Inc., La Jolla, CA, USA) was employed.

All test molecules showed obvious antiviral properties against the replication of HSV-1 (expressed as 50% inhibitory concentration (IC_{50}) value), where the treatment with brassicasterol demonstrated greater anti-HSV-1 activity (IC_{50}: 1.2 µM; selectivity index (SI): 41.7) than ACV (IC_{50}: 2.1 µM; SI: 23.8). Additionally, the potency of anti-HSV-1 activity was improved through the combinatory treatment of brassicasterol with ACV (IC_{50}: 0.7 µM; SI: 71.4) compared with that of ACV as a single treatment.

The effective treatment of HSV remains the greatest global challenge in medicine, where the current pharmacological treatment is complicated by the rapid development of drug resistance. Therefore, and to combat and eliminate drug resistance to antiherpetic drugs, new efficient and safe medicines with the ability to provide less resistance are urgently required to enter the clinical practice [1,15].

The acquired results confirmed that brassicasterol has a promising anti-HSV-1 property via inhibiting the viral replication, and its cellular toxicity on Vero cells was observed at a concentration (>50 µM) higher than its IC_{50} value, which means that this compound has an acceptable level of selectivity (expressed as SI) towards the target virus. It has been previously claimed that combinatory treatment with clinically antiherpetic drugs is a valuable option for improving the treatment efficacy of HSV diseases [27]. Hence, the obtained results support this claim by showing the capacity of brassicasterol to increase the anti-HSV activity of standard ACV via a combinatory treatment.

To date, no studies have claimed the antiherpetic properties of brassicasterol. Therefore, the obtained results by this research could be rationalized with other studies in which various natural products have shown in various preclinical investigations the capability of inducing excellent anti-HSV activities with diverse mechanisms of action that could break barriers to novel anti-HSV drug development. This has been documented in a recent review article in which a large number of natural biomolecules extracted from various natural sources with outstanding activities against HSV infections were comprehensively reviewed [28].

3.2. Assessment of Antituberculosis Activity

Brassicasterol was examined for antituberculosis activity by microdilution susceptibility assay. The in vitro susceptibility test was processed with ten clinical isolates of Mtb along with a standard strain. Brassicasterol displayed an adequate level of inhibitory effects on the growth of all Mtb strains tested with MIC values ranging from 1.9 to 2.4 µM (Table 2), while the MIC values for the standard antitubercular drug rifampicin were also recorded.

Table 2. Antituberculosis activity (MIC, µM) of test compounds.

Mycobacterial Strains	MIC (µM)	
	Brassicasterol	Rifampicin
Mtb [a]	1.9 ± 0.12	0.1 ± 0.01
Mtb-CI1 [b]	2.0 ± 0.13	0.2 ± 0.02
Mtb-CI2 [b]	2.4 ± 0.15	0.2 ± 0.03
Mtb-CI3 [b]	2.2 ± 0.14	0.3 ± 0.02
Mtb-CI4 [b]	2.1 ± 0.14	0.3 ± 0.02
Mtb-CI5 [b]	1.9 ± 0.13	0.1 ± 0.02
Mtb-CI6 [b]	1.9 ± 0.13	0.3 ± 0.01
Mtb-CI7 [b]	2.1 ± 0.14	0.2 ± 0.01
Mtb-CI8 [b]	1.9 ± 0.11	0.4 ± 0.03
Mtb-CI9 [b]	2.1 ± 0.13	0.3 ± 0.02
Mtb-CI10 [b]	2.0 ± 0.15	0.1 ± 0.01

All recorded values are means ± standard deviation (SD) of three independent experiments assayed in triplicate. [a] Mtb: *Mycobacterium tuberculosis* (reference strain; H37Rv CNCTC My 331-88/ATCC 27294); [b] Mtb: *Mycobacterium tuberculosis* clinical strains; MIC: minimum inhibitory concentration. All presented data were processed by PRISM software (GraphPad Software, Inc., La Jolla, CA, USA; version 8.0).

Although substantial advancements have been achieved during the past few decades in the diagnosis and treatment of TB, the problem of antibiotic resistance remains a challenge [29]. In the present study, brassicasterol showed apparent antitubercular properties via inhibiting the growth of all Mtb strains tested, while no bactericidal effect was observed. In further investigation, and to improve the anti-Mtb activity of brassicasterol, combinatory treatment with standard drug rifampicin was performed. Unfortunately, no positive outcomes were detected to reveal any synergy, additive, or even antagonistic effects.

While several phytosterols derived from marine algae and plants were observed with a slight to moderate degree of antimicrobial actions on Mtb [30–33], their mechanisms of action remain poorly examined. This could be related to their low potency as antitubercular agents, which in turn limits performing further investigations to unveil the mechanisms of action. To the best of the author's knowledge, this research reports the first finding on the anti-Mtb effect of brassicasterol.

3.3. Evaluation of Anti-Angiotensin-Converting Enzyme Activity

The inhibition of human ACE activity by brassicasterol was measured by the release of hippuric acid from the enzyme reaction. The activity of ACE was markedly diminished by brassicasterol at a concentration of 12.3 µg/mL with 91.2% inhibition compared with that of standard captopril (99.1% at a concentration of 12.3 µg/mL) (Table 3).

Table 3. Inactivation properties of test compounds against the human angiotensin-converting enzyme.

Compounds	% Inhibition
Brassicasterol	91.2 ± 0.43
Captopril (standard)	99.1 ± 0.12
ACE-catalyzed reaction (no inhibition)	-

All exhibited values are the mean ± standard deviation (SD) ($n = 3$). ACE: Angiotensin-converting enzyme. The presented data were processed by PRISM software version 8.0 (GraphPad Software, Inc., La Jolla, CA, USA).

ACE inhibitors are known to decrease the production of angiotensin-II, leading to lowering blood pressure, and hence are essential for curing hypertension, heart failure, and other cardiovascular and renal diseases [15]. The re-emerging interest in finding new ACE inhibitors has become urgent, due to the occurrence of undesirable side effects associated with treatment with clinically ACE inhibitors such as captopril, lisinopril, and benazepril [34]. Phytosterols have previously been claimed for their ability to control ACE levels without direct inhibition of ACE. For instance, fucosterol was observed to reduce the ACE levels in endothelial cells by impeding the synthesis of glucocorticoid receptors involved in the regulation of enzyme levels [35]. On the other hand, the current study documents the first investigation on brassicasterol as a direct inhibitor of ACE activity.

3.4. Molecular Docking Evaluation

3.4.1. Brassicasterol with Enzymes Involved in Viral Replication

As depicted in Figure 2, the docking results revealed the substantial ability of brassicasterol to suitably bind to the active sites of HSV-1 DNA polymerase, HSV-1 thymidine kinase (HSV-1 TK) and human cyclin-dependent kinase 2 (CDK2) with detected binding energy values −8.0, −3.3, and −6.5 kcal/mol, respectively. The molecular interactions have been established by forming several fundamental interactions with functional groups of brassicasterol and the interacting amino acid residues of the active sites of target enzymes. These interactions were observed to be hydrogen bond, carbon-hydrogen bond, and hydrophobic (alkyl hydrophobic) along with van der Waals contacts.

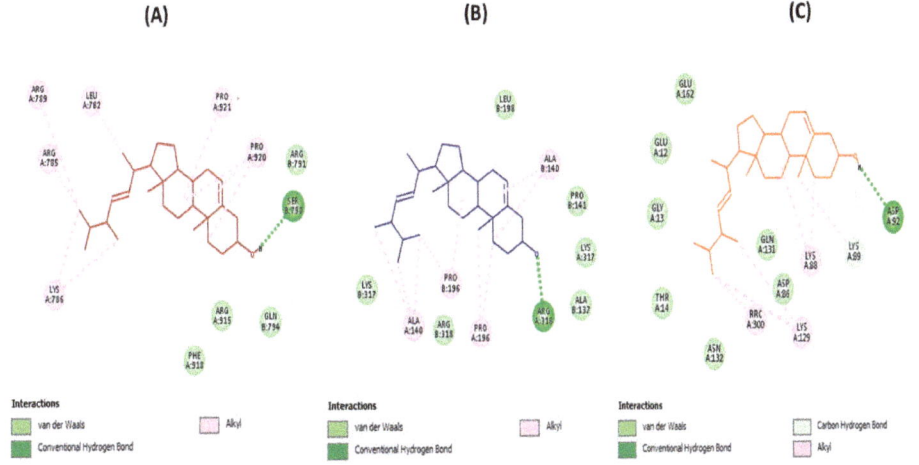

Figure 2. Molecular docking analyses show the molecular interactions and the binding modes of brassicasterol with the active sites of HSV-1 DNA polymerase (**A**), HSV-1 thymidine kinase (**B**), and human cyclin-dependent kinase 2 (**C**), where interactions (hydrogen bond, carbon-hydrogen bond, alkyl hydrophobic, and van der Waals interactions) are presented in a two-dimensional model. Interacting amino acid residues of enzymes active sites with the key functional groups of brassicasterol are shown.

Targeting viral and cellular enzymes that perform significant functions during the HSV-1 replication cycle could help the development of effective broad-spectrum antiherpetic drugs. For instance, HSV-1 DNA polymerase was reported to be an essential enzyme required for viral replication [3], while HSV-1 TK is an important enzyme that catalyzes the transfer of the gamma-phospho group of ATP to thymidine to generate dTMP in the salvage pathway of pyrimidine synthesis, and hence the dTMP serves as a substrate for DNA polymerase during viral DNA replication [36].

It has also been reported that cellular proteins are potential targets for antiviral therapy since most viruses depend on specific cellular proteins for replication. Particularly, CDK2 has been described as a potential target for designing novel anti-HSV-1 drugs [37,38]. According to the currently available evidence, CDK2 was observed to be involved in viral replication and its inhibitors displayed notable anti-HSV-1 activities [39–41]. An additional study unveiled that HSV-1 reactivated in neurons expressing CDK2, and the level of this protein is implicated in the reactivation process [42]. Given together the available data, CDK2 was therefore selected as a target for performing the molecular docking investigations. On the other hand, additional in vitro and in silico studies are necessary to be performed against all CDK families to verify the selectivity of brassicasterol against CDK2.

Unlike the critical role in the viral infection cycle, CDK2 belongs to protein kinases that play a vital role in the eukaryotic cell division cycle. Inhibition of this protein poses a central role in DNA damage-induced cell cycle arrest and DNA repair; however, some negative effects could also be generated [43]. CDK2 is one of the most significant molecular targets identified for cancer-drug discovery and inhibitors of this protein are considered promising chemotherapeutics to combat various types of cancer [44].

3.4.2. Brassicasterol with UDP-Galactopyranose Mutase

UDP-galactopyranose mutase (UGM) is a critical enzyme implicated in the metabolism of galactofuranose, which is known to be a key component of the Mtb cell wall [45]. The docking result of the brassicasterol-UGM complex revealed notable binding mode (Figure 3) with binding energy (−8.1 kcal/mol). The molecular interaction was revealed, where the functional groups of brassicasterol have formed with the interacting amino acid residues of UGM active site several crucial interactions such as hydrogen bond, hydrophobic (alkyl hydrophobic), and van der Waals interactions.

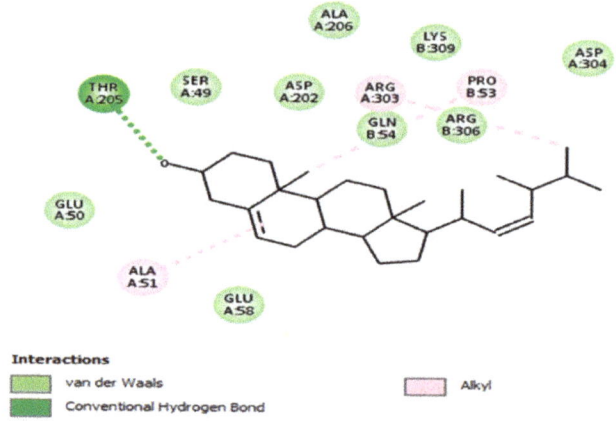

Figure 3. Molecular docking analysis reveals the molecular interaction and the binding mode of brassicasterol with the active site of UDP-galactopyranose mutase (UGM; from *Mycobacterium tuberculosis*), where interactions (hydrogen bond, alkyl hydrophobic, and van der Waals interactions) are shown in a two-dimensional model. Interacting amino acid residues of UGM active site with the key functional groups of brassicasterol are displayed.

Inhibition of mycobacterial cell wall biosynthesis is one of the most effective mechanisms of action of various antibiotics. Mycobacterial cell wall contains a variety of enzymes that play a significant role in its biosynthesis. Therefore, targeting these enzymes is a striking approach for designing effective anti-Mtb drugs [46].

3.4.3. Brassicasterol with Angiotensin-Converting Enzyme

The molecular interaction of brassicasterol with the active site of the angiotensin-converting enzyme (ACE) was explored (Figure 4). The brassicasterol-ACE complex was created with a binding energy value of −9.9 kcal/mol by establishing important hydrogen bond, hydrophobic, and van der Waals interactions. It has been ascertained that zinc is important to the catalytic action of ACE [47], however, brassicasterol was observed to bind to different active pockets than the zinc active-site. Such an outcome may indicate that this compound has a specific type of inhibition that needs to be disclosed in further in vitro investigation.

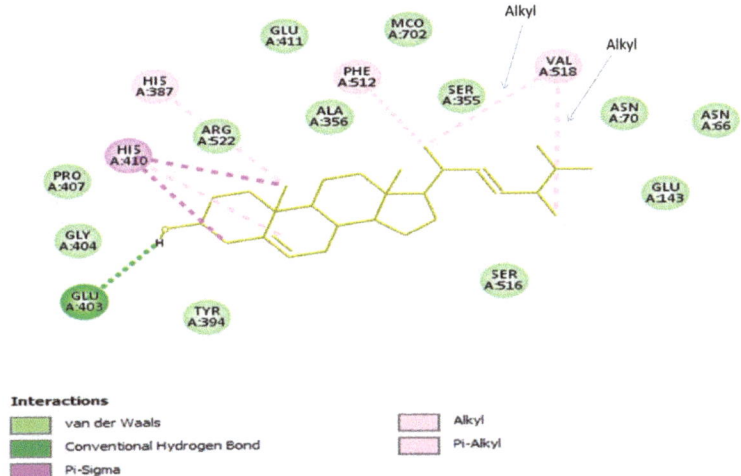

Figure 4. Molecular docking analysis discloses the molecular interaction and the binding mode of brassicasterol with the active site of human angiotensin-converting enzyme (ACE), where interactions (hydrogen bond, alkyl, Pi-alkyl, and Pi-sigma hydrophobic, and van der Waals interactions) are displayed in a two-dimensional model. Interacting amino acid residues of ACE active site with the key functional groups of brassicasterol are shown.

4. Conclusions

In addition to the nutritional and biological values induced by brassicasterol, the outcome of this work has drawn attention to the novel biological properties of this compound, in which anti-infective actions against HSV-1 and Mtb along with cardiovascular protective effects (through inhibition of ACE activity) were ascertained by in vitro and in silico molecular docking studies. Although brassicasterol showed in vitro promising therapeutic values against the investigated targets, further in-depth in vivo investigations are required to validate the obtained results and to unveil the mechanisms of action along with integrated pharmacokinetic and pharmacodynamic studies. Moreover, additional in vitro studies are also necessary to confirm the findings achieved by molecular docking studies.

Funding: This research was partially supported by the Internal Grant Agency (IGA) of the Faculty of Environmental Sciences, Czech University of Life Sciences Prague, Czech Republic. Project No. 20154247/2015 and by the internal fund of the Department of Natural Drugs, Faculty of Pharmacy, University of Veterinary and Pharmaceutical Sciences Brno, Czech Republic.

Conflicts of Interest: The author declares no conflict of interest. The funders had no role in the design of the study; in the collection, analyses, or interpretation of data; in the writing of the manuscript, or in the decision to publish the results.

References

1. Hassan, S.T.; Masarčíková, R.; Berchová, K. Bioactive natural products with anti-herpes simplex virus properties. *J. Pharm. Pharmacol.* **2015**, *67*, 1325–1336. [CrossRef] [PubMed]
2. Brezáni, V.; Leláková, V.; Hassan, S.T.S.; Berchová-Bímová, K.; Nový, P.; Klouček, P.; Maršík, P.; Dall'Acqua, S.; Hošek, J.; Šmejkal, K. Anti-Infectivity against Herpes Simplex Virus and Selected Microbes and Anti-Inflammatory Activities of Compounds Isolated from *Eucalyptus globulus* Labill. *Viruses* **2018**, *10*, 360. [CrossRef] [PubMed]

3. Hassan, S.T.S.; Šudomová, M.; Berchová-Bímová, K.; Šmejkal, K.; Echeverría, J. Psoromic Acid, a Lichen-Derived Molecule, Inhibits the Replication of HSV-1 and HSV-2, and Inactivates HSV-1 DNA Polymerase: Shedding Light on Antiherpetic Properties. *Molecules* **2019**, *24*, 2912. [CrossRef] [PubMed]
4. Čulenová, M.; Sychrová, A.; Hassan, S.T.S.; Berchová-Bímová, K.; Svobodová, P.; Helclová, A.; Michnová, H.; Hošek, J.; Vasilev, H.; Suchý, P.; et al. Multiple In vitro biological effects of phenolic compounds from *Morus alba* root bark. *J. Ethnopharmacol.* **2020**, *248*, 112296. [CrossRef] [PubMed]
5. Hassan, S.T.S.; Šudomová, M.; Masarčíková, R. Herpes simplex virus infection: An overview of the problem, pharmacologic therapy and dietary measures. *Ceska Slov. Farm.* **2017**, *66*, 95–102.
6. Hassan, S.T.S.; Berchová-Bímová, K.; Petráš, J.; Hassan, K.T.S. Cucurbitacin B interacts synergistically with antibiotics against *Staphylococcus aureus* clinical isolates and exhibits antiviral activity against HSV-1. *S. Afr. J. Bot.* **2017**, *108*, 90–94. [CrossRef]
7. Widener, R.W.; Whitley, R.J. Herpes simplex virus. *Handb. Clin. Neurol.* **2014**, *123*, 251–263.
8. Hassan, S.T.S.; Švajdlenka, E.; Berchová-Bímová, K. *Hibiscus sabdariffa* L. and Its Bioactive Constituents Exhibit Antiviral Activity against HSV-2 and Anti-enzymatic Properties against Urease by an ESI-MS Based Assay. *Molecules* **2017**, *22*, 722. [CrossRef]
9. Šudomová, M.; Shariati, M.A.; Echeverría, J.; Berindan-Neagoe, I.; Nabavi, S.M.; Hassan, S.T.S. A Microbiological, Toxicological, and Biochemical Study of the Effects of Fucoxanthin, a Marine Carotenoid, on *Mycobacterium tuberculosis* and the Enzymes Implicated in Its Cell Wall: A Link Between Mycobacterial Infection and Autoimmune Diseases. *Mar. Drugs* **2019**, *17*, 641. [CrossRef]
10. Bell, L.C.K.; Noursadeghi, M. Pathogenesis of HIV-1 and *Mycobacterium tuberculosis* co-infection. *Nat. Rev. Microbiol.* **2018**, *16*, 80–90. [CrossRef]
11. Shingadia, D. The diagnosis of tuberculosis. *Pediatr. Infect. Dis. J.* **2012**, *31*, 302–305. [CrossRef] [PubMed]
12. Hassan, S.T.S.; Šudomová, M.; Berchová-Bímová, K.; Gowrishankar, S.; Rengasamy, K.R.R. Antimycobacterial, Enzyme Inhibition, and Molecular Interaction Studies of Psoromic Acid in *Mycobacterium tuberculosis*: Efficacy and Safety Investigations. *J. Clin. Med.* **2018**, *7*, 226. [CrossRef] [PubMed]
13. Dookie, N.; Rambaran, S.; Padayatchi, N.; Mahomed, S.; Naidoo, K. Evolution of drug resistance in *Mycobacterium tuberculosis*: A review on the molecular determinants of resistance and implications for personalized care. *J. Antimicrob. Chemother.* **2018**, *73*, 1138–1151. [CrossRef] [PubMed]
14. World Health Organization. Fact Sheet on Tuberculosis (2020). Available online: https://www.who.int/news-room/fact-sheets/detail/tuberculosis (accessed on 25 March 2020).
15. Hassan, S.T.S.; Berchová-Bímová, K.; Šudomová, M.; Malaník, M.; Šmejkal, K.; Rengasamy, K.R.R. In Vitro Study of Multi-Therapeutic Properties of *Thymus bovei* Benth. Essential Oil and Its Main Component for Promoting Their Use in Clinical Practice. *J. Clin. Med.* **2018**, *7*, 283. [CrossRef]
16. Li, X.; Chang, P.; Wang, Q.; Hu, H.; Bai, F.; Li, N.; Yu, J. Effects of Angiotensin-Converting Enzyme Inhibitors on Arterial Stiffness: A Systematic Review and Meta-Analysis of Randomized Controlled Trials. *Cardiovasc. Ther.* **2020**, *2020*, 7056184. [CrossRef]
17. Peng, H.; Carretero, O.A.; Vuljaj, N.; Liao, T.D.; Motivala, A.; Peterson, E.L.; Rhaleb, N.E. Angiotensin-converting enzyme inhibitors: A new mechanism of action. *Circulation* **2005**, *112*, 2436–2445. [CrossRef]
18. Izzo, J.L., Jr.; Weir, M.R. Angiotensin-converting enzyme inhibitors. *J. Clin. Hypertens. (Greenwich)* **2011**, *13*, 667–675. [CrossRef]
19. Vanmierlo, T.; Popp, J.; Kölsch, H.; Friedrichs, S.; Jessen, F.; Stoffel-Wagner, B.; Bertsch, T.; Hartmann, T.; Maier, W.; von Bergmann, K.; et al. The plant sterol brassicasterol as additional CSF biomarker in Alzheimer's disease. *Acta Psychiatr. Scand.* **2011**, *124*, 184–192. [CrossRef]
20. Bianconi, V.; Mannarino, M.R.; Sahebkar, A.; Cosentino, T.; Pirro, M. Cholesterol-Lowering Nutraceuticals Affecting Vascular Function and Cardiovascular Disease Risk. *Curr. Cardiol. Rep.* **2018**, *20*, 53. [CrossRef]
21. CFR-Code Federal Regulations: Title 21 (2019). Available online: https://www.accessdata.fda.gov/scripts/cdrh/cfdocs/cfcfr/CFRSearch.cfm?fr=101.83 (accessed on 25 March 2020).
22. Liland, N.S.; Pittman, K.; Whatmore, P.; Torstensen, B.E.; Sissener, N.H. Fucosterol Causes Small Changes in Lipid Storage and Brassicasterol Affects some Markers of Lipid Metabolism in Atlantic Salmon Hepatocytes. *Lipids* **2018**, *53*, 737–747. [CrossRef]

23. Liland, N.S.; Espe, M.; Rosenlund, G.; Waagbø, R.; Hjelle, J.I.; Lie, Ø.; Fontanillas, R.; Torstensen, B.E. High levels of dietary phytosterols affect lipid metabolism and increase liver and plasma TAG in Atlantic salmon (*Salmo salar* L.). *Br. J. Nutr.* **2013**, *110*, 1958–1967. [CrossRef] [PubMed]
24. Clinical and Laboratory Standards Institute. *Laboratory Detection and Identification of Mycobacteria*, 1st ed.; Approved Guideline; CLSI Document M48-A.; Clinical and Laboratory Standards Institute: Wayne, PA, USA, 2008.
25. Clinical and Laboratory Standards Institute. *Susceptibility Testing of Mycobacteria, Nocardiae, and Other Aerobic Actinomycetes*, 2nd ed.; Approved Standard M24-A2; CLSI: Wayne, PA, USA, 2011.
26. Hassan, S.T.S.; Švajdlenka, E. Biological Evaluation and Molecular Docking of Protocatechuic Acid from *Hibiscus sabdariffa* L. as a Potent Urease Inhibitor by an ESI-MS Based Method. *Molecules* **2017**, *22*, 1696. [CrossRef] [PubMed]
27. Field, H.J.; Vere Hodge, R.A. Recent developments in anti-herpesvirus drugs. *Br. Med. Bull.* **2013**, *106*, 213–249. [CrossRef] [PubMed]
28. Treml, J.; Gazdová, M.; Šmejkal, K.; Šudomová, M.; Kubatka, P.; Hassan, S.T.S. Natural Products-Derived Chemicals: Breaking Barriers to Novel Anti-HSV Drug Development. *Viruses* **2020**, *12*, 154. [CrossRef] [PubMed]
29. Jung, Y.E.G.; Schluger, N.W. Advances in the diagnosis and treatment of latent tuberculosis infection. *Curr. Opin. Infect. Dis.* **2020**, *33*, 166–172. [CrossRef]
30. Wächter, G.A.; Franzblau, S.G.; Montenegro, G.; Hoffmann, J.J.; Maiese, W.M.; Timmermann, B.N. Inhibition of *Mycobacterium tuberculosis* growth by saringosterol from *Lessonia nigrescens*. *J. Nat. Prod.* **2001**, *64*, 1463–1464. [CrossRef]
31. Tan, M.A.; Takayama, H.; Aimi, N.; Kitajima, M.; Franzblau, S.G.; Nonato, M.G. Antitubercular triterpenes and phytosterols from *Pandanus tectorius* Soland. var. laevis. *J. Nat. Med.* **2008**, *62*, 232–235. [CrossRef]
32. Olugbuyiro, J.A.; Moody, J.O.; Hamann, M.T. Phytosterols from *Spondias mombin* Linn with Antimycobacterial Activities. *Afr. J. Biomed. Res.* **2013**, *16*, 19–24.
33. Chinsembu, K.C. Tuberculosis and nature's pharmacy of putative anti-tuberculosis agents. *Acta Trop.* **2016**, *153*, 46–56. [CrossRef]
34. Šudomová, M.; Hassan, S.T.S.; Khan, H.; Rasekhian, M.; Nabavi, S.M. A Multi-Biochemical and In Silico Study on Anti-Enzymatic Actions of Pyroglutamic Acid against PDE-5, ACE, and Urease Using Various Analytical Techniques: Unexplored Pharmacological Properties and Cytotoxicity Evaluation. *Biomolecules* **2019**, *9*, 392. [CrossRef]
35. Hagiwara, H.; Wakita, K.; Inada, Y.; Hirose, S. Fucosterol decreases angiotensin converting enzyme levels with reduction of glucocorticoid receptors in endothelial cells. *Biochem. Biophys. Res. Commun.* **1986**, *139*, 348–352. [CrossRef]
36. Xie, Y.; Wu, L.; Wang, M.; Cheng, A.; Yang, Q.; Wu, Y.; Jia, R.; Zhu, D.; Zhao, X.; Chen, S.; et al. Alpha-Herpesvirus Thymidine Kinase Genes Mediate Viral Virulence and Are Potential Therapeutic Targets. *Front. Microbiol.* **2019**, *10*, 941. [CrossRef] [PubMed]
37. Schang, L.M.; St Vincent, M.R.; Lacasse, J.J. Five years of progress on cyclin-dependent kinases and other cellular proteins as potential targets for antiviral drugs. *Antivir. Chem. Chemother.* **2006**, *17*, 293–320. [CrossRef] [PubMed]
38. Viegas, D.J.; Edwards, T.G.; Bloom, D.C.; Abreu, P.A. Virtual screening identified compounds that bind to cyclin dependent kinase 2 and prevent herpes simplex virus type 1 replication and reactivation in neurons. *Antiviral. Res.* **2019**, *172*, 104621. [CrossRef] [PubMed]
39. Schang, L.M. The cell cycle, cyclin-dependent kinases, and viral infections: New horizons and unexpected connections. *Prog. Cell. Cycle Res.* **2003**, *5*, 103–124.
40. Schang, L.M.; Phillips, J.; Schaffer, P.A. Requirement for cellular cyclin-dependent kinases in herpes simplex virus replication and transcription. *J. Virol.* **1998**, *72*, 5626–5637. [CrossRef]
41. Davido, D.J.; Leib, D.A.; Schaffer, P.A. The cyclin-dependent kinase inhibitor roscovitine inhibits the transactivating activity and alters the posttranslational modification of herpes simplex virus type 1 ICP0. *J. Virol.* **2002**, *76*, 1077–1088. [CrossRef]
42. Schang, L.M.; Bantly, A.; Schaffer, P.A. Explant-induced reactivation of herpes simplex virus occurs in neurons expressing nuclear cdk2 and cdk4. *J. Virol.* **2002**, *76*, 7724–7735. [CrossRef]

43. Wang, H.; Kim, N.H. CDK2 Is Required for the DNA Damage Response During Porcine Early Embryonic Development. *Biol. Reprod.* **2016**, *95*, 31. [CrossRef]
44. Tadesse, S.; Caldon, E.C.; Tilley, W.; Wang, S. Cyclin-Dependent Kinase 2 Inhibitors in Cancer Therapy: An Update. *J. Med. Chem.* **2019**, *62*, 4233–4251. [CrossRef]
45. Soltero-Higgin, M.; Carlson, E.E.; Gruber, T.D.; Kiessling, L.L. A unique catalytic mechanism for UDP-galactopyranose mutase. *Nat. Struct. Mol. Biol.* **2004**, *11*, 539–543. [CrossRef] [PubMed]
46. Abrahams, K.A.; Besra, G.S. Mycobacterial cell wall biosynthesis: A multifaceted antibiotic target. *Parasitology* **2018**, *145*, 116–133. [CrossRef] [PubMed]
47. Natesh, R.; Schwager, S.L.; Evans, H.R.; Sturrock, E.D.; Acharya, K.R. Structural details on the binding of antihypertensive drugs captopril and enalaprilat to human testicular angiotensin I-converting enzyme. *Biochemistry* **2004**, *43*, 8718–8724. [CrossRef] [PubMed]

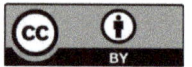

© 2020 by the author. Licensee MDPI, Basel, Switzerland. This article is an open access article distributed under the terms and conditions of the Creative Commons Attribution (CC BY) license (http://creativecommons.org/licenses/by/4.0/).

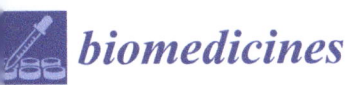

Article

Identification of Key Phospholipids That Bind and Activate Atypical PKCs

Suresh Velnati [1,2,*], Sara Centonze [1,2], Federico Girivetto [1,2], Daniela Capello [1,3], Ricardo M. Biondi [4,5], Alessandra Bertoni [1], Roberto Cantello [1], Beatrice Ragnoli [6], Mario Malerba [1,6], Andrea Graziani [7,8] and Gianluca Baldanzi [1,2]

1. Department of Translational Medicine, University of Piemonte Orientale, 28100 Novara, Italy; sara.centonze@uniupo.it (S.C.); 20020549@studenti.uniupo.it (F.G.); daniela.capello@uniupo.it (D.C.); alessandra.bertoni@med.uniupo.it (A.B.); roberto.cantello@med.uniupo.it (R.C.); mario.malerba@uniupo.it (M.M.); gianluca.baldanzi@med.uniupo.it (G.B.)
2. Center for Translational Research on Allergic and Autoimmune Diseases (CAAD), University of Piemonte Orientale, 28100 Novara, Italy
3. UPO Biobank, University of Piemonte Orientale, 28100 Novara, Italy
4. Department of Internal Medicine 1, Goethe University Hospital Frankfurt, 60590 Frankfurt, Germany; dabiondi@yahoo.co.uk
5. Biomedicine Research Institute of Buenos Aires—CONICET—Partner Institute of the Max Planck Society, Buenos Aires C1425FQD, Argentina
6. Respiratory Unit, Sant'Andrea Hospital, 13100 Vercelli, Italy; beatrice.ragnoli@hotmail.it
7. Molecular Biotechnology Center, Department of Molecular Biotechnology and Health Sciences, University of Torino, 10126 Turin, Italy; andrea.graziani@unito.it
8. Division of Oncology, Università Vita-Salute San Raffaele, 20132 Milan, Italy
* Correspondence: suresh.velnati@med.uniupo.it

Citation: Velnati, S.; Centonze, S.; Girivetto, F.; Capello, D.; Biondi, R.M.; Bertoni, A.; Cantello, R.; Ragnoli, B.; Malerba, M.; Graziani, A.; et al. Identification of Key Phospholipids That Bind and Activate Atypical PKCs. *Biomedicines* **2021**, *9*, 45. https://doi.org/10.3390/biomedicines9010045

Received: 30 November 2020
Accepted: 1 January 2021
Published: 6 January 2021

Publisher's Note: MDPI stays neutral with regard to jurisdictional claims in published maps and institutional affiliations.

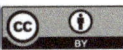

Copyright: © 2021 by the authors. Licensee MDPI, Basel, Switzerland. This article is an open access article distributed under the terms and conditions of the Creative Commons Attribution (CC BY) license (https://creativecommons.org/licenses/by/4.0/).

Abstract: PKCζ and PKCι/λ form the atypical protein kinase C subgroup, characterised by a lack of regulation by calcium and the neutral lipid diacylglycerol. To better understand the regulation of these kinases, we systematically explored their interactions with various purified phospholipids using the lipid overlay assays, followed by kinase activity assays to evaluate the lipid effects on their enzymatic activity. We observed that both PKCζ and PKCι interact with phosphatidic acid and phosphatidylserine. Conversely, PKCι is unique in binding also to phosphatidylinositol-monophosphates (e.g., phosphatidylinositol 3-phosphate, 4-phosphate, and 5-phosphate). Moreover, we observed that phosphatidylinositol 4-phosphate specifically activates PKCι, while both isoforms are responsive to phosphatidic acid and phosphatidylserine. Overall, our results suggest that atypical Protein kinase C (PKC) localisation and activity are regulated by membrane lipids distinct from those involved in conventional PKCs and unveil a specific regulation of PKCι by phosphatidylinositol-monophosphates.

Keywords: membrane; lipid-protein interaction; lipid signalling; kinase regulation; phosphatidylinositols

1. Introduction

Protein kinase C (PKC) is a family of multidomain Ser/Thr kinases that regulate cell growth, differentiation, apoptosis, and motility. Considering their protein structure and their biochemical characteristics, these kinases are classified into the classical or conventional PKCs (α, β, and γ isoforms; cPKCs); the novel PKCs (δ, θ, ε, and η isoforms; nPKCs); and the atypical PKCs (ζ and λ (mouse)/ι (human) isoforms; aPKCs). In physiological conditions, both atypical PKCs play a vital role in cell polarity and signalling. Indeed, these kinases regulate the subcellular localisation of a wide range of polarity proteins by phosphorylating them [1,2]. The PAR6-PAR3-aPKCs trimeric complex is fundamental to modulate the polarity of the epithelial cells and to determinate the cell fate through the orientation of the apical/basal cell asymmetric division [3–5]. Both the aPKCs are also known to enhance the cell migration, invasion, and epithelial–mesenchymal transition in multiple cancer cell types [6–8]. However, it is fascinating to observe that the two aPKCs isotypes may have specific functions in different cancer cell types. For instance, the PKCι/λ isoform promotes cancer growth and metastasis in triple-negative breast cancers [9], while PKCζ is the isoform required for the head and neck squamous cell carcinoma growth and development [10]. Nevertheless, establishing a specific isoform contribution in tumour development is made difficult by the high degree of homology between the PKCζ and PKCι sequences and the lack of specific tools to evaluate a distinct isotype activation.

All these PKC enzymes are characterised by the presence of a kinase domain in the C-terminal region and a regulatory domain placed in the N-terminal region. cPKC regulatory domains also contain a C2 domain that binds anionic phospholipids in a calcium-dependent manner. Conversely, the nPKCs C2 domain is Ca^{2+}-independent but still diacylglycerol (DAG)-sensitive. aPKCs do not possess a C2 domain, whereas they contain a single DAG-insensitive C1 domain. Interestingly, the aPKCs C1 domain (C1 A in cPKCs and nPKCs) is preceded by a basic pseudosubstrate region (PSR) [11]. The PSR binds at the substrate-binding site in an inactive conformation and participates in keeping the kinase inactive in the absence of second messengers. In aPKCs, the C1 domain also participates in the inhibition of the catalytic domain by interactions with the small lobe [12]. In the process of activation, the PSR and the C1 domain must be released from their interactions with the catalytic domain. aPKCs further contain a Phox and Bem1 (PB1) domain located in the N-terminus. This domain extends about 85 amino acids and binds to other PB1 domain-containing proteins, such as zeta-PKC-interacting protein (ZIP/p62), Partitioning-defective Protein 6 (PAR-6) or Mitogen-Activated Protein Kinase 5 (MAPK5) through a homologous PB1–PB1 domain interaction [13].

Although not DAG-sensitive, aPKCs are recruited to membranes upon cell stimulation through protein–protein and protein–lipid interactions [14–18]. The contribution of lipid binding to aPKC localisation is still obscure. Limatola et al. reported that phosphatidic acid (PA), but not other anionic phospholipids, directly binds and activates PKCζ using a gel-shift assay [19]. Building upon this, Pu et al. noted that, compared with the DAG/phorbol ester-sensitive C1 domains, the rim of the binding cleft of the aPKCs C1 domains possesses four additional positively charged arginine residues (at positions 7, 10, 11, and 20) that may be responsible for PA binding. Indeed, mutations of those residues to the corresponding residues in the PKCδ C1b domain conferred a response to phorbol ester [20]. The importance of PA for aPKC regulation is underscored by our previous findings that PA production by diacylglycerol kinase alpha (DGKα) at cell-ruffling sites recruits aPKCs at the plasma membrane where their activity is necessary for protrusion extension and cell migration [14,15,21]. PKCζ is also reported to interact with ceramide (CE), which specifically binds to and regulates its kinase activity in a biphasic manner with high- and low-affinity binding sites characterised by Bmax values of 60 and 600 nM and Kd values of 7.5 and 320 nM, respectively [22]. Using CE overlay assays with proteolytic fragments of PKCζ and vesicle-binding assays with ectopically expressed protein, Wang et al. 2009 showed that a protein fragment comprising the carboxyl-terminal 20-kDa sequence of PKCζ (amino acids 405–592, distinct from the C1 domain) bound to C16:0 ceramide [23]. This interaction with CE activates PKCζ and promotes the local proapoptotic complex formation with PAR-4 [18]. Moreover, an analogous interaction was observed also between sphingosine-1-phosphate (S1P) and PKCζ. Indeed, S1P is suggested to bind the kinase domain of PKCζ constituted by R_{375} and K_{399} and reliving an autoinhibitory constrain [24]. While the PSR and C1 domain participates in the autoinhibition of catalytic activity, the PSR was found to be key for the activation by a lipid mix [11]. NMR studies suggested that phosphatidylinositol-3,4,5-trisphosphate (PI(3,4,5)P$_3$) binds directly to the basic residues in the pseudosubstrate sequence of PKCζ, displacing it from the substrate-binding site during kinase activation [25]. This finding is controversial, as later studies indicated that PI(3,4,5)P$_3$ does not directly regulate PKCζ activity [26]. More recently, an interesting work by Dong and colleagues suggested a membrane-targeting mechanism based on electrostatic binding between the PI(4)P, PI(4,5)P$_2$, and aPKCs PSR polybasic domains. In PKCζ, this binding requires the formation of a complex with PAR-6 through the PB1 domain and regulates localisation but not activity [27].

Although phosphorylation by phosphoinositide-dependent kinase-1 (PDK1) [28] and by mTORC2 (target of rapamycin complex 2) [29] are required for aPKC activity, it is widely considered that, upon phosphorylation (maturation), the aPKCs remain in an inactive conformation stabilised by the PSR and the C1 domain. Signalling lipids activate in vitro its kinase activity, reminiscent of conventional PKC. Activators include acidic phospholipids such PA and phosphatidylserine (PS) [19], PI(3,4,5)P$_3$ [30], S1P [24], and CE [22,31]. Altogether, these shreds of evidence support the possibility of the direct regulation of PKCζ by lipids, while no information is available for PKCι, which is generally assumed to share regulatory models based on high homology with PKCζ. However, a full understanding of how lipid signalling contributes to the control of aPKC localisation and activity is made difficult by the presence of heterogeneous results obtained with different assays. In here, we used a lipid overlay assay and ELISA technique by using Cova phosphatidylinositol monophosphate (PIP) screening plates to evaluate systematically the lipid-binding specificity and luminescent kinase activity assays to assess the activation of purified human PKCζ and PKCι in the presence of various lipids. We observed that both aPKC isoforms bind to PS and PA. Conversely, only PKCι specifically associates with phosphatidylinositol monophosphates. Likewise, we found that PA and PS activate both aPKCs, while only PKCι is PI(4)P-sensitive.

2. Results

To explore systematically the lipid-binding properties of aPKCs, initially, we decided to perform lipid overlay assays that probe highly purified lipids spotted on solid supports to screen for lipid binding in a stable way to recombinant tagged aPKC. The lipid overlay assay technique allows to assay in parallel several lipid species and has been used extensively to study the specificity of lipid-binding domains [32].

2.1. PKCζ Selectively Binds to PA and PS

At first, we tested human FLAG-PKCζ purified by immunoprecipitation, against the main signalling lipids present in the cell membrane. Specifically, on a lipid PIP strip P-6001, that has been spotted with 100 pmol of all eight phosphoinositides (PI, PI(3)P, PI(4)P, PI (5)P, PI(3,4)P$_2$, PI(3,5)P$_2$, PI(4,5)P$_2$, and PI(3,4,5)P$_3$) and seven other biological important lipids (lysophosphatidic acid (LPA), lysophosphocoline (LPC), phosphatidylethanolamine (PE), phosphatidylcholine (PC), S1P, PA, and PS). Interestingly, we can confirm the reported interaction of PKCζ with PA and PS [19], but no direct binding to PI(3,4,5)P$_3$ or other phosphatidylinositols was detected (Figure 1A).

Following, to establish the relative affinity for PA and PS, we used the membrane lipid array P-6003 that has been spotted with DAG, PA, PS, PI, PE, PC, phosphatidylglycerol (PG), and sphingomyelin (SM) in a concentration gradient (100–1.56 pmol). We provided evidence of selective and comparable binding to PS and PA and a very modest binding to PG (Figure 1C,D). As ceramide and S1P were reported to interact with the PKCζ C-terminal region [18], using FLAG-PKCζ, we also probed a sphingolipid array S-6001 that has been spotted with a concentration gradient of eight different sphingolipids, but we observed no specific association to any of them (Figure 1B).

To summarise, among all the lipids tested in our assay, full-length PKCζ binds selectively to PA and PS (Figure 1 and Table 1). Conversely, we did not observe binding to any phosphatidylinositol or sphingolipids.

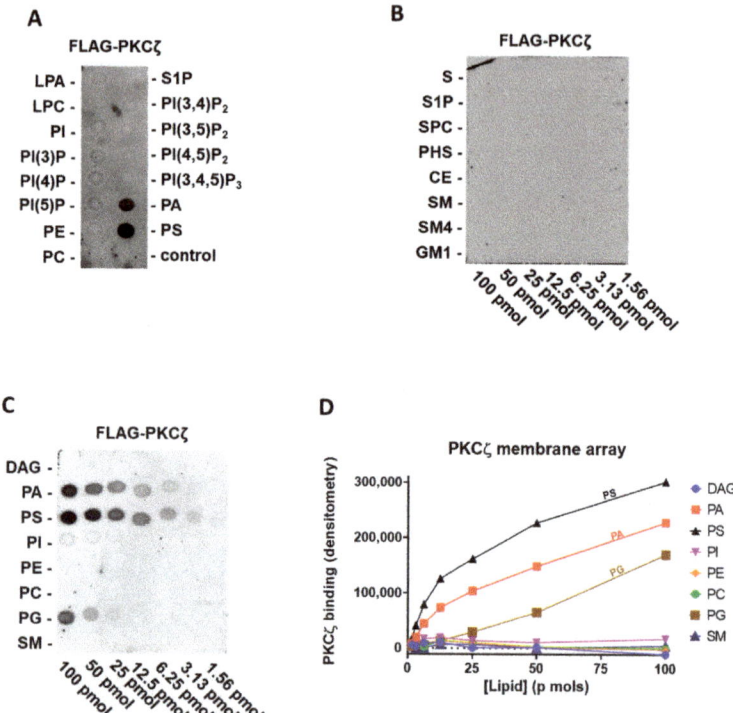

Figure 1. PKCζ selectively binds phosphatidic acid (PA) and phosphatidylserine (PS) and weakly to phosphatidylglycerol (PG) (**A**) Batch purified FLAG-PKCζ was incubated with a phosphatidylinositol monophosphate (PIP) strip overnight, and after washing detected with anti-FLAG antibody, a representative experiment out of three performed is shown. (**B**) Batch purified FLAG-PKCζ was incubated with a sphingo array overnight and, after washing, detected with anti-FLAG antibody. (**C**) Batch purified with FLAG-PKCζ was incubated with a membrane lipid array overnight and, after washing, detected with anti-FLAG antibody (left). (**D**) Quantification by densitometry of (**C**). DAG: diacylglycerol, PE: phosphatidylethanolamine, PC: phosphatidylcholine, SM: sphingomyelin, PKC: protein kinase C, LPA: lysophosphatidic acid, LPC: lysophosphocoline, S: sphingosine, S1P: sphingosine-1-phosphate, SPC: sphingosylphosphorycholine, PHS: phytosphingosine, CE: ceramide, SM4: sulfatide, and GM1: monosialoganglioside.

2.2. PKCι Binds to Phosphatidylinositol Monophosphates, along with PA and PS

To explore the lipid-binding specificity of the highly homologous human PKCι, we used a highly purified commercial preparation of FLAG-PKCι in the same assay. Like PKCζ, we tested purified FLAG-PKCι on the previously described PIP strip P-6001, representing the main signalling lipids present in the cell membrane. We observed that PKCι also interacts with PA and PS but not with PI (Figure 2A). Surprisingly, PKCι also selectively binds to phosphatidylinositol monophosphates (PIPs, e.g., PI(3)P, PI(4)P, and PI(5)P), regardless of the phosphorylation position. Interestingly, PKCι neither binds to the phosphatidylinositol diphosphates nor triphosphates, which was already indicative of a very selective interaction mechanism.

Table 1. Protein/lipid interactions detected by the lipid overlay assay.

	PKCζ	PKCι
PI	−	−
PI(3)P	−	++
PI(4)P	−	++
PI(5)P	−	++
PI(3,4)P$_2$	−	−
PI(3,5)P$_2$	−	−
PI(4,5)P$_2$	−	−
PI(3,4,5)P$_3$	−	−
PA	++	++
LPA	−	−
PC	−	−
LPC	−	−
PS	++	++
PE	−	−
PG	+	+
DAG	−	−
S	−	−
S1P	−	−
SPC	−	−
PHS	−	−
CE	−	−
SM	−	−
SM4	−	+
GM1	−	−

++ strong signal, + weak signal, and − no signal. PKC: protein kinase C, PIP: phosphatidylinositol monophosphate, PA: phosphatidic acid, LPA: lysophosphatidic acid, PC: phosphatidylcholine, LPC: lysophosphocholine, PS: phosphatidylserine, PE: phosphatidylethanolamine, PG: phosphatidylglycerol, DAG: diacylglycerol, S: sphingosine, S1P: sphingosine-1-phosphate, SPC: sphingosylphosphorycholine, PHS: phytosphingosine, CE: ceramide, SM: sphingomyelin, SM4: sulfatide, and GM1: monosialoganglioside.

Using the membrane lipid array P-6003 that has been spotted with DAG, PA, PS, PI, PE, PC, PG, and SM in a concentration gradient, we can confirm that also PKCι binds to PS and PA with a comparable affinity (Figure 2C,D). Moreover, to further investigate the relative affinity in PIP binding, we used a PIP array P-6100 that has been spotted with a concentration gradient of all eight phosphoinositides, i.e., PI, PI(3)P, PI(4)P, PI(5)P, PI(3,4)P$_2$, PI(3,5)P$_2$, PI(4,5)P$_2$, and PI(3,4,5)P$_3$. We confirmed the binding to phosphatidylinositol monophosphates and a lack of selectivity for the phosphate position in the PIPs (Figure 2E,F) since purified FLAG-PKCι binds to PI(3)P, PI(4)P, and PI(5)P to a similar extent. Similar to FLAG-PKCζ, we did not observe any interaction between purified FLAG-PKCι and sphingolipids, apart from a weak binding to sulfatide (SM4), which, however, could be due to its structural similarity in charge and dimensions to PIPs (Figure 2B).

To conclude, PKCι also binds to PA and PS. Furthermore, unlike PKCζ, PKCι selectively binds to PIPs without any specificity for the phosphate position (Figure 2 and Table 1).

2.3. PKCι Binds to PI(3)P and PI(4)P through the Catalytic Domain

To further confirm the data obtained through lipid overlay assays and to identify the aPKC domains responsible for binding, we performed the ELISA technique using Cova PIP screening plates that were precoated with 20 nmols of either PI(3)P or PI(4)P per well, preblocked and ready for the addition of the proteins. On those plates, we used in-house purified GST-tagged full-length aPKCs and their deletion mutants and detected their binding using anti-GST antibodies. The constructs used are described in Figure 3A [12]. We used the same concentrations of purified GST as in the negative control.

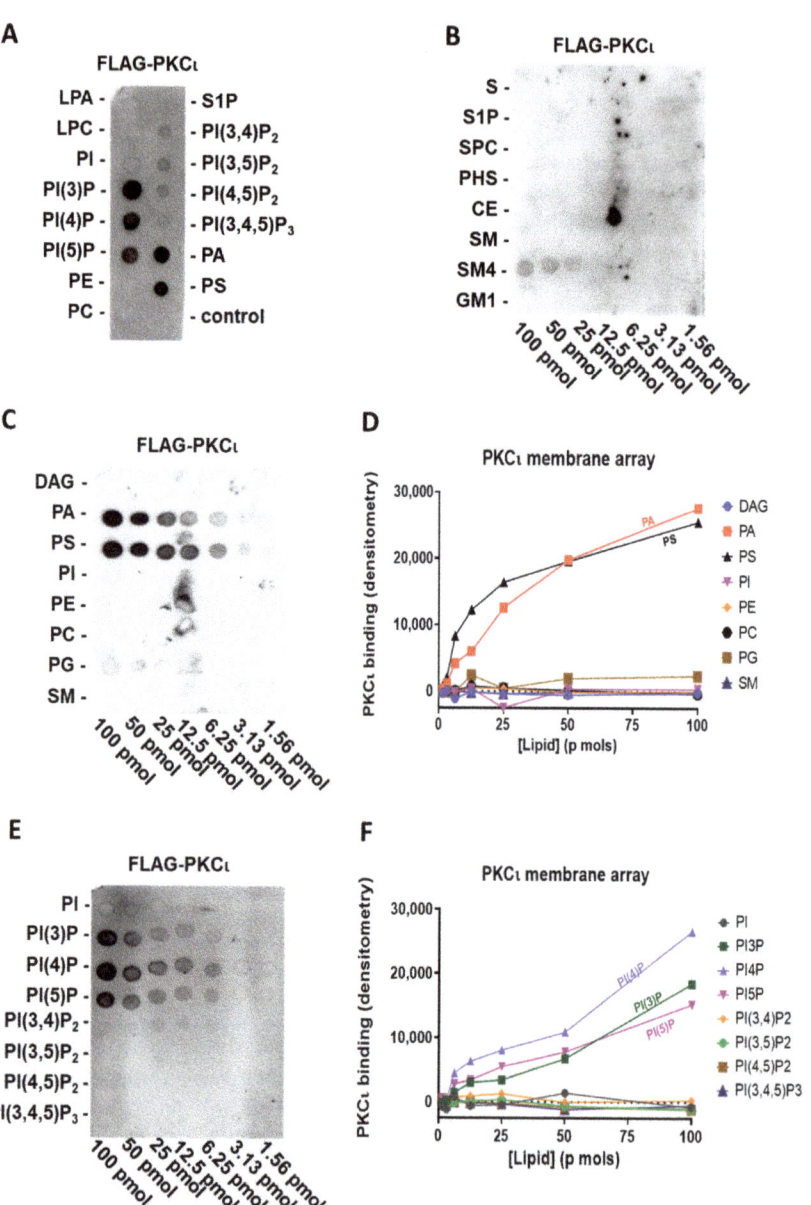

Figure 2. PKCι binds PIPs, PA, and PS (**A**) Highly purified FLAG-PKCι was incubated with a PIP strip overnight and, after washing, detected with anti-FLAG antibody. (**B**) Highly purified FLAG-PKCι was incubated with sphingolipid array overnight and, after washing, detected with anti-FLAG antibody. (**C**) Highly purified FLAG-PKCι was incubated with a membrane lipid array overnight and, after washing, detected with anti-FLAG antibody (left). (**D**) Quantification by densitometry of (**C**). (**E**) Highly purified FLAG-PKCι was incubated with a PIP array overnight and after, washing detected, with anti-FLAG antibody (left). (**F**) Quantification by densitometry of (**E**).

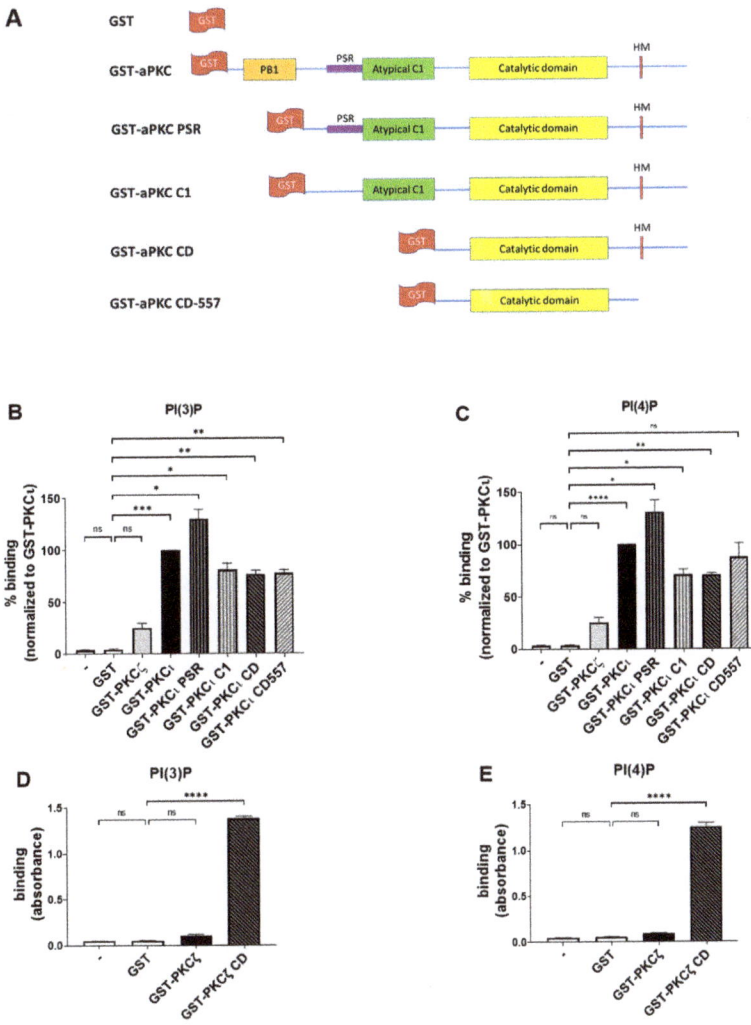

Figure 3. PKCι, but not PKCζ, binds selectively to both PI(3)P and PI(4)P. (**A**) Schematic domain structure of GST tagged PKCζ, PKCι, and the deletion mutants used in this study. (**B**) GST-PKCζ, GST-PKCι, and deletion mutants binding on Cova PIP screening plates coated with PI(3)P. Purified GST was used as a negative control. Data are the mean ± SEM of three independent experiments. (**C**) GST-PKCζ, GST-PKCι, and deletion mutants binding on Cova PIP screening plates coated with PI(4)P. Purified GST was used as a negative control. Data are the mean ± SEM of three independent experiments. (**D**) GST-PKCζ and GST-PKCζ CD binding on Cova PIP screening plates coated with PI(3)P. Purified GST was used as a negative control. Data are the mean ± SEM of three independent experiments. (**E**) GST-PKCζ and GST-PKCζ CD binding on Cova PIP screening plates coated with PI(4)P. Purified GST was used as a negative control. Data are the mean ± SEM of three independent experiments. A single, double, triple and four asterisks denote their significance of p-value ≤ 0.05, ≤ 0.01, ≤ 0.001 and ≤ 0.0001 respectively, ns mean No significant.

While the GST alone gave no detectable binding, as expected, the PKCι isoform strongly bound to both PI(3)P and PI(4)P (Figure 3B,C), in line with our previous findings. Conversely, PKCζ neither bound to PI(3)P nor PI(4)P (Figure 3B,C). Those data indicate that, similar to what we observed in the lipid overlay assays, the binding of PKCι to PIPs is isoform-specific and does not require the presence of additional proteins.

Besides, all the truncated forms of PKCι resulted in some binding to both PI(3)P and PI(4)P, suggesting that a relevant lipid binding takes place in the catalytic domain (CD) as it is the only domain common to all those truncated proteins. On the other hand, we observed an increased binding signal towards PI(3)P and PI(4)P when testing the PKCι PSR. Indeed, the PSR is a polybasic domain, enriched with Arg and Lys residues, which confers to the protein the ability to bind directly the phosphoinositides such as PI(4)P but is masked when the protein is not involved in interactions with PAR-6 [27]. It may be possible that removing the PB1 region makes the PSR domain more accessible to the electrostatic binding to the lipids, resulting in a stronger signal when compared to the full-length protein.

Moreover, we observed a strong binding of both PI(3)P and PI(4)P to PKCζ CD, a truncated mutant lacking the N-terminal PB1, PSR, and C1 domains. Interestingly, the full-length PKCζ remained unbound (Figure 3D,E), indicating that the N-terminal domains inhibited the interaction and that the PI(3)P and PI(4)P interacting region is located within evolutionarily conserved regions in the CD region of PKCζ and PKCι.

Overall, these data indicate that full-length PKCι readily binds selectively to PI(3)P and PI(4)P, while the CD appears as a primary binding site for phosphatidylinositol monophosphates. In PKCζ, this binding is masked by the presence of N-terminal regulatory domains.

2.4. PS and PA Activates Both aPKCs, While PI(4)P Activates PKCι Selectively

To evaluate the effect of lipid binding on the catalytic activity of human aPKC, we performed kinase activity assays using highly purified commercial PKCι and PKCζ, incubated with PS, PA, and PI(4)P at a final concentration of 50 µg/mL. Following, the ADP produced was detected using the ADP-Glow luminescence kit. Those assays were run following the preoptimised conditions suggested by the provider; in those conditions, the basal PKCζ activity is quite low. This might be due to the low concentrations of the enzyme (0.1 ng/µL of PKCζ) (four times less enzyme when compared to PKCι—0.4 ng/µL). In similar experimental conditions, the PKCι activity is evidently higher compared to the background (Supplementary Figure S1). However, we can easily observe the expected stimulation of PKCζ in the presence of either PA or PS, while PI4P is ineffective (Figure 4A). Those data are in line with previous reports in the literature [19,27].

Conversely, we can easily measure the basal activity of unstimulated PKCι, which is at least 10x when compared to the background. The PKCι basal activity is strongly stimulated by PA, followed by PS (Figure 4B). Interestingly, PI(4)P acts an allosteric activator selective for PKCι, as we observed no activation of highly purified commercial PKCζ by this lipid (Figure 4A,B). These data suggest that the previously reported binding of aPKC to PS, PA, and PIPs enhanced enzyme activity putatively, promoting the switch to the open more active conformation.

To further investigate the domains involved in lipid-mediated PKCι activation, we performed the kinase activity assays by using in-house purified full-length GST-tagged PKCι and its truncated forms (PKCι C1 and PKCι CD) in the presence of PS, PA, or PI(4)P. Similar to what we observed before, full-length GST-PKCι is strongly activated with PA and PI(4)P, whereas PS activation is still significant but less strong (Figure 4C). The CD is not further activated by lipid mixes in vitro [11]. Even though we noticed some binding of PI(4)P to the PKCι CD mutant, no further activation of the CD was detected in kinase activity assays. The PKCι C1 mutant, which lacks the PB1 and PSR, is considerably inhibited by the C1 domain [12]. The PKCι C1 mutant retained the ability to respond to PA and PI(4P), indicating that the PSR is not required for the activation by these lipids (Figure 4C). Together, the results indicate that the activation by PA and PI(4) is linked to the release of autoinhibition by the C1 domain.

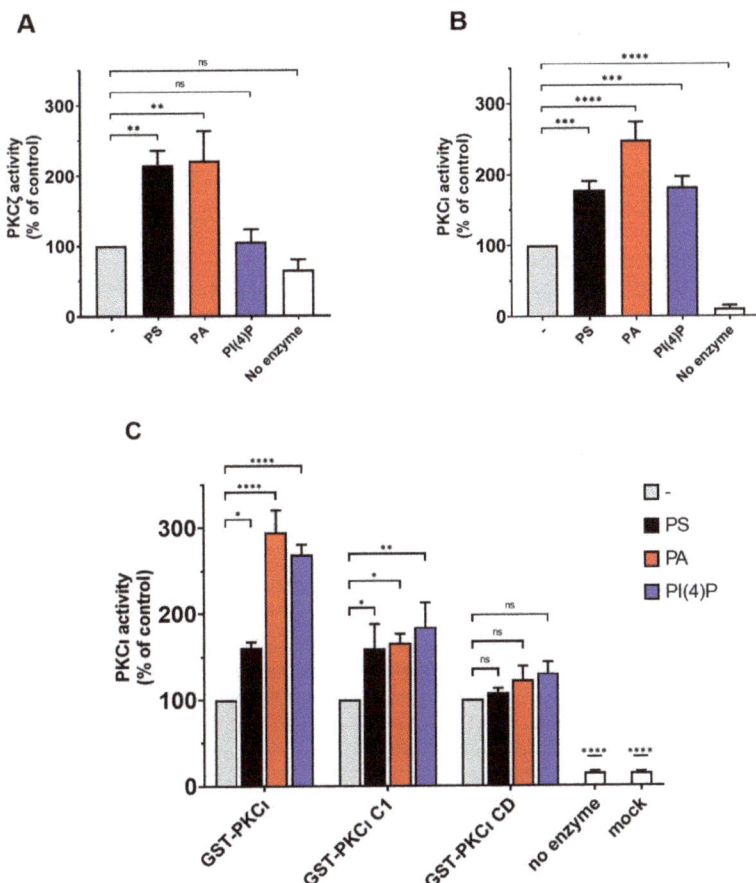

Figure 4. PKCι is activated by PS, PA, and PI(4)P. (**A**) The activity of commercial purified GST-PKCζ was measured in the presence of 50-μg/mL PS or PA or PI(4)P. A complete reaction without an enzyme is considered as the negative control. (**B**) The activity of commercial purified GST-PKCι was measured in presence of 50-μg/mL PS or PA or PI(4)P. A complete reaction without an enzyme is considered as the negative control. (**C**) The activity of in-house purified GST-PKCι and deletion mutants was measured in presence of 0.5-ng/mL PS or PA or PI(4)P. Mock purification and no enzyme conditions are used as negative controls. Data are the mean ± SEM of at least 4 independent experiments performed in triplicate. A single, double, triple and four asterisks denote their significance of p-value ≤ 0.05, ≤ 0.01, ≤ 0.001 and ≤ 0.0001 respectively, ns mean No significant.

3. Discussion

Among the three PKCs subfamilies, the aPKCs (PKCζ and PKCλ/ι) do require neither calcium nor DAG for their activation, but many shreds of evidence indicate that their interactions with lipids may contribute to the control of aPKCs localisation and activity. In order to further understand their mechanisms of regulation and explore their isotype-specific lipid activators, the present work aims to estimate the lipid-binding specificity and activation of the human aPKCs isozymes through a systematic approach.

By performing lipid overlay assays, we observed that aPKCs can selectively bind PA and PS, and this binding results in a relevant increase in aPKCs activity. Those findings are in line with previous results obtained with a lipid motility shift assay [19]. Previously, our group demonstrated that DGKα-produced PA is required to localise the aPKCs to the plasma membrane, where their activity leads to cytoskeletal remodelling and membrane ruffles formation, two essential processes required for cell migration [14,15,21]. These findings indicate that PA provides a key signal to recruit and activate aPKCs at specific membrane compartments. This PA can be derived from DAG through DGK activity or else from PC through phospholipase D (PLD) hydrolysing activity. Indeed, through PA-mediated mechanisms, PLD modulates small GTPases, playing an essential role in membrane homeostasis and cytoskeletal remodelling [33], such as antigen-stimulated membrane ruffling [34]. Interestingly, PLD-generated PA is required for sorbitol-induced activation of aPKCs and GLUT4 translocation/glucose transport [35]. Besides PA, we identified binding to PS, a lipid constitutively present at membranes. We hypothesise that PA, together with PS, recruits and activates aPKC to specific membrane domains. In this manner, DGKα and PLD, modulating PA availability, may be potential regulators of aPKCs localisation and activation. However, the information regarding the spatial and temporal PA distribution in subcellular compartments is still limited. Nishioka et al., using a Phosphatidic Acid indicator (Pii) biosensor based on the FRET technique, observed a divergence in PA content among various cell types and an individual heterogeneity within the same cell line [36]. The authors reported that, upon EGF stimulation, PA level increases rapidly at the plasma membrane, and it seems that this PA production is due mostly to PLD rather than DGK [36]. Similar results were obtained by Zhang and colleagues using a Phosphatidic Acid biosensor with Superior Sensitivity (PASS), and interestingly, their data seem to suggest that EGF triggers a sequential activation of PLD and DGK in distinct membrane nanodomains [37].

Interestingly, our findings demonstrated that, unlike PKCζ, PKCι interacts directly with phosphatidylinositol monophosphates (PI(3)P, PI(4)P, and PI(5)P) in a specific and dose-dependent manner. This binding is, at least in part, mediated by the PKCι catalytic domain and results in enzyme activation. Polyphosphoinositides derivatives represent a crucial membrane-localised signal in the control of essential cellular processes by driving the subcellular localisation and activation of specific effector proteins [38]. Indeed, they feature specific subcellular localisation with PI(4)P mainly at the plasma membrane and Golgi apparatus; PI(3)P at the plasma membrane, early endosomal surface and autophagosome; and PI(5)P in very low concentrations at the plasma membrane, the nucleus, Golgi complex, and sarco/endoplasmic reticulum [39,40]. They also feature specific biologic functions: PI(3)P induces autophagy [41], whereas PI(4)P is associated with endosomal trafficking, endoplasmic reticulum (ER) export, autophagy, signalling at the plasma membrane, cytokinesis, and actin dynamics [39,42]. The role of PI(5)P is not completely understood, despite many pieces of evidence suggesting its involvement in the cell cycle, stress response, T-cell activation, and chromatin remodelling [43].

The biological significance of this differential lipid regulation between these two highly homologous isoforms relies on their distinct functions. Even if PKCζ and PKCι display 72% amino acid sequence homology, several reports demonstrated functional differences among them. PKCζ is more efficiently involved in the NF-κB activation pathway when compared to PKCι/λ [44,45]. Interestingly, PKCι is frequently overexpressed and mislocalised in human tumours when compared to PKCζ. This involvement results in a consequent loss of cell polarity, which represents the first crucial step towards cell motility and invasiveness [45,46]. In particular, it has been reported that PKCι is often mislocalised to the cytoplasm and the nucleus of the transformed cancer cells [47–50], but fascinatingly, despite the loss of its restricted localisation within the membrane, PKCι seems to remain in complex with PAR-6 in tumour cells [51–53], indicating that this association, along with the PKCι activity, is somehow important for the maintenance of the cancer cell phenotypes [51,54–56].

While this work was in preparation, Dong et al. demonstrated that PKCζ is capable of PI(4)P binding only when engaged in a complex with PAR-6, which unmasks the polybasic PSR. This PKCζ-PI(4)P binding is important for the localisation of the complex but not for enzyme activity [27]. Remarkably, our results suggest the existence of a further binding site in the PKCι catalytic domain that is not affected by the phosphorylation position on the inositol ring. While full-length PKCι readily interacted with phosphatidylinositol monophosphates, only the construct comprising the isolated CD of PKCζ showed an interaction with phosphatidylinositol monophosphates. This finding suggests that the CD of both isoforms possess the ability to bind phosphatidylinositol monophosphates but that differences at the N-terminal region hinder the interaction of full-length PKCζ with the phosphatidylinositol monophosphates. In line with this hypothesis, the removal of N-terminal regulatory domains enables PI(4)P and PI(3)P binding to the PKCζ catalytic domain (Figure 3D,E). The small differences in the ability to interact with phosphatidylinositol monophosphates suggest that PKCζ would require binding to PS or PA to "open" the structure of the kinase and expose the catalytic domain that holds the binding site to phosphatidylinositol monophosphates. In a physiological context, those binding sites could be exposed upon PB1 binding to proteins as PAR-6. However, a constitutively active truncated version of PKCζ consisting of the catalytic domain is normally expressed in neuronal cells and is potentially localised by PIPs [57].

Though further studies are yet to be conducted regarding this binding, we can speculate that PI(3)P and PI(4)P binding may contribute to the reported recruitment of PKCι at specific membrane compartments, such as the reported localisations at lysosomes [58] or the apical domains of epithelial cells [50]. In the case of PKCζ, it may require recruitment by other lipids, and the binding to phosphatidylinositol monophosphates may support the activity once the protein is recruited to the specific membrane location.

The lipid overlay assay used in our work is a very stringent assay in which the protein must remain bound for the relatively long period of washings; therefore, it detects only high-affinity interactions with relatively low off rates. Indeed, even if PI(3,4,5)P$_3$ has been reported as aPKC activator [25,59], we and others were unable to detect any binding suggesting an indirect interaction between aPKC and PI(3,4,5)P$_3$ [26]. We also observed no direct binding of aPKC to CE, which was reported to bind PKCζ [22], resulting in recruitment to lipid raft and enzyme activation [60,61]. Recently, by using CE-binding assays and lipid vesicle-binding assays, Wang and colleagues demonstrated that PKCζ can bind to C16:0 CE in a specific manner [18,23]. Similarly, recent studies highlighted a specific interaction between aPKCs and S1P, which is a bioactive lipid obtained by the deacylation of ceramide [24]. In contrast with these data, our approach by lipid overlay assay did not reveal any binding between PKCζ or PKCι and CE or S1P. The discrepancies between our data and those of others could be due to the higher off rates of the interactions with CE or S1P. Alternatively, it is possible that our solid-phase/overlay binding assays may not be suitable to identify proteins that bind to ceramide [62], possibly due to the different conformations of ceramide integrated into a lipid membrane compared to a solid phase. Moreover, to perform the overlay assay, Wang et al. used PKCζ proteolytic fragments, while we used full-length proteins where the CE-binding site may be hidden, as shown for the PI(4)P-binding site. All in vitro studies have limitations, because it is not easy to recapitulate all lipid components and other protein interacting partners in the test tube. Therefore, the study may miss some relevant lipids and protein partners that may be physiologically significant. On the other hand, the assays reported here in two different binding formats and in activity assays were a strong indication that the aPKCs can bind with high affinity and high selectivity to the identified lipids and that they can regulate the activity of PKCι.

Whereas PS is considered to bind to the C1 domain, S1P [24] and PIPs bind to the catalytic domain. The binding of lipids at two different sites on aPKCs provides a means for synergistic binding when two lipids are present. The binding site for PIPs on the catalytic domain has not been determined. However, we can exclude the substrate/pseudosubstrate-binding site as a possible interaction site for PIPs, because the binding there would compete with substrate binding and would be inhibitory. We can speculate that S1P and PIPs could bind at the same region on the small lobe of the catalytic domain where the C1 domain binds. In such a scenario, the activation would be promoted by lipids competing for the two sites of the inhibitory interaction of the C1 domain onto the catalytic domain.

Finally, in the overlay assay, we report the interaction of PKCι to sulfatide. The interaction was comparably lower, and we did not validate the binding using a second methodology. However, we would like to note that human and yeast PDK1 bind sulfatide as well [63], and PDK1 has also been described to bind to PS [64]. The simultaneous binding of upstream kinase PDK1 and its aPKC substrate to sulfatide and PS could potentially be relevant for the phosphorylation of aPKCs at the activation loop during the maturation stage or as a regulatory event.

In brief, through lipid overlay assays and kinase assays, we observed that both PKCζ and PKCι bind to PA and PS, and the sole PKCι also binds to PI(3)P, PI(4)P, and PI(5)P. Moreover, those interactions result in a selective enhancement of aPKC activity. These data suggest a differential regulation of these two highly homologous isoforms by membrane lipids in line with the reported overlapping but different biological roles.

4. Materials and Methods

4.1. Reagents

Anti-FLAG M2 for immunoprecipitation is from Sigma Aldrich, St. Louis, MO, USA (A2220). Horseradish peroxidase-labelled anti-DDK (FLAG) tag is from Origene, Rockville, MD, USA (A190-101P). Secondary antibodies HRP-mouse and HRP-rabbit were from Perkin Elmer.

Unless specified, all chemical reagents, including protease inhibitors mix and protein G agarose are from Sigma Aldrich.

4.2. Constructs

The FLAG-PKCζ construct used in Figure 1 was kindly provided by Dr Alex Toker (Boston, MA, USA) [20].

Recombinant human PKCι with C-terminal DDK (FLAG) tag purified ≥ 80% from human HEK293 cells used in Figure 2 is from Origene, Rockville, USA (TP305379).

GST-PKCζ, GST-PKCι, and their truncated forms were previously described in Zang H et al. [12].

4.3. Protein Purification

For lipid overlay assays with lipid arrays, recombinant proteins were obtained by transfecting 293T cells (5 × 10 cm dishes) with the corresponding constructs using lipofectamine 3000 (Thermo Fisher Scientific, Waltham, MA, USA) according to the manufacturer's instruction. After 48 h, cells in each plate were lysed in 0.5 mL of lysis buffer (25-mM HEPES, pH 8, 150-mM NaCl, 1% Nonidet P-40, 5-mM EDTA, 2-mM EGTA, 50-mM NaF, 10% glycerol supplemented with fresh 1-mM Na_3VO_4, and protease inhibitors) and clarified after centrifugation for 15 min at 12,000 rpm at 4 °C.

FLAG-tagged recombinant proteins were batch-purified by overnight immunoprecipitation with 50-μg antibody against the protein tag and 100-μL protein-agarose beads. After 4 washes in lysis buffer and 2 in phosphate-buffered saline (PBS—137-mM NaCl, 2.68-mM KCl, 4.3-mM Na_2HPO_4, and 1.47-mM KH_2PO_4, pH 7.3), the immunoprecipitated protein was eluted twice with 100 μL of 0.1-M glycine (pH 3.5) and immediately neutralised with 10× tris buffer saline (0.5-M tris and 1.2-M NaCl, pH 7.4).

For purification of GST-tagged recombinant proteins, lysis buffer was supplemented with 2-mM dithiothreitol. GST-tagged proteins were batch-purified upon 4 h of immunoprecipitation with 200-μL glutathione-agarose beads (GE healthcare). After 4 washes in lysis buffer and 2 in phosphate-buffered saline (PBS), the immunoprecipitated protein was eluted with 200-μL elution buffer (100-mM Tris HCl, pH 8.0, 10-mM NaCl, 5% glycerol supplemented with fresh 2-mM DTT, and glutathione 10 mM).

Purified proteins were further subjected to SDS-PAGE for purity evaluation and protein quantification against a BSA calibration curve.

4.4. Lipid Overlay Assay

Lipid arrays (Echelon Biosciences, Salt Lake City, UT, USA) used in this work are PIP Strip (P6001), Membrane Lipid Strip (P6002), Membrane Lipid Array (P6003), PIP Array (P6100), and Sphingo Array (S6001). After saturation (3% bovine serum albumin and 0.1% Tween 20 in TBS buffer), membranes were incubated overnight with 5 mL of the protein of interest dissolved in the same buffer. After 4 washes with 0.1% Tween 20 in TBS buffer, the lipid-bound protein was detected upon 1-h incubation with the relevant HRP-labelled anti-tag antibody, followed by a further 4 washes. Detection antibodies were visualised and quantified using Western Lightning Chemiluminescence Reagent Plus (Perkin Elmer, Waltham, MA, USA) and a ChemiDoc imager (Bio-Rad, Hercules, CA, USA). The software automatically checks saturation and auto-scaled images to optimise signal/noise.

4.5. Cova PIP ELISA Assay

Proteins of interest were diluted in TBS supplemented with 1% BSA (1 µg/mL in a final volume of 100 µL per well) and added to Cova PIP screening plates (provided by Echelon Bioscience, H-6203; H-6204), followed by overnight incubation with gentle agitation at 4°C.

After 3 washes using 0.1% Tween 20 in TBS buffer, primary antibody anti-GST (Santa Cruz Biotechnology cat # SC-459, 1:1000 dilution in TBS + 1% BSA) was added and incubated at room temperature for 1 h with gentle agitation. Post-incubation, 3 washes with 0.1% Tween 20 in TBS buffer were performed before adding the secondary antibody diluted 1:5000 in TBS + 1% BSA for 1 h at room temperature on a plate shaker. Later, the plates were washed for 5 additional times before adding 100 µL/well of peroxidase substrate: 3,3',5,5'-Tetramethylbenzidine liquid substrate (TMB) and stopped the reaction by adding 50 µL/well of 0.5-M H_2SO_4 when significant blue colour developed. The absorbance was read with a Tecan Spark instrument plate reader at 450-nm wavelength immediately after adding the stop solution.

4.6. aPKC Activity Assay

Protein kinase assays were performed using the PKCι Kinase Enzyme System (Promega; Catalogue #: V3751) and PKCζ Kinase Enzyme System (Promega; Catalogue #: V2781) and ADP-Glo Kinase Assay kit (Promega; Catalogue #: V9101). The reaction was performed in a final volume of 25 µL containing 5 µL of stock solution reaction buffer A supplemented with 2.5-µL DTT (final concentration 50 µM); 5-µL active full-length PKCι (final concentration 4 nM) and 5-µL active full-length PKCζ (final concentration 1 nM); 5 µL of CREBtide substrate stock solution; 2.5 µL of ATP (final concentration 50 µM); 2.5 µL of DMSO (10%); 2.5 µL of lipid activator (10×); or PS, PA, and PI(4)P (dissolved by sonication in MOPS; final concentration 50 µg/mL).

The assay was carried out in 96-well luminescent white plates by incubating the reaction mixture at 30 °C for 20 min. After this incubation period, the ADP-Glo™ Reagent was added to simultaneously terminate the kinase reaction and deplete the remaining ATP. The plate was then incubated for 40 min at room temperature before adding 50 µL of Kinase Detection Reagent to convert ADP to ATP and incubated again for a further 30 min at room temperature. The luminescence of the 96-well reaction plate was finally read using the Tecan Spark 10 M Multimode Plate Reader.

Controls were set up including all the assay components by replacing the enzyme with equal volume of water (negative control). Lipids were replaced with equal volume of MOPS (for both positive and negative controls).

4.7. Data Processing and Statistical Analysis

The binding spots obtained on membrane strips or arrays were acquired with the ChemiDoc imager and quantified by using Image lab 6.0 software (Bio-Rad). Data obtained from PIP arrays and membrane arrays were collected as Excel files and analysed using

GraphPad Prism 9.0 software. We analysed our data using one-way ANOVA analysis with Dunnett's multiple comparisons for ELISA assays (Figure 3B,C), and for kinase activation assays (Figure 4A,B). For Figure 4C of the kinase activation assays, we used two-way ANOVA with Dunnett's multiple comparisons.

Supplementary Materials: The following are available online at https://www.mdpi.com/2227-9059/9/1/45/s1.

Author Contributions: A.B., R.C., M.M., D.C., B.R., A.G., R.M.B. and G.B.: study design and funding and S.V., S.C. and F.G.: performed experiments. All authors contributed to the manuscript preparation and data analysis under SV and GB coordination. All authors have read and agreed to the published version of the manuscript.

Funding: This study was funded by the National Ministry of University and research PRIN 2017 (grant 201799WCRH to GB) by the Italian Ministry of Education, University and Research (MIUR) program "Departments of Excellence 2018–2022", AGING Project—Department of Translational Medicine, Università del Piemonte Orientale (DC), FAR-2017 (DC and GB), and by Consorzio Interuniversitario di Biotecnologie (CIB) call "Network-CIB: Catalisi dell'Innovazione nelle Biotecnologie" (GB).

Institutional Review Board Statement: Not applicable.

Informed Consent Statement: Not applicable.

Data Availability Statement: The data presented in this study are available by the authors. For any further request contact the corresponding author.

Conflicts of Interest: The authors declare no conflicts of interest. The funders had no role in the design of the study; in the collection, analyses, or interpretation of data; in the writing of the manuscript, or in the decision to publish the results.

Abbreviations

LPA	lysophosphatidic acid
LPC	lysophosphocoline
PI	phosphatidylinositol
$PI(3)P$	phosphatidylinositol 3-phosphate
$PI(4)P$	phosphatidylinositol 4-phosphate
$PI(5)P$	phosphatidylinositol 5-phosphate
$PI(3,4)P_2$	phosphatidylinositol 3,4-bisphosphate
$PI(3,5)P_2$	phosphatidylinositol 3,5-bisphosphate
$PI(4,5)P_2$	phosphatidylinositol 4,5-bisphosphate
$PI(3,4,5)P_3$	phosphatidylinositol 3,4,5-trisphosphate
DAG	diacylglycerol
PA	phosphatidic acid
PS	phosphatidylserine
PE	phosphatidylethanolamine
PC	phosphatidylcholine
PG	phosphatidylglycerol
S	sphingosine
S1P	sphingosine-1-phosphate
SM	sphingomyelin
SPC	sphingosylphosphorycholine
PHS	phytosphingosine
CE	ceramide
SM4	sulfatide
GM1	monosialoganglioside
TAG	triacylglycerol
CL	cardiolipin
CH	Cholesterol

References

1. Hong, Y. aPKC: The Kinase that Phosphorylates Cell Polarity. *F1000Research* **2018**, *7*, 903. [CrossRef] [PubMed]
2. Xiao, H.; Liu, M. Atypical protein kinase C in cell motility. *Cell. Mol. Life Sci.* **2012**, *70*, 3057–3066. [CrossRef] [PubMed]
3. Chen, J.; Zhang, M. The Par3/Par6/aPKC complex and epithelial cell polarity. *Exp. Cell Res.* **2013**, *319*, 1357–1364. [CrossRef]
4. Vorhagen, S.; Niessen, C.M. Mammalian aPKC/Par polarity complex mediated regulation of epithelial division orientation and cell fate. *Exp. Cell Res.* **2014**, *328*, 296–302. [CrossRef] [PubMed]
5. Drummond, M.L.; Prehoda, K.E. Molecular Control of Atypical Protein Kinase C: Tipping the Balance between Self-Renewal and Differentiation. *J. Mol. Biol.* **2016**, *428*, 1455–1464. [CrossRef]
6. Reina-Campos, M.; Diaz-Meco, M.T.; Moscat, J. The Dual Roles of the Atypical Protein Kinase Cs in Cancer. *Cancer Cell* **2019**, *36*, 218–235. [CrossRef]
7. Du, G.-S.; Qiu, Y.; Wang, W.-S.; Peng, K.; Zhang, Z.-C.; Li, X.-S.; Xiao, W.; Yang, H. Knockdown on aPKC-ι inhibits epithelial-mesenchymal transition, migration and invasion of colorectal cancer cells through Rac1-JNK pathway. *Exp. Mol. Pathol.* **2019**, *107*, 57–67. [CrossRef]
8. Qian, Y.; Yao, W.; Yang, T.; Yang, Y.; Liu, Y.; Shen, Q.; Zhang, J.; Qi, W.; Wang, J. aPKC-ι/P-Sp1/Snail signaling induces epithelial-mesenchymal transition and immunosuppression in cholangiocarcinoma. *Hepatology* **2017**, *66*, 1165–1182. [CrossRef]
9. Paul, A.; Gunewardena, S.; Stecklein, S.R.; Saha, B.; Parelkar, N.; Danley, M.; Rajendran, G.; Home, P.; Ray, S.; Jokar, I.; et al. PKCλ/ι signaling promotes triple-negative breast cancer growth and metastasis. *Cell Death Differ.* **2014**, *21*, 1469–1481. [CrossRef]
10. Cohen, E.E.W.; Lingen, M.W.; Zhu, B.; Zhu, H.; Straza, M.W.; Pierce, C.; Martin, L.E.; Rosner, M.R. Protein Kinase Cζ Mediates Epidermal Growth Factor–Induced Growth of Head and Neck Tumor Cells by Regulating Mitogen-Activated Protein Kinase. *Cancer Res.* **2006**, *66*, 6296–6303. [CrossRef]
11. Lopez-Garcia, L.A.; Schulze, J.O.; Fröhner, W.; Zhang, H.; Süss, E.; Weber, N.; Navratil, J.; Amon, S.; Hindie, V.; Zeuzem, S.; et al. Allosteric Regulation of Protein Kinase PKCζ by the N-Terminal C1 Domain and Small Compounds to the PIF-Pocket. *Chem. Biol.* **2011**, *18*, 1463–1473. [CrossRef] [PubMed]
12. Zhang, H.; Neimanis, S.; Lopez-Garcia, L.A.; Arencibia, J.M.; Amon, S.; Stroba, A.; Zeuzem, S.; Proschak, E.; Stark, H.; Bauer, A.F.; et al. Molecular Mechanism of Regulation of the Atypical Protein Kinase C by N-terminal Domains and an Allosteric Small Compound. *Chem. Biol.* **2014**, *21*, 754–765. [CrossRef] [PubMed]
13. Corbalán-García, S.; Gómez-Fernández, J.C. Protein kinase C regulatory domains: The art of decoding many different signals in membranes. *Biochim. Biophys. ActaMol. Cell Biol. Lipids* **2006**, *1761*, 633–654. [CrossRef] [PubMed]
14. Chianale, F.; Rainero, E.; Cianflone, C.; Bettio, V.; Pighini, A.; Porporato, P.E.; Filigheddu, N.; Serini, G.; Sinigaglia, F.; Baldanzi, G.; et al. Diacylglycerol kinase mediates HGF-induced Rac activation and membrane ruffling by regulating atypical PKC and RhoGDI. *Proc. Natl. Acad. Sci. USA* **2010**, *107*, 4182–4187. [CrossRef] [PubMed]
15. Rainero, E.; Cianflone, C.; Porporato, P.E.; Chianale, F.; Malacarne, V.; Bettio, V.; Ruffo, E.; Ferrara, M.; Benecchia, F.; Capello, D.; et al. The Diacylglycerol Kinase α/Atypical PKC/β1 Integrin Pathway in SDF-1α Mammary Carcinoma Invasiveness. *PLoS ONE* **2014**, *9*, e97144. [CrossRef]
16. Dang, P.M.-C.; Fontayne, A.; Hakim, J.; El Benna, J.; Périanin, A. Protein Kinase C ζ Phosphorylates a Subset of Selective Sites of the NADPH Oxidase Component p47phoxand Participates in Formyl Peptide-Mediated Neutrophil Respiratory Burst. *J. Immunol.* **2001**, *166*, 1206–1213. [CrossRef]
17. Akimoto, K.; Takahashi, R.; Moriya, S.; Nishioka, N.; Takayanagi, J.; Kimura, K.; Fukui, Y.; Osada, S.-I.; Mizuno, K.; Hirai, S.-I.; et al. EGF or PDGF receptors activate atypical PKClambda through phosphatidylinositol 3-kinase. *EMBO J.* **1996**, *15*, 788–798. [CrossRef]
18. Wang, G.; Silva, J.; Krishnamurthy, K.; Tran, E.; Condie, B.G.; Bieberich, E. Direct Binding to Ceramide Activates Protein Kinase Cζ before the Formation of a Pro-apoptotic Complex with PAR-4 in Differentiating Stem Cells. *J. Biol. Chem.* **2005**, *280*, 26415–26424. [CrossRef] [PubMed]
19. Limatola, C.; Schaap, D.; Moolenaar, W.H.; Van Blitterswijk, W.J. Phosphatidic acid activation of protein kinase C-ζ overexpressed in COS cells: Comparison with other protein kinase C isotypes and other acidic lipids. *Biochem. J.* **1994**, *304*, 1001–1008. [CrossRef]
20. Pu, Y.; Peach, M.L.; Garfield, S.H.; Wincovitch, S.; Marquez, V.E.; Blumberg, P.M. Effects on Ligand Interaction and Membrane Translocation of the Positively Charged Arginine Residues Situated along the C1 Domain Binding Cleft in the Atypical Protein Kinase C Isoforms. *J. Biol. Chem.* **2006**, *281*, 33773–33788. [CrossRef]
21. Chianale, F.; Cutrupi, S.; Rainero, E.; Baldanzi, G.; Porporato, P.E.; Traini, S.; Filigheddu, N.; Gnocchi, V.F.; Santoro, M.M.; Parolini, O.; et al. Diacylglycerol Kinase-α Mediates Hepatocyte Growth Factor-induced Epithelial Cell Scatter by Regulating Rac Activation and Membrane Ruffling. *Mol. Biol. Cell* **2007**, *18*, 4859–4871. [CrossRef] [PubMed]
22. Müller, G.; Ayoub, M.; Storz, P.; Rennecke, J.; Fabbro, D.; Pfizenmaier, K. PKC zeta is a molecular switch in signal transduction of TNF-alpha, bifunctionally regulated by ceramide and arachidonic acid. *EMBO J.* **1995**, *14*, 1961–1969. [CrossRef]
23. Wang, G.; Krishnamurthy, K.; Umapathy, N.S.; Verin, A.D.; Bieberich, E. The Carboxyl-terminal Domain of Atypical Protein Kinase Cζ Binds to Ceramide and Regulates Junction Formation in Epithelial Cells. *J. Biol. Chem.* **2009**, *284*, 14469–14475. [CrossRef] [PubMed]
24. Kajimoto, T.; Caliman, A.D.; Tobias, I.S.; Okada, T.; Pilo, C.A.; Van, A.-A.N.; McCammon, J.A.; Nakamura, S.-I.; Newton, A.C. Activation of atypical protein kinase C by sphingosine 1-phosphate revealed by an aPKC-specific activity reporter. *Sci. Signal.* **2019**, *12*, eaat6662. [CrossRef] [PubMed]

25. Ivey, R.A.; Sajan, M.P.; Farese, R.V. Requirements for Pseudosubstrate Arginine Residues during Autoinhibition and Phosphatidylinositol 3,4,5-(PO4)3-dependent Activation of Atypical PKC. *J. Biol. Chem.* **2014**, *289*, 25021–25030. [CrossRef] [PubMed]
26. Tobias, I.S.; Kaulich, M.; Kim, P.K.; Simon, N.; Jacinto, E.; Dowdy, S.F.; King, C.C.; Newton, A.C. Protein kinase Cζ exhibits constitutive phosphorylation and phosphatidylinositol-3,4,5-triphosphate-independent regulation. *Biochem. J.* **2016**, *473*, 509–523 [CrossRef] [PubMed]
27. Dong, W.; Lu, J.; Zhang, X.; Wu, Y.; Lettieri, K.; Hammond, G.R.; Hong, Y. A polybasic domain in aPKC mediates Par6-dependent control of membrane targeting and kinase activity. *J. Cell Biol.* **2020**, *219*. [CrossRef]
28. Chou, M.M.; Hou, W.; Johnson, J.; Graham, L.K.; Lee, M.H.; Chen, C.-S.; Newton, A.C.; Schaffhausen, B.S.; Toker, A. Regulation of protein kinase C ζ by PI 3-kinase and PDK-1. *Curr. Biol.* **1998**, *8*, 1069–1078. [CrossRef]
29. Li, X.; Gao, T. mTORC 2 phosphorylates protein kinase Cζ to regulate its stability and activity. *EMBO Rep.* **2014**, *15*, 191–198. [CrossRef]
30. Nakanishi, H.; Brewer, K.; Exton, J.H. Activation of the zeta isozyme of protein kinase C by phosphatidylinositol 3,4,5-trisphosphate. *J. Biol. Chem.* **1993**, *268*, 13–16. [CrossRef]
31. Wang, Y.M.; Seibenhener, M.L.; Vandenplas, M.L.; Wooten, M.W. Atypical PKC zeta is activated by ceramide, resulting in coactivation of NF-kappaB/JNK kinase and cell survival. *J. Neurosci. Res.* **1999**, *55*, 293–302. [CrossRef]
32. Dowler, S.; Kular, G.; Alessi, D.R. Protein Lipid Overlay Assay. *Sci. Signal.* **2002**, *2002*, pl6. [CrossRef] [PubMed]
33. Gomez-Cambronero, J.; Morris, A.; Henkels, K. PLD Protein–Protein Interactions With Signaling Molecules and Modulation by PA. In *Methods in Enzymology*; Academic Press: Cambridge, MA, USA, 2017; Volume 583, pp. 327–357. [CrossRef]
34. O'Luanaigh, N.; Pardo, R.; Fensome, A.; Allen-Baume, V.; Jones, D.; Holt, M.R.; Cockcroft, S. Continual Production of Phosphatidic Acid by Phospholipase D Is Essential for Antigen-stimulated Membrane Ruffling in Cultured Mast Cells. *Mol. Biol. Cell* **2002**, *13*, 3730–3746. [CrossRef] [PubMed]
35. Sajan, M.P.; Bandyopadhyay, G.; Kanoh, Y.; Standaert, M.L.; Quon, M.J.; Reed, B.C.; Dikic, I.; Farese, R.V. Sorbitol activates atypical protein kinase C and GLUT4 glucose transporter translocation/glucose transport through proline-rich tyrosine kinase-2, the extracellular signal-regulated kinase pathway and phospholipase D. *Biochem. J.* **2002**, *362*, 665–674. [CrossRef] [PubMed]
36. Nishioka, T.; Frohman, M.A.; Matsuda, M.; Kiyokawa, E. Heterogeneity of Phosphatidic Acid Levels and Distribution at the Plasma Membrane in Living Cells as Visualized by a Förster Resonance Energy Transfer (FRET) Biosensor. *J. Biol. Chem.* **2010**, *285*, 35979–35987. [CrossRef] [PubMed]
37. Zhang, F.; Wang, Z.; Lu, M.; Yonekubo, Y.; Liang, X.; Zhang, Y.; Wu, P.; Zhou, Y.; Grinstein, S.; Hancock, J.F.; et al. Temporal Production of the Signaling Lipid Phosphatidic Acid by Phospholipase D2 Determines the Output of Extracellular Signal-Regulated Kinase Signaling in Cancer Cells. *Mol. Cell. Biol.* **2014**, *34*, 84–95. [CrossRef]
38. De Matteis, M.A.; Di Campli, A.; Godi, A. The role of the phosphoinositides at the Golgi complex. *Biochim. Biophys. Acta Bioenerg* **2005**, *1744*, 396–405. [CrossRef]
39. De Craene, J.-O.; Bertazzi, D.L.; Bär, S.; Friant, S. Phosphoinositides, Major Actors in Membrane Trafficking and Lipid Signaling Pathways. *Int. J. Mol. Sci.* **2017**, *18*, 634. [CrossRef]
40. Phan, T.K.; Williams, S.; Bindra, G.K.; Lay, F.T.; Poon, I.K.H.; Hulett, M.D. Phosphoinositides: Multipurpose cellular lipids with emerging roles in cell death. *Cell Death Differ.* **2019**, *26*, 781–793. [CrossRef]
41. Nascimbeni, A.C.; Codogno, P.; Morel, E. Phosphatidylinositol-3-phosphate in the regulation of autophagy membrane dynamics. *FEBS J.* **2017**, *284*, 1267–1278. [CrossRef]
42. De Matteis, M.A.; Wilson, C.; D'Angelo, G. Phosphatidylinositol-4-phosphate: The Golgi and beyond. *BioEssays* **2013**, *35*, 612–622. [CrossRef] [PubMed]
43. Poli, A.; Zaurito, A.E.; Abdul, S.; Fiume, R.; Faenza, I.; Divecha, N. Phosphatidylinositol 5 Phosphate (PI5P): From Behind the Scenes to the Front (Nuclear) Stage. *Int. J. Mol. Sci.* **2019**, *20*, 2080. [CrossRef] [PubMed]
44. Soloff, R.S.; Katayama, C.; Lin, M.Y.; Feramisco, J.R.; Hedrick, S.M. Targeted Deletion of Protein Kinase C λ Reveals a Distribution of Functions between the Two Atypical Protein Kinase C Isoforms. *J. Immunol.* **2004**, *173*, 3250–3260. [CrossRef] [PubMed]
45. Murray, N.R.; Kalari, K.R.; Fields, A.P. Protein kinase Cι expression and oncogenic signaling mechanisms in cancer. *J. Cell. Physiol.* **2010**, *226*, 879–887. [CrossRef] [PubMed]
46. Parker, P.J.; Justilien, V.; Riou, P.; Linch, M.; Fields, A.P. Atypical Protein Kinase Cι as a human oncogene and therapeutic target. *Biochem. Pharmacol.* **2014**, *88*, 1–11. [CrossRef]
47. Regala, R.P.; Weems, C.; Jamieson, L.; Khoor, A.; Edell, E.S.; Lohse, C.M.; Fields, A.P. Atypical Protein Kinase Cι Is an Oncogene in Human Non–Small Cell Lung Cancer. *Cancer Res.* **2005**, *65*, 8905–8911. [CrossRef]
48. Eder, A.M.; Sui, X.; Rosen, D.G.; Nolden, L.K.; Cheng, K.W.; Lahad, J.P.; Kango-Singh, M.; Lu, K.H.; Warneke, C.L.; Atkinson, E.N.; et al. Atypical PKCι contributes to poor prognosis through loss of apical-basal polarity and Cyclin E overexpression in ovarian cancer. *Proc. Natl. Acad. Sci. USA* **2005**, *102*, 12519–12524. [CrossRef]
49. Du, G.; Wang, J.-M.; Lu, J.-X.; Li, Q.; Ma, C.-Q.; Du, J.-T.; Zou, S.-Q. Expression of P-aPKC-ι, E-Cadherin, and β-Catenin Related to Invasion and Metastasis in Hepatocellular Carcinoma. *Ann. Surg. Oncol.* **2009**, *16*, 1578–1586. [CrossRef]
50. Kojima, Y.; Akimoto, K.; Nagashima, Y.; Ishiguro, H.; Shirai, S.; Chishima, T.; Ichikawa, Y.; Ishikawa, T.; Sasaki, T.; Kubota, Y.; et al. The overexpression and altered localization of the atypical protein kinase C λ/ι in breast cancer correlates with the pathologic type of these tumors. *Hum. Pathol.* **2008**, *39*, 824–831. [CrossRef]

41. Justilien, V.; Fields, A.P. Ect2 links the PKCι–Par6α complex to Rac1 activation and cellular transformation. *Oncogene* **2009**, *28*, 3597–3607. [CrossRef]
42. Regala, R.P.; Weems, C.; Jamieson, L.; Copland, J.A.; Thompson, E.A.; Fields, A.P. Atypical Protein Kinase Cι Plays a Critical Role in Human Lung Cancer Cell Growth and Tumorigenicity. *J. Biol. Chem.* **2005**, *280*, 31109–31115. [CrossRef] [PubMed]
43. Erdogan, E.; Lamark, T.; Stallings-Mann, M.; Jamieson, L.; Pellechia, M.; Thompson, E.A.; Johansen, T.; Fields, A.P. Aurothiomalate Inhibits Transformed Growth by Targeting the PB1 Domain of Protein Kinase Cι. *J. Biol. Chem.* **2006**, *281*, 28450–28459. [CrossRef] [PubMed]
44. Frederick, L.; Matthews, J.; Jamieson, L.; Justilien, V.; Thompson, E.; Radisky, D.C.; Fields, A.P. Matrix metalloproteinase-10 is a critical effector of protein kinase Cι-Par6α-mediated lung cancer. *Oncogene* **2008**, *27*, 4841–4853. [CrossRef] [PubMed]
45. Justilien, V.; Jameison, L.; Der, C.J.; Rossman, K.L.; Fields, A.P. Oncogenic Activity of Ect2 Is Regulated through Protein Kinase Cι-mediated Phosphorylation. *J. Biol. Chem.* **2010**, *286*, 8149–8157. [CrossRef]
46. Aranda, V.; Haire, T.; Nolan, M.E.; Calarco, J.P.; Rosenberg, A.Z.; Fawcett, J.P.; Pawson, T.; Muthuswamy, S.K. Par6–aPKC uncouples ErbB2 induced disruption of polarized epithelial organization from proliferation control. *Nat. Cell Biol.* **2006**, *8*, 1235–1245. [CrossRef]
47. Hernández, A.I.; Blace, N.; Crary, J.F.; Serrano, P.A.; Leitges, M.; Libien, J.M.; Weinstein, G.; Tcherapanov, A.; Sacktor, T.C. Protein Kinase Mζ Synthesis from a Brain mRNA Encoding an Independent Protein Kinase Cζ Catalytic Domain. *J. Biol. Chem.* **2003**, *278*, 40305–40316. [CrossRef]
48. Sánchez-Gómez, P.; De Cárcer, G.; Sandoval, I.V.; Moscat, J.; Diaz-Meco, M.T. Localization of Atypical Protein Kinase C Isoforms into Lysosome-Targeted Endosomes through Interaction with p62. *Mol. Cell. Biol.* **1998**, *18*, 3069–3080. [CrossRef]
49. Standaert, M.L.; Bandyopadhyay, G.; Kanoh, Y.; Sajan, M.P.; Farese, R.V. Insulin and PIP3 Activate PKC-ζ by Mechanisms That Are Both Dependent and Independent of Phosphorylation of Activation Loop (T410) and Autophosphorylation (T560) Sites. *Biochemistry* **2001**, *40*, 249–255. [CrossRef]
50. Fox, T.E.; Houck, K.L.; Oneill, S.M.; Nagarajan, M.; Stover, T.C.; Pomianowski, P.T.; Unal, O.; Yun, J.K.; Naides, S.J.; Kester, M. Ceramide Recruits and Activates Protein Kinase C ζ (PKCζ) within Structured Membrane Microdomains. *J. Biol. Chem.* **2007**, *282*, 12450–12457. [CrossRef]
51. Bourbon, N.A.; Yun, J.K.; Kester, M. Ceramide Directly Activates Protein Kinase C ζ to Regulate a Stress-activated Protein Kinase Signaling Complex. *J. Biol. Chem.* **2000**, *275*, 35617–35623. [CrossRef]
52. Chalfant, C.E.; Szulc, Z.; Roddy, P.; Bielawska, A.; Hannun, Y.A. The structural requirements for ceramide activation of serine-threonine protein phosphatases. *J. Lipid Res.* **2003**, *45*, 496–506. [CrossRef] [PubMed]
53. Pastor-Flores, D.; Schulze, J.O.; Bahí, A.; Süß, E.; Casamayor, A.; Biondi, R.M. Lipid regulators of Pkh2 in Candida albicans, the protein kinase ortholog of mammalian PDK1. *Biochim. Biophys. Acta Mol. Cell Biol. Lipids* **2016**, *1861*, 249–259. [CrossRef] [PubMed]
54. Heras-Martínez, G.D.L.; Calleja, V.; Bailly, R.; Dessolin, J.; Larijani, B.; Requejo-Isidro, J. A Complex Interplay of Anionic Phospholipid Binding Regulates 3′-Phosphoinositide-Dependent-Kinase-1 Homodimer Activation. *Sci. Rep.* **2019**, *9*, 1–18. [CrossRef] [PubMed]

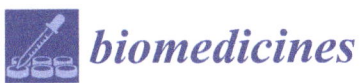

Article

The Minimal Effect of Linker Length for Fatty Acid Conjugation to a Small Protein on the Serum Half-Life Extension

Jinhwan Cho [1,†], Junyong Park [2,†], Giyoong Tae [1], Mi Sun Jin [3] and Inchan Kwon [1,2,*]

1. School of Materials Science and Engineering, Gwangju Institute of Science and Technology (GIST), Gwangju 61005, Korea; kroea2002@gist.ac.kr (J.C.); gytae@gist.ac.kr (G.T.)
2. Department of Biomedical Science and Engineering, GIST, Gwangju 61005, Korea; happydragon@gist.ac.kr
3. School of Life Science, GIST, Gwangju 61005, Korea; misunjin@gist.ac.kr
* Correspondence: inchan@gist.ac.kr; Tel.: +82-62-715-2312
† These authors contributed equally to this work.

Received: 9 April 2020; Accepted: 23 April 2020; Published: 26 April 2020

Abstract: Conjugation of serum albumin or one of its ligands (such as fatty acid) has been an effective strategy to prolong the serum half-lives of drugs via neonatal Fc receptor (FcRn)–mediated recycling of albumin. So far, fatty acid (FA) has been effective in prolonging the serum half-lives for therapeutic peptides and small proteins, but not for large therapeutic proteins. Very recently, it was reported a large protein conjugated to FA competes with the binding of FcRn with serum albumin, leading to limited serum half-life extension, because primary FA binding sites in serum albumin partially overlap with FcRn binding sites. In order to prevent such competition, longer linkers between FA and the large proteins were required. Herein, we hypothesized that small proteins do not cause substantial competition for FcRn binding to albumin, resulting in the extended serum half-life. Using a small protein (28 kDa), we investigated whether the intramolecular distance in FA-protein conjugate affects the FcRn binding with albumin and serum half-life using linkers with varying lengths. Unlike with the FA-conjugated large protein, all FA-conjugated small proteins with different linkers exhibited comparable the FcRn binding to albumin and extended serum half-life.

Keywords: serum half-life extension; fatty acid conjugation; FcRn-mediated recycling; serum albumin

1. Introduction

Therapeutic proteins have been widely used for the treatment of human diseases [1]. However, therapeutic proteins are rapidly eliminated from the blood of patients due to several mechanisms, including renal filtration, proteolysis, intracellular degradation, and immune responses, which result in short serum half-lives [2,3]. Such short serum half-lives of therapeutic proteins result in the need for frequent administration [2–4]. Therefore, the extension of the serum half-life of therapeutic proteins is very important in developing new therapeutic proteins [2,4,5]. Conventionally, polyethylene glycol (PEG) chains have been conjugated to therapeutic proteins for serum half-life extension in order to reduce renal filtration and proteolysis [6]. However, recently several concerns have been raised about PEG conjugation, including PEG accumulation due to its poor degradability in the body and reduced efficacy resulting from immune responses to PEG [7].

As an alternative to PEG, human serum albumin (HSA) has been investigated as a half-life extender [8]. In contrast to PEG, HSA is biodegradable and minimally immunogenic [9,10]. Furthermore, HSA has an exceptionally long serum half-life (more than two weeks) partly due to evasion from intracellular degradation via neonatal Fc receptor (FcRn)–mediated recycling [2,3,10–13]. Direct coupling of therapeutic protein to HSA via either genetic fusion or chemical conjugation led to a significant extension of therapeutic protein serum half-life in vivo [11,12,14–17]. Recently, indirect coupling of therapeutics to HSA using albumin ligands such as fatty acids has received much attention, because fatty acids are cheaper than HSA and exhibit a much higher conjugation yield than HSA [9]. Furthermore, fatty acids are biocompatible and not immunogenic [18].

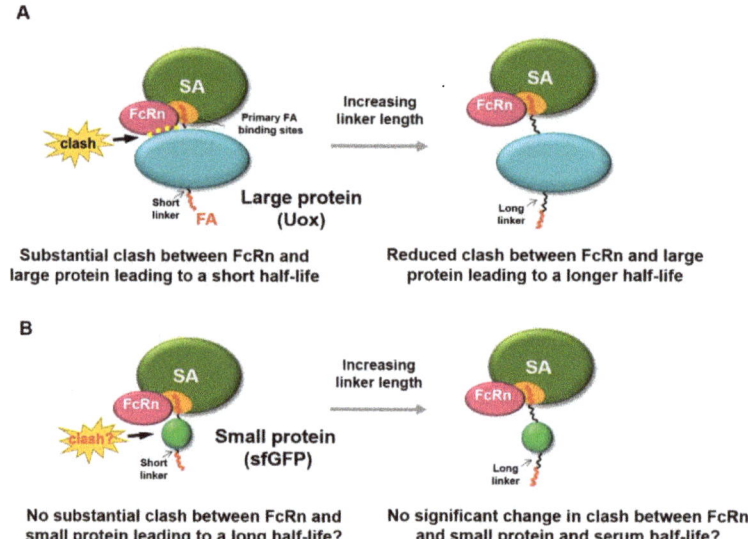

Figure 1. Effect of protein size of fatty acid-conjugated protein on the binding of FcRn with serum albumin. (**A**) For a large protein (Uox, 140 kDa), conjugation of fatty acid with a short linker leads to steric hindrance to binding of FcRn to serum albumin, due to its large size. Increasing the linker length reduces the steric hindrance to binding of FcRn to serum albumin, resulting in longer serum half-life. (**B**) For a small protein (superfolder green fluorescent protein [sfGFP], 28 kDa), conjugation of a fatty acid with a short linker may not exhibit substantial steric hindrance to binding of FcRn to serum albumin, due to its small size. Therefore, increasing linker length may not substantially alter the steric hindrance to the binding of FcRn to serum albumin.

Despite the numerous reports of serum half-life extension via fatty acid conjugation, its molecular mechanism was not yet fully revealed. It is noteworthy that fatty acid conjugation was effective for serum half-life extension of therapeutic peptides and small proteins (less than 28 kDa) [17,19–24]. Considering that a majority of therapeutic proteins and other candidates have molecular weights greater than 28 kDa [25], it is important to understand whether there is any protein size–dependent factor in serum half-life extension via fatty acid conjugation. Regarding this, a very recent report showed that fatty acid conjugation extends the serum half-life of urate oxidase (Uox) (140 kDa) [26], a large therapeutic protein used to treat hyperuricemia [27–31]. In this report, the conventional short linker between fatty acid (palmitic acid) and large protein (Uox) was shown not to be able to substantially extend the serum half-life of Uox, due to compromised FcRn binding to serum albumin. In order to avoid competition with FcRn binding and achieve the substantial serum half-life extension, longer linkers between fatty acid and Uox were required (Figure 1A) [26]. There are seven palmitic acid (PA) binding sites on serum albumin (FA1 to FA7) [32]. Two dominant PA binding sites at domain III of serum albumin (FA4 and FA5) [33–38] overlap with FcRn binding sites. With a short linker, PA-conjugated Uox (Uox-PA) was expected to be located near domain III of serum albumin. Therefore, the existence of bulky Uox near domain III was attributed to the significant reduction of FcRn binding to serum albumin in vitro, resulting in limited extension in serum half-life in vivo [26]. In contrast, longer linkers were expected to locate Uox-PA away from domain III, leading to the recovery of FcRn binding affinity to serum albumin in vitro and substantial extension of serum half-life in vivo [26].

Considering that fatty acid conjugation led to significant serum half-life extension of therapeutic peptides and small proteins [17,19–23], we hypothesized that small proteins exhibit minimal steric hindrance to binding of FcRn to serum albumin. Therefore, herein we investigated whether fatty acid conjugation to a small protein with linkers with various lengths affects binding of FcRn with serum albumin in vitro and serum half-life in vivo. For a small protein, if linkers with varying lengths do not substantially affect the binding affinity of FcRn to serum albumin in vitro and serum half-life in vivo (Figure 1B), that would demonstrate that protein size is an important factor in serum half-life extension via fatty acid conjugation. These results would facilitate our understanding of the molecular mechanism of fatty acid conjugation–mediated serum half-life extension of proteins.

2. Materials and Methods

2.1. Materials

Ampicillin; palmitic acid N-hydroxysuccinimide (NHS-PA); 3,3',5,5'-tetramethylbenzidine (TMB); sinapinic acid; and deoxycholate (DCA) were obtained from Sigma-Aldrich (St. Louis, MO, USA). Mouse serum albumin (MSA) was obtained from Equitech-Bio Inc. (Kerrville, TX, USA). Isopropyl β-D-1-thiogalactopyranoside (IPTG), amine-binding plate, and phosphate-buffered saline (PBS) were obtained from Thermo Fisher Scientific (Waltham, MA, USA). Tween-20 was obtained from Bio-Rad (Hercules, CA, USA). Nickel-nitrilotriacetic acid (Ni-NTA) agarose beads and polypropylene columns were obtained from Qiagen Inc (Valencia, CA, USA). PD-10 column was obtained from GE Health care (Piscataway, NJ, USA). Vivaspin centrifugal concentrators with molecular weight cut-off (MWCO) of 10 kDa were purchased from Sartorius Corporation (Bohemia, NY, USA). Dibenzocyclooctyne (DBCO)-amine, DBCO-PEG4-amine, azidoacetic acid N-hydroxysuccinimide (NHS) ester, and azido-PEG4-NHS ester were obtained from Click Chemistry Tools LLC (Scottsdale, AZ, USA). 6×His tag antibody and horseradish peroxidase (HRP)–conjugated anti-rabbit Immunoglobulin G (IgG) were obtained from Cell Signaling Technology (Beverly, MA, USA). ZipTip with C18 resin was purchased from Millipore Corporation (Billerica, MA, USA). Protein Standard II was obtained from Bruker Daltonics (Bremen, Germany). Mouse FcRn was obtained from ACRO Biosystems (Newark, DE, USA).

2.2. Preparation of Purified Superfolder Green Fluorescent Protein (sfGFP) from E. coli

In order to obtain purified sfGFP using E. coli, cloning, expression, and purification of sfGFP were conducted as previously described [23]. Briefly, the pQE80-sfGFP plasmid was transformed into TOP10 E. coli competent cells. The transformed colony was precultured into 2×·YT medium containing 100 µg/mL ampicillin. After 8 h incubation at 37 °C, the precultured cells were inoculated into a 2×·YT medium containing 100 µg/mL ampicillin and incubated at 37 °C for the main culture. When the optical density at 600 nm reached 0.5, 1 mM IPTG was added to the main culture for sfGFP induction. After 5 h incubation at 37 °C, cells were collected by pellet down at 5000 g for 10 min. The cell pellets were stored at −80 °C until further use. In order to start the purification of sfGFP, the cell pellets were resuspended with lysis buffer (pH 7.4, 10 mM imidazole) by complete vortexing. The resuspended cell pellets were broken down by sonication for 1 h. Cell debris was removed by centrifugation at 12,000 rpm for 30 min. The supernatant was mixed with Ni-NTA agarose beads thoroughly and incubated at 15 °C and 220 rpm for 1 h, then was poured into a polypropylene column, followed by washing with washing buffer (pH 7.4, 20 mM imidazole) to remove impurities. The sfGFP was eluted with elution buffer (pH 7.4, 250 mM imidazole), and then was immediately subjected to buffer exchange into PBS buffer (pH 7.4) using a PD-10 column. Finally, the purified sfGFP was concentrated to a proper concentration with a Vivaspin column (MWCO: 10 kDa) according to the supplier's manual and stored at 4 °C before use. The molar extinction coefficient at 280 nm value of sfGFP was calculated to be 19,035 M^{-1} cm^{-1} by the following equation: ε_{280} = (5500 × number of tryptophan residues) + (1490 × number of tyrosine residues) + (125 × number of disulfide bonds) [39]. The concentration of sfGFP was then determined using the Beer-Lambert law.

2.3. Preparation of sfGFP-PA Conjugates with Various Linkers

The sfGFP-PA conjugates with various linker lengths were prepared as previously reported, except sfGFP was used instead of Uox [26]. The chemical structures of intermediates and linkers (LK01, 02, 03, and 04) are shown in Figure 2A and Figure S1 in Supplementary Materials. Briefly, each DBCO-amine or DBCO-PEG4-amine (180 µM) was reacted with NHS-PA (900 µM) at 37 °C for 20 h to make DBCO-PA or DBCO-PEG4-PA, respectively. The unreacted NHS-PA was quenched with excess Tris base (100 mM, pH 7.4). The sfGFP-PA conjugates with various linker lengths (SP01, SP02, SP03, and SP04) were generated using three different PA-containing reagents (NHS-PA, DBCO-PA, and DBCO-PEG4-PA). First, sfGFP (50 µM) and NHS-PA (500 µM) were reacted in PBS containing 0.40% (w/v) DCA at room temperature for 3 h, yielding SP01. Second, sfGFP (50 µM) and azidoacetic acid NHS ester (1500 µM) were reacted in PBS on ice for 2 h and quenched with excess Tris base (150 mM, pH 7.4) to make sfGFP-azides intermediate. After desalting and concentration by Vivaspin (MWCO: 10 kDa), the concentration of sfGFP-azides intermediate was measured using the Beer-Lambert law. sfGFP-azides intermediate (50 µM) was reacted with DBCO-PA (100 µM) in PBS with 0.80% (w/v) DCA at room temperature for 3 h, yielding SP02. Third, sfGFP (50 µM) and azido-PEG4-NHS ester (1500 µM) were reacted in PBS on ice for 2 h and quenched with excess Tris base (150 mM, pH 7.4) to make sfGFP-PEG4-azides intermediate. After desalting and concentration by Vivaspin (MWCO: 10 kDa), the concentration of sfGFP-PEG4-azides was measured using the Beer-Lambert law. sfGFP-PEG4-azides (50 µM) was reacted with DBCO-PA (100 µM) in PBS with 0.80% (w/v) DCA at room temperature for 3 h, yielding SP03. Fourth, sfGFP-PEG4-azides (50 µM) was reacted with DBCO-PEG4-PA (100 µM) in PBS with 0.80% (w/v) DCA at room temperature for 3 h, yielding SP04. Finally, all sfGFP-PA conjugates were desalted to PBS buffer (pH 7.4) using a PD-10 column and stored at 4 °C until required for use.

2.4. Matrix-Assisted Laser Desorption Ionization/Time-of-Flight (MALDI-TOF) Analysis of the sfGFP and sfGFP-PA Conjugates

In order to analyze the intact mass of the sfGFP or sfGFP-PA conjugate, the sample was desalted on a ZipTip C18 according to the manufacturer's (Millipore Corporation) protocol. The first layer applied to a polished steel plate using sinapinic acid in absolute ethanol. The desalted sfGFP or sfGFP-PA conjugate was mixed with 1:1 of sinapinic acid in TA30 solution (0.1% Trifluoroacetic acid:acetonitrile = 7:3) and then applied to the first layer prior to mass analysis via Microflex MALDI-TOF (Bruker Daltonics; Bremen, Germany). The MALDI-TOF was calibrated using a Protein Standard II (20–90 kDa) before measurement according to the manufacturer's instructions. The average masses of sfGFP, SP01, SP02, SP03, and SP04 were obtained by multiplying each area and its corresponding mass of all peaks and then dividing its average value by the average area of all peaks. The average numbers of conjugated PAs at SP01, SP02, SP03, and SP04 were obtained by using the molecular weight of the PA containing linker from the mass shift from sfGFP, sfGFP-azides, and sfGFP-PEG4-azides.

2.5. In Vitro Serum Albumin Binding Assay

MSA (10 µg/mL) in 100 µL of PBS (pH 7.4) was applied to amine-binding plates at 4 °C overnight. 5% skim milk in PBS containing 0.05% (v/v) of Tween-20 (PBS-T) (pH 7.4) was used for blocking nonspecific binding at room temperature for 2 h. sfGFP and sfGFP-PA conjugates (14 µM) in 50 µL of PBS were incubated on the plate at room temperature for 2 h. The amount of sfGFP bound was determined by enzyme-linked immunosorbent assay (ELISA) using the anti-6×His antibody. After that, the anti-6×His antibody (1:1000 diluted) was incubated at room temperature for 2 h and washed. Immediately after, HRP-conjugated anti-rabbit IgG (1:1000 diluted) was added and incubated for 1 h.

After washing, the TMB substrate was added, incubated for the appropriate time, and stopped with 1 M sulfuric acid. Absorbance at 450 nm was monitored using a Synergy H1 multimode microplate reader. (BioTek; Winooski, VT, USA).

2.6. sfGFP Fluorescence Assay

The fluorescence of sfGFP or sfGFP-PA conjugate was measured using a Synergy H1 multimode microplate reader. Each sfGFP or sfGFP-PA conjugate (1.7 µM) in 100 µL of PBS was added to a 96-well plate, and then the fluorescence was measured at an excitation wavelength of 480 nm and an emission wavelength of 510 nm. The relative fluorescence of sfGFP-PA conjugate was normalized by that of sfGFP.

2.7. Serum Half-Life Determination in Mice

The amounts of sfGFP and sfGFP-PA conjugate in vivo were investigated by injecting each protein (10 µM) in 200 µL of PBS into the tail veins of 9-week-old female BALB/c mice (n = 5). Experiments on mice were performed according to the guidelines of the Animal Care and Use Committee of the Gwangju Institute of Science and Technology (GIST) (GIST-2019-071). Blood samples (below 50 µL) were collected at 10, 20, 30, 40, and 50 min for sfGFP; 10 min and 1, 2, and 4 h for sfGFP-PA conjugates. Collected blood samples were allowed to clot at room temperature for 30 min, then centrifuged at 1500 rpm for 10 min at 4 °C to obtain the serum from the blood. The separated serum was stored at −20 °C until required for use. The concentrations of sfGFP and sfGFP-PA conjugates in the serum samples were measured by using a GFP ELISA kit according to the manufacturer's (Cell Biolabs Inc; San Diego, CA, USA) protocol.

2.8. FcRn/Serum Albumin/sfGFP-PA Tertiary Complex Formation Assay

Mouse FcRn (10 µg/mL) in 100 µL of PBS (pH 6.0) applied to an amine-binding plate at 4 °C overnight. In order to block nonspecific binding, 5% skim milk in PBS-T (pH 6.0) was added and incubated at room temperature for 2 h. MSA (1 mg/mL) in 100 µL of PBS (pH 6.0) was added at room temperature for 2 h. After washing, 14 µM of sfGFP or sfGFP-PA conjugates in 50 µL of PBS (pH 6.0) was added and incubated at room temperature for 2 h. After that, 100 µL of anti-6×His antibody (1:1000 diluted) was incubated at room temperature for 2 h. After washing, HRP-conjugated anti-rabbit IgG (1:1000 diluted) was added and incubated at room temperature for 1 h. Then, the TMB substrate was added, incubated for the appropriate time, and stopped with 1 M sulfuric acid. Absorbance at 450 nm was monitored with a Synergy H1 multimode microplate reader.

3. Results and Discussion

3.1. PA-Conjugated sfGFP Conjugates with Various Linker Lengths

We chose sfGFP as a small model protein to investigate the competition to binding of FcRn to serum albumin and the serum half-life extension upon fatty acid conjugation. Although green fluorescent protein is not a therapeutic protein, it has been widely used in biomedical applications [40–44]. In particular, its unique spectral properties including fluorescence and biocompatibility, make sfGFP a great surrogate for a therapeutic protein in drug delivery studies [41,42]. In order to investigate the protein-size dependency of serum half-life extension via fatty acid conjugation, a model protein should be much smaller than Uox (140 kDa). Considering that the molecular weight of sfGFP with an anti-hexahistidine (6×His) tag used in this study is about 28 kDa, sfGFP was suitable as a small model protein. Purified sfGFP was prepared as described previously [8,23,45]. Briefly, the gene of sfGFP was overexpressed in TOP 10 *E. coli* cells. Then, the recombinant sfGFP was purified via metal affinity chromatography using its 6×His tag. The band of purified sfGFP was observed in the Coomassie blue–stained protein gel (Figure 2B, lane 1), indicating that the purity of sfGFP was greater than 95%.

Next, four linkers with various lengths (LK01, 02, 03, and 04) were conjugated to sfGFP to generate sfGFP-PA conjugates (SP01, 02, 03, and 04) (Figure 2A). The same four linkers were previously used to prepare Uox-PA conjugates [26]. In general, properties of the fatty acid linker, such as solubility and length, may affect serum albumin binding affinity. However, for Uox-PA conjugates, the linkers did not exhibit substantial differences in serum albumin binding affinity [26]. Therefore, in order to minimize the effects of fatty acid linkers on serum albumin binding, we chose the same set of linkers for sfGFP-PA conjugates. The lengths of linkers were estimated as 0.25, 1.5, 2.8, and 4.8 nm, respectively [26]. Since these linker lengths were estimated at a maximal stretch, the actual linker lengths could be shorter than those theoretical values. The four sfGFP-PA conjugates (SP01, 02, 03, and 04) were prepared similarly to those of Uox-PA [26]. Briefly, for SP01, NHS-PA (Figure S1a in Supplementary Materials) was directly conjugated to lysine residues of sfGFP via NHS-amine reaction (Figure S1b in Supplementary Materials). In the case of SP02, azidoacetic acid NHS ester (Figure S1c in Supplementary Materials) was reacted with lysine residues of sfGFP to generate sfGFP-azides. DBCO-amine (Figure S1d in Supplementary Materials) was reacted with NHS-PA to generate an intermediate (DBCO-PA) (Figure S1e in Supplementary Materials). Then, DBCO-PA was reacted with sfGFP-azides via strain-promoted alkyne-azide cycloaddition (SPAAC) reactions (Figure S1f in Supplementary Materials) to obtain SP02. In the case of SP03, azido-PEG4-NHS (Figure S1g in Supplementary Materials) was reacted with lysine residues of sfGFP to generate sfGFP-PEG4-azides. Then, DBCO-PA was reacted with sfGFP-PEG4-azides to generate SP03. Finally, for SP04, NHS-PA was reacted with DBCO-PEG4-amine (Figure S1h in Supplementary Materials) to generate DBCO-PEG4-PA (Figure S1i in Supplementary Materials). Then, DBCO-PEG4-PA was reacted with sfGFP-PEG4-azides to generate SP04.

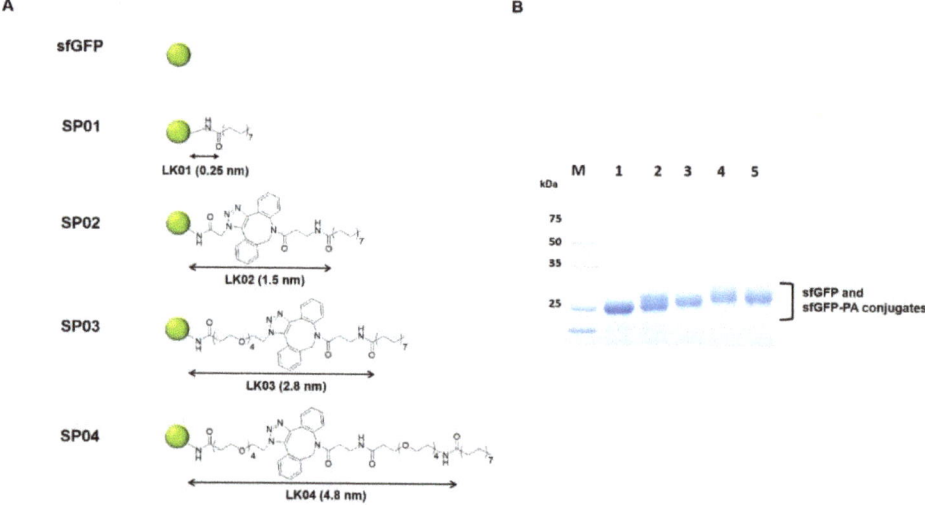

Figure 2. The structures and characterization of sfGFP-PA conjugates with various linker lengths. (**A**) sfGFP is represented as a green circle. The length of each linker was measured between the ε-carbon in a lysine residue of sfGFP and carbonyl carbon of PA when the linker was maximally stretched using Chem3D software and marked with black arrows. (**B**) Coomassie blue–stained protein gel image of purified sfGFP and sfGFP-PA conjugates was taken by Bio-Rad ChemiDoc XRS+. Lane M, molecular weight markers; Lane 1, sfGFP; Lane 2, SP01; Lane 3, SP02; Lane 4, SP03; Lane 5, SP04.

PA conjugation to the four sfGFP-PA conjugates was verified by protein band shifts in the protein gel and mass shifts in MALDI-TOF mass spectra (Figure 2B and Figure S2 in Supplementary Materials). In the protein gel, the bands of sfGFP-PA conjugates (SP01, 02, 03, and 04) were shifted up from the band of unmodified sfGFP, indicating the mass of sfGFP increased upon PA conjugation. Furthermore, we performed a MALDI-TOF spectrometric analysis of sfGFP and sfGFP-PA conjugates. The mass of unmodified sfGFP determined by MALDI-TOF analysis was 27,705 Da, which was consistent with its theoretical value (27,604 Da), with a 0.37% error. For sfGFP-PA conjugates, peaks were right-shifted, indicating that the mass of sfGFP increased upon PA conjugation. For all four sfGFP-PA conjugates, the mass differences between sfGFP-PA conjugate and unmodified sfGFP indicated that the average number of PA conjugated to single sfGFP was about one. Therefore, we speculated that the property differences among sfGFP-PA conjugates resulting from the different number of conjugated PAs were minimal.

3.2. Serum Albumin Binding Affinity of sfGFP-PA Conjugates

Using the sfGFP-PA conjugates, we first performed serum albumin binding assays at pH 7.4. 96-well plate was coated with MSA. Then, either the purified sfGFP-PA conjugate or unmodified sfGFP was incubated in a well. The amount of either sfGFP-PA conjugate or unmodified sfGFP bound MSA on the plate was analyzed by ELISA using anti-6×His antibody. The binding affinities sfGFP-PA conjugates (SP01, 02, 03, and 04) were comparable but significantly greater than that of unmodified sfGFP (Figure 3A). These results indicate that PA conjugation to sfGFP retained the albumin binding capacity. Furthermore, although linker properties may affect serum albumin binding affinity, the set of linkers used in this study did not substantially alter serum albumin binding affinity for all sfGFP-PA conjugates; this was consistent with the results for Uox-PA conjugates [26].

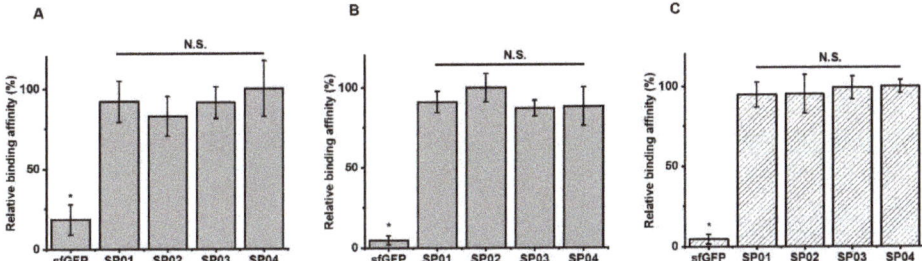

Figure 3. Relative albumin binding affinities of sfGFP-PA conjugate and tertiary complex formation of FcRn/MSA/sfGFP-PA conjugates. The amount of sfGFP or sfGFP-PA conjugate bound on MSA without mouse FcRn at pH 7.4 (**A**) or pH 6.0 (**B**). The amount of sfGFP or sfGFP-PA conjugate complexed with MSA and mouse FcRn at pH 6.0 (**C**). The amount of sfGFP or sfGFP-PA conjugate bound on the plate was normalized based on the highest signal to calculate relative binding affinity. The graph represents the mean ± standard deviations (SD) (n = 3). * $p < 0.01$; N.S.: not significant (two-tailed student t-test).

3.3. Fluorescence of sfGFP-PA Conjugates

Next, we investigated whether PA conjugation to sfGFP affected the fluorescence intensity of sfGFP. All sfGFP-PA conjugates (SP01, SP02, SP03, and SP04) exhibited about 20% reduction in fluorescence intensity compared to that of sfGFP (Figure S3 in Supplementary Materials). However, the fluorescence intensities of all sfGFP-PA conjugates were comparable. Such a reduction in fluorescence intensity is likely attributable to the use of DCA to increase the solubility of PAs during conjugation reaction [9,26]. Since DCA is a well-known detergent, it may perturb the folded structure of sfGFP, resulting in reduced fluorescence. Such a moderate reduction in fluorescence intensity of sfGFP-PA conjugate was not problematic in determining the serum half-life of sfGFP-PA because relative residual amounts of sfGFP-PA in serum were analyzed.

3.4. Serum Half-Lives of sfGFP-PA Conjugates

Then, the half-lives of sfGFP and sfGFP-PA conjugates were determined from the studies on mice. As reported previously [45], the percentages of residual sfGFP amounts were fitted to a two-phase model (Figure 4A). It was reported that FcRn-mediated recycling affects beta-phase in pharmacokinetics [46]. Therefore, beta-phase half-lives were plotted for sfGFP or sfGFP-PA conjugates in the order of increasing linker length. The half-life of sfGFP (single-phase) was 0.13 h. The beta-phase half-lives of sfGFP-PA conjugates were between 1.34 and 1.57 h, more than 10 times longer than that of sfGFP. This trend was notably different from that of Uox-PA conjugates [26]. In the case of Uox-PA conjugates up to a certain linker length, the half-life of Uox-PA conjugate increased as linker length increased (Figure 4B, light gray). However, the half-lives of sfGFP-PA conjugates were comparable, demonstrating that all linkers allow effective half-life extension of sfGFP in vivo (Figure 4B, dark gray). These results support our hypothesis that, for a small protein such as sfGFP, the distance between PA and small protein does not substantially alter serum half-life extension in vivo.

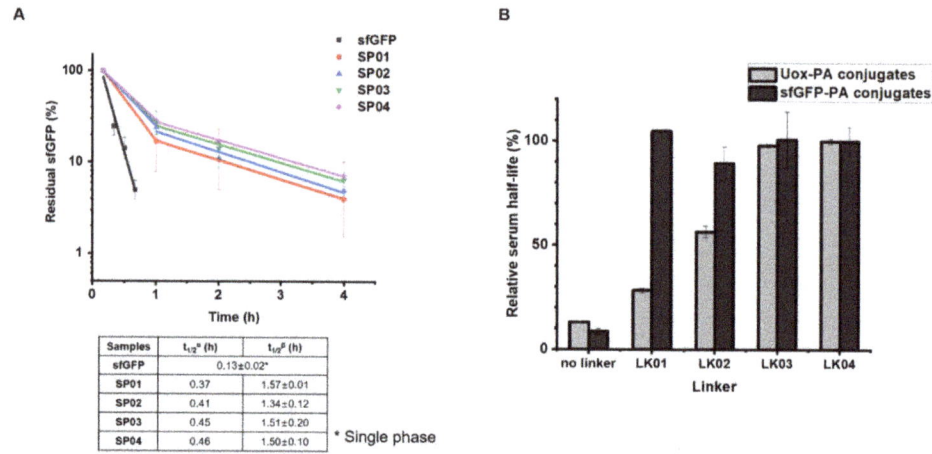

Figure 4. Pharmacokinetic studies of sfGFP and sfGFP-PA conjugates in mice. (**A**) Either purified sfGFP or sfGFP-PA conjugate was intravenously injected into the tail vein of a female Balb/c mouse (n = 4). The concentrations of sfGFP and sfGFP-PA conjugates were measured from blood samples taken at different time points: 10, 20, 30, 40, and 50 min for sfGFP; 10 min and, 1, 2, and 4 h for sfGFP-PA conjugates. The residual sfGFP amounts in serum were plotted on a logarithmic scale. Each data point represents the mean ± SD (n = 4). $t_{1/2}{}^{\alpha}$ and $t_{1/2}{}^{\beta}$ indicate the serum half-lives in the α- and β-phase, respectively. The serum half-lives of sfGFP and sfGFP-PA conjugates are summarized in the below table. (**B**) Comparison of relative serum half-lives of either Uox-PA (light gray) or sfGFP-PA conjugates (dark gray) versus corresponding linkers. The serum half-lives of unmodified protein and PA conjugates were normalized using those of PA conjugates with the LK04 linker. The serum half-life data of Uox and Uox-PA conjugates were obtained from the literature [26].

3.5. FcRn Binding Assays of sfGFP-PA Conjugates

In order to investigate whether sfGFP-PA conjugates compete with the binding of FcRn to serum albumin depending on linker length, we performed FcRn binding assays. The assays for sfGFP-PA conjugates were based on the formation of FcRn/serum albumin/sfGFP-PA tertiary structure, as reported previously for Uox-PA conjugates [26]. The dissociation constant between mouse FcRn and MSA was reported to be 546 nM [47]. Therefore, the tertiary structure formation should be dependent of binding of sfGFP-PA with MSA. The pH value of 6.0 was often used to confirm the interaction of albumin with FcRn [45,48]. Hu et al. reported that endo-lysosomal pH varies from 4.5 to 6.5 [49]. Therefore, we chose pH 6.0 for FcRn binding assays in our study. In order to evaluate albumin binding affinities of sfGFP-PA conjugates, the amount of sfGFP-PA bound on MSA was first determined. The albumin binding affinities of all four sfGFP-PA conjugates were comparable at pH 6.0 but significantly greater than that of unmodified sfGFP (Figure 3B). Then, we performed the FcRn binding assays. As expected for a small protein, all sfGFP-PA conjugates (SP01, 02, 03, and 04) showed the comparable formation of FcRn/MSA/sfGFP-PA tertiary complex (Figure 3C), indicating that none of the sfGFP-PA conjugates substantially interfere with FcRn binding to serum albumin in vitro. Combined with the FcRn/serum albumin/sfGFP-PA tertiary complex formation results, the sfGFP-PA conjugate, even with a short linker, does not hinder the FcRn binding to serum albumin; the result is effective half-life extension in vivo. Therefore, the results of sfGFP-PA conjugates support our previous results: Uox requires a long linker in the PA conjugate in order to achieve effective half-life extension in vivo for mitigating the steric hindrance between Uox and FcRn due to its large size. In view of the pharmacokinetics and FcRn binding assay results of large protein Uox-PA conjugates [26] and small protein sfGFP-PA conjugates, it can be concluded that the protein size is the dominating factor to consider for fatty acid conjugation.

4. Conclusions

In conclusion, our results showed that, for a small protein (sfGFP, 28 kDa), PA conjugation does not compromise the binding of FcRn to serum albumin in vitro or the serum half-life extension in vivo regardless of linker length. Combined with the previous results for a large protein (Uox, 140 kDa) [24], our results supported that the protein size in the fatty acid–protein conjugate is an important factor for effective binding of FcRn with serum albumin leading to prolonged serum half-life in vivo. We believe our findings can contribute to the successful design of other fatty acid–conjugated therapeutic proteins for serum half-life extension.

Supplementary Materials: The following are available online at http://www.mdpi.com/2227-9059/8/4/96/s1. Figure S1: The chemical structures of linkers and scheme of reactions for linker preparation. Figure S2: MALDI-TOF mass spectra of sfGFP and sfGFP-PA conjugates. Figure S3: Relative fluorescence of sfGFP and sfGFP-PA conjugates.

Author Contributions: Conceptualization, J.C. and I.K.; Formal analysis, J.C., J.P., G.T. and M.S.J.; Funding acquisition, I.K.; Investigation, J.C. and J.P.; Supervision, G.T. and I.K.; Visualization, M.S.J.; Writing—original draft, J.C., J.P., G.T. and I.K.; Writing—review & editing, M.S.J. and I.K. All authors have read and agreed to the published version of the manuscript.

Funding: This work was supported by the National Research Foundation of Korea (NRF), funded by the Ministry of Science and ICT (Grant No. 2019R1A2C1084910 and and 2018R1A4A1024963). This work was also supported by GIST Research Institute (GRI) grant funded by the GIST in 2020.

Conflicts of Interest: The authors declare no conflict of interest.

References

1. Agyei, D.; Ahmed, I.; Akram, Z.; MN Iqbal, H.; K Danquah, M. Protein and peptide biopharmaceuticals: An overview. *Protein Pept. Lett.* **2017**, *24*, 94–101. [CrossRef] [PubMed]
2. Kontermann, R.E. Strategies for extended serum half-life of protein therapeutics. *Curr. Opin. Biotechnol.* **2011**, *22*, 868–876. [CrossRef] [PubMed]
3. Kontermann, R.E. Strategies to Extend Plasma Half-Lives of Recombinant Antibodies. *BioDrugs* **2009**, *23*, 93–109. [CrossRef] [PubMed]
4. Jevševa, S.; Kunstelj, M.; Porekar, V.G. PEGylation of therapeutic proteins. *Biotechnol. J.* **2010**, *5*, 113–128. [CrossRef] [PubMed]
5. Lim, H.-K.; Hong, S.H.; Bae, S.M.; Choi, I.Y.; Kim, H.H. A Liquid Formulation of a Long-acting Erythropoietin Conjugate. *Biotechnol. Bioprocess Eng.* **2020**, *25*, 117–125. [CrossRef]
6. Pelegri-O'Day, E.M.; Lin, E.-W.; Maynard, H.D. Therapeutic Protein–Polymer Conjugates: Advancing Beyond PEGylation. *J. Am. Chem. Soc.* **2014**, *136*, 14323–14332. [CrossRef]
7. Verhoef, J.J.F.; Anchordoquy, T.J. Questioning the use of PEGylation for drug delivery. *Drug Deliv. Transl. Res.* **2013**, *3*, 499–503. [CrossRef]

8. Yang, B.; Lim, S.I.; Kim, J.C.; Tae, G.; Kwon, I. Site-Specific Albumination as an Alternative to PEGylation for the Enhanced Serum Half-Life in Vivo. *Biomacromolecules* **2016**, *17*, 1811–1817. [CrossRef]
9. Cho, J.; Lim, S.I.; Yang, B.S.; Hahn, Y.S.; Kwon, I. Generation of therapeutic protein variants with the human serum albumin binding capacity via site-specific fatty acid conjugation. *Sci. Rep.* **2017**, *7*, 18041. [CrossRef]
10. Bern, M.; Sand, K.M.K.; Nilsen, J.; Sandlie, I.; Andersen, J.T. The role of albumin receptors in regulation of albumin homeostasis: Implications for drug delivery. *J. Control. Release* **2015**, *211*, 144–162. [CrossRef]
11. Sleep, D.; Cameron, J.; Evans, L.R. Albumin as a versatile platform for drug half-life extension. *Biochim. Biophys. Acta-Gen. Subj.* **2013**, *1830*, 5526–5534. [CrossRef] [PubMed]
12. Lim, S.I.; Hahn, Y.S.; Kwon, I. Site-specific albumination of a therapeutic protein with multi-subunit to prolong activity in vivo. *J. Control. Release* **2015**, *207*, 93–100. [CrossRef] [PubMed]
13. Zaman, R.; Islam, R.A.; Ibnat, N.; Othman, I.; Zaini, A.; Lee, C.Y.; Chowdhury, E.H. Current strategies in extending half-lives of therapeutic proteins. *J. Control. Release* **2019**, *301*, 176–189. [CrossRef]
14. Kratz, F. Albumin as a drug carrier: Design of prodrugs, drug conjugates and nanoparticles. *J. Control. Release* **2008**, *132*, 171–183. [CrossRef] [PubMed]
15. Madsbad, S.; Kielgast, U.; Asmar, M.; Deacon, C.F.; Torekov, S.S.; Holst, J.J. An overview of once-weekly glucagon-like peptide-1 receptor agonists-available efficacy and safety data and perspectives for the future. *Diabetes Obes. Metab.* **2011**, *13*, 394–407. [CrossRef] [PubMed]
16. Rosenstock, J.; Reusch, J.; Bush, M.; Yang, F.; Stewart, M.; Albiglutide Study Group, for the A.S. Potential of albiglutide, a long-acting GLP-1 receptor agonist, in type 2 diabetes: A randomized controlled trial exploring weekly, biweekly, and monthly dosing. *Diabetes Care* **2009**, *32*, 1880–1886. [CrossRef]
17. Elsadek, B.; Kratz, F. Impact of albumin on drug delivery—New applications on the horizon. *J. Control. Release* **2012**, *157*, 4–28. [CrossRef]
18. Carta, G.; Murru, E.; Banni, S.; Manca, C. Palmitic Acid: Physiological Role, Metabolism and Nutritional Implications. *Front. Physiol.* **2017**, *8*, 902. [CrossRef]
19. Knudsen, L.B.; Nielsen, P.F.; Huusfeldt, P.O.; Johansen, N.L.; Madsen, K.; Pedersen, F.Z.; Thøgersen, H.; Wilken, M.; Agersø, A. Potent Derivatives of Glucagon-like Peptide-1 with Pharmacokinetic Properties Suitable for Once Daily Administration. *J. Med. Chem.* **2000**, *43*, 1664–1669. [CrossRef]
20. Lee, J.; Lee, C.; Kim, I.; Moon, H.R.; Kim, T.H.; Oh, K.T.; Lee, E.S.; Lee, K.C.; Youn, Y.S. Preparation and evaluation of palmitic acid-conjugated exendin-4 with delayed absorption and prolonged circulation for longer hypoglycemia. *Int. J. Pharm.* **2012**, *424*, 50–57. [CrossRef]
21. Ramírez-Andersen, H.S.; Behrens, C.; Buchardt, J.; Fels, J.J.; Folkesson, C.G.; Jianhe, C.; Nørskov-Lauritsen, L.; Nielsen, P.F.; Reslow, M.; Rischel, C. Long-acting human growth hormone analogue by noncovalent albumin binding. *Bioconjug. Chem.* **2018**, *29*, 3129–3143. [CrossRef] [PubMed]
22. Shechter, Y.; Sasson, K.; Lev-Goldman, V.; Rubinraut, S.; Rubinstein, M.; Fridkin, M. Newly Designed Modifier Prolongs the Action of Short-Lived Peptides and Proteins by Allowing Their Binding to Serum Albumin. *Bioconjug. Chem.* **2012**, *23*, 1577–1586. [CrossRef] [PubMed]
23. Lim, S.I.; Mizuta, Y.; Takasu, A.; Hahn, Y.S.; Kim, Y.H.; Kwon, I. Site-specific fatty acid-conjugation to prolong protein half-life in vivo. *J. Control. Release* **2013**, *170*, 219–225. [CrossRef]
24. Gil, M.S.; Cho, J.; Thambi, T.; Giang Phan, V.H.; Kwon, I.; Lee, D.S. Bioengineered robust hybrid hydrogels enrich the stability and efficacy of biological drugs. *J. Control. Release* **2017**, *267*, 119–132. [CrossRef]
25. Milo, R.; Phillips, R. *Cell Biology by the Numbers*; Garland Science: New York, NY, USA, 2015. ISBN 1317230698.
26. Cho, J.; Park, J.; Kim, S.; Kim, J.C.; Tae, G.; Jin, M.S.; Kwon, I. Intramolecular distance in the conjugate of urate oxidase and fatty acid governs FcRn binding and serum half-life in vivo. *J. Control. Release* **2020**, *321*, 49–58. [CrossRef] [PubMed]
27. Vogt, B. Urate oxidase (rasburicase) for treatment of severe tophaceous gout. *Nephrol. Dial. Transplant.* **2005**, *20*, 431–433. [CrossRef]
28. Wang, L.-Y.; Shih, L.-Y.; Chang, H.; Jou, S.-T.; Lin, K.-H.; Yeh, T.-C.; Lin, S.-F.; Liang, D.-C. Recombinant Urate Oxidase (Rasburicase) for the Prevention and Treatment of Tumor Lysis Syndrome in Patients with Hematologic Malignancies. *Acta Haematol.* **2006**, *115*, 35–38. [CrossRef] [PubMed]
29. Richette, P.; Bardin, T. Successful treatment with rasburicase of a tophaceous gout in a patient allergic to allopurinol. *Nat. Clin. Pract. Rheumatol.* **2006**, *2*, 338–342. [CrossRef]
30. Edwards, N.L. Treatment-failure gout: A moving target. *Arthritis Rheum.* **2008**, *58*, 2587–2590. [CrossRef]

31. Fels, E.; Sundy, J.S. Refractory gout: What is it and what to do about it? *Curr. Opin. Rheumatol.* **2008**, *20*, 198–202. [CrossRef]
32. Bhattacharya, A.A.; Grüne, T.; Curry, S. Crystallographic analysis reveals common modes of binding of medium and long-chain fatty acids to human serum albumin. *J. Mol. Biol.* **2000**, *303*, 721–732. [CrossRef] [PubMed]
33. Curry, S.; Brick, P.; Franks, N.P. Fatty acid binding to human serum albumin: New insights from crystallographic studies. *Biochim. Biophys. Acta-Mol. Cell Biol. Lipids* **1999**, *1441*, 131–140. [CrossRef]
34. Simard, J.R.; Zunszain, P.A.; Hamilton, J.A.; Curry, S. Location of High and Low Affinity Fatty Acid Binding Sites on Human Serum Albumin Revealed by NMR Drug-competition Analysis. *J. Mol. Biol.* **2006**, *361*, 336–351. [CrossRef] [PubMed]
35. Fujiwara, S.; Amisaki, T. Identification of High Affinity Fatty Acid Binding Sites on Human Serum Albumin by MM-PBSA Method. *Biophys. J.* **2008**, *94*, 95–103. [CrossRef]
36. Fujiwara, S.; Amisaki, T. Fatty acid binding to serum albumin: Molecular simulation approaches. *Biochim. Biophys. Acta-Gen. Subj.* **2013**, *1830*, 5427–5434. [CrossRef]
37. Rizzuti, B.; Bartucci, R.; Sportelli, L.; Guzzi, R. Fatty acid binding into the highest affinity site of human serum albumin observed in molecular dynamics simulation. *Arch. Biochem. Biophys.* **2015**, *579*, 18–25. [CrossRef]
38. Hamilton, J.A. NMR reveals molecular interactions and dynamics of fatty acid binding to albumin. *Biochim. Biophys. Acta-Gen. Subj.* **2013**, *1830*, 5418–5426. [CrossRef]
39. Pace, C.N.; Vajdos, F.; Fee, L.; Grimsley, G.; Gray, T. How to measure and predict the molar absorption coefficient of a protein. *Protein Sci.* **1995**, *4*, 2411–2423. [CrossRef]
40. Pédelacq, J.-D.; Cabantous, S.; Tran, T.; Terwilliger, T.C.; Waldo, G.S. Engineering and characterization of a superfolder green fluorescent protein. *Nat. Biotechnol.* **2006**, *24*, 79–88. [CrossRef]
41. Feng, G.; Mellor, R.H.; Bernstein, M.; Keller-Peck, C.; Nguyen, Q.T.; Wallace, M.; Nerbonne, J.M.; Lichtman, J.W.; Sanes, J.R. Imaging Neuronal Subsets in Transgenic Mice Expressing Multiple Spectral Variants of GFP. *Neuron* **2000**, *28*, 41–51. [CrossRef]
42. Okabe, M.; Ikawa, M.; Kominami, K.; Nakanishi, T.; Nishimune, Y. 'Green mice' as a source of ubiquitous green cells. *FEBS Lett.* **1997**, *407*, 313–319. [CrossRef]
43. Jung, S.-K. A Review of Image Analysis in Biochemical Engineering. *Biotechnol. Bioprocess Eng.* **2019**, *24*, 65–75. [CrossRef]
44. Ahn, G.; Yu, G.; Abdullah, A.; Kim, Y.; Lee, D. Controlling the Release Profile Through Phase Control of Calcium Phosphate-Alginate Core-shell Nanoparticles in Gene Delivery. *Macromol. Res.* **2019**, *27*, 579–585. [CrossRef]
45. Yang, B.; Kim, J.C.; Seong, J.; Tae, G.; Kwon, I. Comparative studies of the serum half-life extension of a protein via site-specific conjugation to a species-matched or-mismatched albumin. *Biomater. Sci.* **2018**, *6*, 2092–2100. [CrossRef] [PubMed]
46. Datta-Mannan, A. Mechanisms Influencing the Pharmacokinetics and Disposition of Monoclonal Antibodies and Peptides. *Drug Metab. Dispos.* **2019**, *47*, 1100–1110. [CrossRef] [PubMed]
47. Nilsen, J.; Bern, M.; Sand, K.M.K.; Grevys, A.; Dalhus, B.; Sandlie, I.; Andersen, J.T. Human and mouse albumin bind their respective neonatal Fc receptors differently. *Sci. Rep.* **2018**, *8*, 14648. [CrossRef]
48. Seijsing, J.; Lindborg, M.; Höidén-Guthenberg, I.; Bönisch, H.; Guneriusson, E.; Frejd, F.Y.; Abrahmsén, L.; Ekblad, C.; Löfblom, J.; Uhlén, M.; et al. An engineered affibody molecule with pH-dependent binding to FcRn mediates extended circulatory half-life of a fusion protein. *Proc. Natl. Acad. Sci. USA* **2014**, *111*, 17110–17115. [CrossRef]
49. Hu, Y.-B.; Dammer, E.B.; Ren, R.-J.; Wang, G. The endosomal-lysosomal system: From acidification and cargo sorting to neurodegeneration. *Transl. Neurodegener.* **2015**, *4*, 18. [CrossRef]

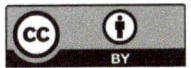

© 2020 by the authors. Licensee MDPI, Basel, Switzerland. This article is an open access article distributed under the terms and conditions of the Creative Commons Attribution (CC BY) license (http://creativecommons.org/licenses/by/4.0/).

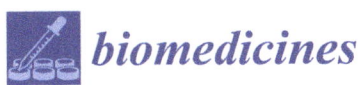

Article

Structure–Activity Analysis and Molecular Docking Studies of Coumarins from *Toddalia asiatica* as Multifunctional Agents for Alzheimer's Disease

Pitchayakarn Takomthong [1], Pornthip Waiwut [2], Chavi Yenjai [3], Bungon Sripanidkulchai [1,4], Prasert Reubroycharoen [5], Ren Lai [6], Peter Kamau [6] and Chantana Boonyarat [1,4,*]

1. Faculty of Pharmaceutical Sciences, Khon Kaen University, Khon Kaen 40002, Thailand; ppitcha.t@gmail.com (P.T.); bungorn@kku.ac.th (B.S.)
2. Faculty of Pharmaceutical Sciences, Ubon Ratchathani University, Ubon Ratchathani 34190, Thailand; pwaiwut79@yahoo.com
3. Faculty of Sciences, Khon Kaen University, Khon Kaen 40002, Thailand; chayen@kku.ac.th
4. Center for Research and Development of Herbal Health Products, Khon Kaen University, Khon Kaen 40002, Thailand
5. Department of Chemical Technology, Faculty of science, Chulalongkorn University, Bangkok 10330, Thailand; Prasert.R@chula.ac.th
6. Kunming Institute of Zoology, the Chinese Academy of Sciences, Kunming 650223, China; rlai@mail.kiz.ac.cn (R.L.); kmpeter26@gmail.com (P.K.)
* Correspondence: chaboo@kku.ac.th; Tel.: +66-81-3073313 or +66-43-202305

Received: 4 April 2020; Accepted: 30 April 2020; Published: 2 May 2020

Abstract: Coumarins, naturally occurring phytochemicals, display a wide spectrum of biological activities by acting on multiple targets. Herein, nine coumarins from the root of *Toddalia asiatica* were evaluated for activities related to pathogenesis of Alzheimer's disease (AD). They were examined for acetylcholinesterase (AChE) and AChE- or self-induced amyloid beta (Aβ) aggregation inhibitory activities, as well as neuroprotection against H_2O_2- and $Aβ_{1-42}$-induced human neuroblastoma SH-SY5Y cell damage. Moreover, in order to understand the mechanism, the binding interactions between coumarins and their targets: (i) AChE and (ii) $Aβ_{1-42}$ peptide were investigated *in silico*. All coumarins exhibited mild to moderate AChE and self-induced Aβ aggregation inhibitory actions. In addition, the coumarins substituted with the long alkyl chain at position 6 or 8 illustrated ability to inhibit AChE-induced Aβ aggregation, resulting from their dual binding site at catalytic anionic site and peripheral active site in AChE. Moreover, the most potent multifunctional coumarin, phellopterin, could attenuate neuronal cell damage induced by H_2O_2 and $Aβ_{1-42}$ toxicity. Conclusively, seven out of nine coumarins were identified as multifunctional agents inhibiting the pathogenesis of AD. The structure–activity relationship information obtained might be applied for further optimization of coumarins into a useful drug which may combat AD.

Keywords: acetylcholinesterase; amyloid beta aggregation; neuroprotection; molecular docking; multi-target drug; structure–activity relationship

1. Introduction

Alzheimer's disease (AD), the most common cause of dementia, is a chronic and progressive neurodegenerative disorder. The main clinical manifestation of AD is memory impairment, leading to the progressive loss of attention, emotions, mental capacity, and the ability to learn [1,2]. The molecular mechanisms of AD are still unclear; however, several studies explained that AD is related to cholinergic deficiency [3], amyloid beta peptide (Aβ) aggregation [4], hyperphosphorylation of tau protein [5], and oxidative stress [6].

Several studies suggested that memory impairment results from a decline of acetylcholine (ACh), which is the neurotransmitter that plays roles in the encoding of new memories and information [7]. Therefore, AD treatments are currently based on the inhibition of acetylcholinesterase (AChE). AChE, which locates at post-synaptic membranes, is an enzyme that hydrolyses the ester bond of acetylcholine (ACh) into acetate and choline, leading to termination of the action of ACh [8]. AChE is composed of three binding sites including the catalytic site (CAS), anionic site (AS), and peripheral anionic site (PAS). The CAS has a catalytic triad composed of three principle amino acids including Ser 200, Glu 327, and His 440, which are directly involved in ACh hydrolysis. The AS is located in the middle gorge and consists of Trp84, Tyr130, and Phe330. The PAS at the entry to the gorge is represented by Tyr 70, Asp72, Tyr121, Tyr 334, and Trp279 [8,9]. Interestingly, several studies suggested that AChE was not only involved in the hydrolysis of ACh, but also accelerated the aggregation of Aβ into amyloid fibrils [10–12]. Moreover, researchers indicated that AChE interacts with Aβ and induces Aβ fibril formation at the PAS of AChE. Aβ interacts with the hydrophobic region of AChE to stabilize the AChE–Aβ complex [10]. Therefore, the dual binding agents that interact simultaneously with both the CAS and PAS sites of AChE might exhibit dual inhibition of AChE and Aβ-aggregation.

Aβ aggregation also plays a key role in AD progression [13]. The Aβ peptides in the brain are generated from the amyloid precursor protein (APP) through sequential cleavages by β- and γ-secretase enzyme activities. Aβ is accumulated in the brain and spontaneously aggregates into the oligomers to form insoluble fibrils that turn to amyloid plaques, which initiate mitochondrial oxidative stress and promote hyperphosphorylation of tau proteins [14], resulting in neurotoxicity.

Currently, there are only five drugs approved by the Food and Drug Administration (FDA) for AD treatment. However, the current approved drugs that modulate one target could only enable a palliative treatment instead of curing AD. Due to the multi-pathogenesis of AD, the classical single-target approach may be inadequate. Therefore, searching for candidates that target at multiple sites of the pathologic cascade has become an effective strategy for developing drugs against AD [15–17]. Natural products from plants have been considered as an important medical reservoir holding enormous potential. The natural products possessing multifunction characteristics were found to have a potential for the treatment of AD such as galantamine isolated from *Galanthus woronowii* Losinsk and Huperzine A obtained from *Huperzia serrata* [18,19]. Thus, the natural compounds acting against a wider range of targets associated with pathologic cascade might afford additional benefits for AD therapy.

In the present study, we focused on *Toddalia asiatica* (L.) Lam, which is a medicinal plant of the family Rutaceae. This plant is widely distributed in many countries of Africa and Asia [20]. The plant is used traditionally to treat several diseases including malaria, stomachache, and chest pains [21,22]. Coumarins are the major components found in *T. asiatica*. Coumarins have been studied for various pharmacological effects, such as anti-inflammatory [23], anti-cancer [24], anti-oxidant [25], anti-coagulant [26], and anti-microbial [27] activities, as well as anti-AChE activity [28,29]. They display a wide spectrum of biological activities by acting on multiple targets. Thus, in this study, we focused on the coumarins that can interact with AChE, both of PAS and CAS, to discover the novel therapeutic agents that can increase the amount and duration of acetylcholine (ACh) action, as well as prevent Aβ aggregation. Nine coumarins extracted from the root of *T. asiatica* include phellopterin, isoimpinellin, toddalolactone, toddaculin, toddacoumaquinone, toddalenone, toddanone, artanin, and fraxinol (Figure 1). They were evaluated for biological activities related to AD, including AChE inhibitory and AChE- and self-induced amyloid beta (Aβ) aggregation inhibitory activities. In order to understand the mechanism, the binding interactions between coumarins and their targets AChE and Aβ peptide were investigated *in silico* by molecular docking. Moreover, the most potent multifunctional coumarin was evaluated for neuroprotective effects against H_2O_2- and Aβ-induced cell damage.

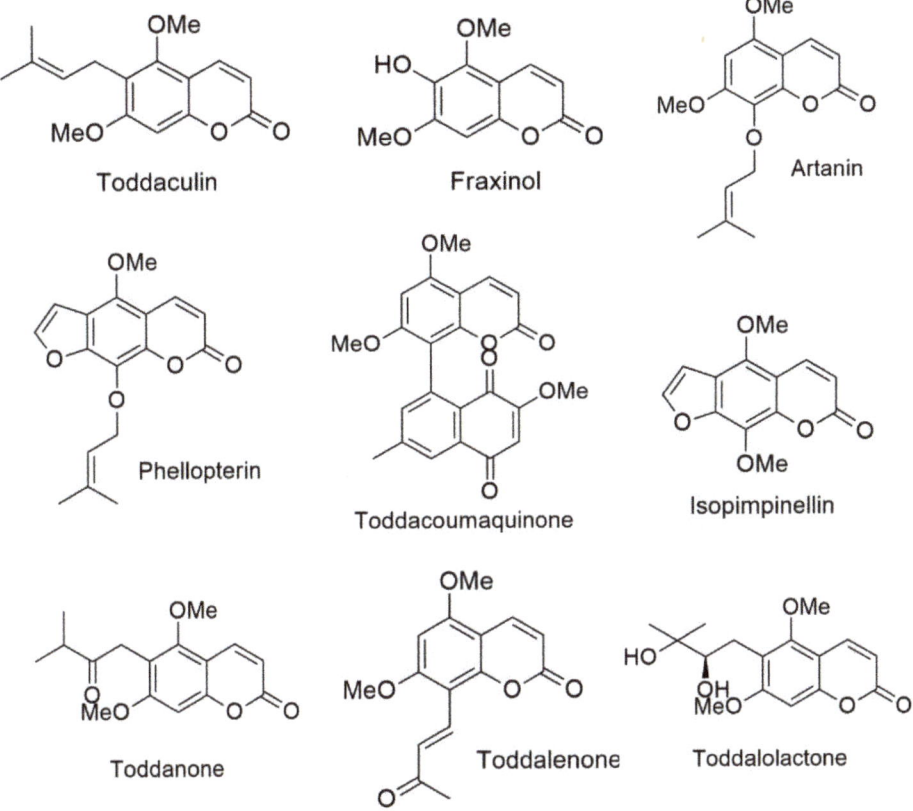

Figure 1. Structures of coumarin derivatives.

2. Materials and Methods

2.1. Coumarin Derivatives

Nine coumarins extracted from the root of *Toddalia asiatica*, including phellopterin, isopimpinellin, toddalolactone, toddaculin, toddacoumaquinone, toddalenone, toddanone, artanin, and fraxinol (Figure 1), were gifted by Chavi Yenjai (Faculty of science, Khon Kaen university, Thailand). The isolation and structural elucidation were explained in a previous report [30,31]. Acetylthiocholine iodide (ATCI), bovine serum albumin (BSA), beta amyloid 1-42 (Aβ1–42), tacrine, trolox, N-acetyl cysteine (NAC), trypsine, fetal bovine serum (FBS), and Dulbecco's modified Eagle medium nutrient mixture F-12 (DMEM/F12) were purchased from Sigma-Aldrich (SM Chemical supplies Co., Ltd., Bangkok, Thailand), Merck (Merck, Bangkok, Thailand), Gibthai (GT Chemical supplies Co., Ltd., Bangkok, Thailand), and Fluka (SM Chemical supplies Co., Ltd., Bangkok, Thailand). AutoDock program version 4.2.6 (the Scripps Research Institute, La Jolla, CA, USA) and BIOVIA Discovery Studio 2017 (BIOVIA, San Diego, CA, USA) were used in the molecular docking study.

2.2. Acetylcholinesterase Inhibitory Activity

Acetylcholinesterase inhibitory activity was determined and modified from Ellman, as described elsewhere [32]. Briefly, the assay mixture consisted of 25 µL of 0.1 M phosphate buffer (pH 7.4), 25 µL of 1 mM substrate (acetylthiocholine iodide solution), 125 µL of 1 mM 5, 5′-dithiobis-(2 nitrobenzoic acid (DTNB), 50 μL of 0.2 Units/mL AChE from *Electrophorus electricus* (type VI-S), and 25 μL of test inhibitors in various concentrations (0–100 μM). The stock solutions of test inhibitors were dissolved in DMSO and diluted with phosphate buffer so that the final concentration of DMSO did not exceed 0.1%. The enzyme activity was measured by the increase in absorbance at 405 nm for 5 min with a METERTECH Accureader M965 microplate reader. The enzyme activity and the percentage inhibition were determined. The compound concentration producing 50% of AChE inhibition (IC_{50}) was calculated from a concentration-inhibition curve using linear regression analysis. All determinations were carried out at least three times and in triplicate wells.

2.3. Inhibition of AChE-Induced Aβ$_{1-42}$ Aggregation

Inhibition of AChE-induced Aβ$_{1-42}$ aggregation was modified and measured using a thioflavin T (ThT) binding assay, as described elsewhere [33,34]. Briefly, Aβ$_{1-42}$ was dissolved in 50 mM phosphate buffer (pH 8.0). Three μL of Aβ$_{1-42}$ (250 μM) and 10 μL of AChE (10 unit/mL) or PBS in the presence and absence of 2 μL of test inhibitors (0–500 μM) were co-incubated for 3 h at 37 °C. To quantify amyloid fibril formation, the mixture was diluted to a final volume of 200 μL with 5 μM ThT in glycine–NaOH buffer (pH 8.5) after the incubation period, and the fluorescence measurement was obtained at the excitation and emission wavelengths of 446 nm and 490 nm, respectively. The fluorescence intensities were recorded, and the percentage of inhibition on aggregation was calculated by using the following equation: (1 − IFi/IFc) * 100%, in which IFi and IFc were the fluorescence of the AChE-induced Aβ$_{1-42}$ aggregation group in the presence and absence of the test compounds, respectively, after subtracting the fluorescence of self Aβ$_{1-42}$ aggregation and the background fluorescence of 5 μM ThT in the blank buffers. The compound concentration producing 50% of inhibition of AChE-induced Aβ$_{1-42}$ aggregation (IC_{50}) was calculated from a concentration-inhibition curve by using linear regression analysis. All determinations were carried out at least three times and in triplicate wells. Curcumin was used as a reference compound.

2.4. Inhibition of Self-Induced Aβ$_{1-42}$ Aggregation

Inhibition of self-induced Aβ$_{1-42}$ aggregation was assayed, as described elsewhere [34]. Briefly, nine microliters of 25 μM of Aβ$_{1-42}$ in 50 mM phosphate buffer, pH 7.4, was incubated with 1 μL of the test compound at various concentrations (0–500 μM) in the dark at 37 °C for 48 h. After incubation, the samples were mixed with 50 μM glycine/NaOH buffer (pH 8.5) containing 5 μM ThT. Fluorescence intensities were measured at an excitation wavelength of 446 nm and an emission wavelength of 490 nm. The fluorescence intensities were recorded, and the percentage of inhibition on aggregation was calculated by using the following equation: (1 − IFi/IFc) * 100% in which IFi and IFc were the fluorescence intensities obtained for Aβ$_{1-42}$ aggregation group in the presence and absence of the test compounds, respectively, after subtracting the background fluorescence of 5 μM ThT in the blank buffers. The compound concentration producing 50% of Aβ$_{1-42}$ aggregation inhibition (IC_{50}) was calculated from a concentration-inhibition curve for each compound using linear regression analysis. The experiment was done in independent triplicates.

2.5. Computational Studies

The target templates AChE and Aβ$_{1-42}$ were constructed by removing water and other solvent molecules, adding all hydrogens, assigning Gasteiger charges, and merging non-polar hydrogen atoms. The AChE template was prepared from a crystal structure of *Tc*AChE bound with the AChE inhibitor, N-[8-(1,2,3,4-tetrahydroacridin-9-ylthio)octyl]-1,2,3,4-tetrahydro acridin-9-amine, 2CEK and validated by crystallographic structures of six AChE inhibitors (2CEK, 1H22, 1ZGB, 2CMF, 1ODC, and 1UT6). The Aβ fibril template was prepared using the X-ray crystal PDB code 2BEG. AutoGrid was used to generate grid maps. The grids were designated to include the active site of AChE and the whole fibril structue. The grid box dimensions were defined with a size of 80 × 70 × 70 and 120 × 60 × 40 Å for AChE and Aβ fibrils, respectively, and the grid spacing was set to 0.375 Å. All ligands were docked by using the Lamarckian genetic algorithm via the AutoDock 4.2.6 program. The Lamarckian genetic algorithm protocol was set using a population size of 100 individuals with 100 ligand orientation runs. Additionally, the energy evaluation was 1,000,000 and the maximum number of evaluation was 27,000. The orientation with the lowest docked energy was considered as the best conformation. After the docking process, the docking complex poses were analyzed for their interactions by using BIOVIA Discovery Studio 2017.

2.6. Neuroprotective Activity against Hydrogen Peroxide (H_2O_2) and $A\beta_{1-42}$ Toxicity

Human neuroblastoma cells (SH-SY5Y) were cultured in Dulbecco's Modified Eagle Medium (DMEM/Ha's F12) containing 50 IU/mL penicillin, 50 g/mL streptomycin, 2 mM L-glutamine, and 10% fetal bovine serum. Cells were maintained at 37 °C in a humidified incubator in an atmosphere of 5% CO_2 For the assay, the SH-SY5Y cells, at a density of 5×10^5 cell/mL, were seeded in a 96-well plate and incubated for 48 h.

For cytotoxicity evaluation, the cells were treated with potential coumarin derivatives in various concentrations for 24 h. After that, cell viability was determined by staining the cells with 3-(4, 5-dimethyl-2-thiazolyl)-2, 5-diphenyl-2H-tetrazolium bromide, and MTT (5 mg/mL in PBS) for 2 h. The optical density of each well was measured at 550 nm in a METERTECH Accureader M965 microplate reader.

For neuroprotection against H_2O_2 investigation, the cells were pretreated with coumarin in various concentrations for 24 h. After removing unabsorbed test compounds by washing with phosphate buffer saline, the cells were treated with 100 μM H_2O_2 for 2 h to induce oxidative stress. Cell viability was determined by the MTT colorimetric method. The optical density of each well was measured at 550 nm. Curcumin at the concentration of 10 μM was used as a reference standard. All data were expressed as a percentage of non-H_2O_2-treated groups (control group). The cell viability of the control group was expressed as 100%. The experiment was done in independent triplicates (4 wells/group).

For neuroprotection against $A\beta_{1-42}$ toxicity, the $A\beta_{1-42}$ preparation was modified from [17]. Briefly, lyophilized $A\beta_{1-42}$ was reconstituted in sterile water and keep at −80 °C until further use. Aliquots were diluted with a culture medium to achieve a final concentration of 25 μM and then incubated at 37 °C for 72 h to form aggregated amyloid. For the assay, SH-SY5Y cells were incubated with aggregated Aβ (25 μM), with or without the test compounds, for 24 h. Cell viability was determined by the MTT colorimetric method. The optical density of each well was measured at 550 nm in a METERTECH Accureader M965 microplate reader. Curcumin (10 μM) was used as a reference standard. All data were expressed as a percentage of non-$A\beta_{1-42}$-treated groups (control group). Cell viability of the control group was expressed as 100%. The experiment was done in independent triplicates (4 wells/group).

The results are expressed as mean ± SD ($n = 3$). Statistical significance was determined by paired t-test (two group comparison). For all statistical analysis, significance levels were set at p value < 0.05.

3. Results and Discussion

3.1. Acetylcholinesterase Inhibition

The inhibitory activity of coumarin derivatives against AChE was evaluated according to the spectrophotometric method of Ellman using tacrine, an AChE inhibitor, as a positive control. The ability of the test compounds to inhibit AChE function was shown as IC_{50}, which is the test compound concentration that resulted in 50% inhibition of AChE activity. The AChE inhibitory activity of coumarins is summarized in Table 1. All coumarins exhibited moderate inhibitory activity with IC_{50} values in the range of 17 to 53 μM. To elucidate the correlation between the inhibitory activity and the substitution groups on the coumarin ring, all compounds were divided into three groups according to substitution on position 6, substitution of furan ring, and substitution on position 8. As indicated in Table 1, fraxinol, which possesses a small hydroxyl group at position 6 of the coumarin ring, showed the highest inhibitory potency toward AChE. It was more potent than toddanone, toddaculin, and toddalolactone, which bear a longer side chain. The replacement of hydroxyl group with long alkyl chain might decrease electrostatic distribution in coumarin ring and might generate the steric hindrance that decrease the binding affinity between coumarin and AChE, resulting in diminished inhibitory activity [16]. The presence of a furan ring at position 6–7 showed an improved inhibitory activity. Apparently, phellopterin (IC$_{50}$ = 38 μM) was more potent than artanin (IC$_{50}$ = 51 μM), which does not bear any furan ring in the coumarin ring. Similarly, the presence of furano- or pyranocoumarins slightly increased the AChE inhibitory activity in natural coumarins [35], which could indicate that the furan ring possessing high electron density might influence the increase in binding affinity with AChE. Our results revealed that phellopterin, which possesses a longer chain substituent at position 8 of the coumarin moiety, showed similar effect with isopimpinellin, which contains a methoxyl group. However, some studies reported that the inhibitory activity of the natural coumarins can be increased when presented with larger substituents at position 8 [35,36]. Our present study showed that the coumarin moiety is the essential part of AChE activity. The presence of bulkier substituents at position 6 influenced a decrease in the activity, which was also found in [15]. Moreover, we suggested that substitution of the furan ring at position 6–7 might improve AChE inhibitory activity by increasing the binding affinity.

Table 1. Biological activities of coumarins related to Alzheimer's disease (AD).

Compound	AChE assay IC$_{50}$ (μM)	AChE-Induce Aβ IC$_{50}$ (μM)	Self-Induced Aβ IC$_{50}$ (μM)
Phellopterin	38 ± 3	97 ± 7	95 ± 3
Isopimpinellin	41 ± 1	IC$_{50}$ > 500 μM	125 ± 13
Toddalolactone	49 ± 5	105 ± 9	220 ± 1
Toddacoumaquinone	46 ± 12	72 ± 5	145 ± 2
Toddanone	46 ± 3	110 ± 2	76 ± 1
Toddaculin	53 ± 9	232 ± 10	143 ± 4
Toddalenone	40 ± 4	211 ± 29	99 ± 1
Artanin	51 ± 2	98 ± 19	124 ± 10
Fraxinol	18 ± 7	IC$_{50}$ > 500 μM	209 ± 21
Tacrine	0.28 ± 0.04	Not detected	Not detected
Curcumin	Not detected	5.8 ± 0.3	5.0 ± 0.1

3.2. AChE-Induced Aβ Aggregation Inhibitory Activity

Several pieces of evidence indicated an association between AChE and Aβ. Apart from enhancing hydrolysis of ACh, AChE also plays a role in Aβ aggregation promotion by forming a complex with Aβ at the hydrophobic region of PAS [12,37]. To explore the effects of nine coumarins on AChE-induced Aβ aggregation inhibitory activity, a ThT-based fluorescence assay was performed, and curcumin was used as a positive control. The inhibitory effects of the test compounds are summarized in Table 1. Seven of nine coumarins showed an ability to inhibit Aβ$_{1-42}$-aggregation induced by AChE. Isopimpinellin and fraxinol did not have inhibitory effects. Among the tested inhibitors, toddacoumaquinone exhibited the most potent activity with IC$_{50}$ value of 72 μM. The substitution at position 6 of the coumarin ring played a vital role, for instance, fraxinol, which bears a small hydroxyl group, did not have an inhibitory effect against AChE-induced Aβ aggregation, while coumarin, which has a longer side chain like todaculin, toddalolactone, and toddanone was active. In addition, the presence of di-hydroxyl or carbonyl groups on the long alkyl chain at position 6, similar to toddalolactone (logP = 1.84, calculated by Swiss ADME program) and toddanone (logP = 2.61), resulted in enhanced activity, comparable to toddaculin (logP = 3.34). The inhibitory activity seemed to relate with hydrophilicity of the substituents at position 6. The presence of a furan ring in the coumarin ring did not affect Aβ aggregation induced by AChE. Apparently, phellopterin and artanin possessed similar inhibitory activities toward the AChE-induced aggregation of Aβ$_{1-42}$. For position 8, substitution with a bulky group enhanced the inhibitory effect against Aβ aggregation induced by AChE. The lipophilicity of the substitution group at position 8 seems to play a role in the inhibitory action. The results showed that toddacoumaquinone (logP = 3.33) possessed better activity than artanin (logP = 3.03) and toddalactone (logP = 3.34), respectively.

3.3. Self-Induced Aβ Aggregation Inhibitory Activity

To determine the inhibition of self-induced $A\beta_{1-42}$ aggregation of coumarins, we used a ThT fluorescence assay to monitor and quantify aggregation of Aβ, and curcumin was used as the reference compound. All coumarins exhibited inhibitory effects with IC_{50} values ranging from 76 to 220 µM (Table 1). Toddanone, phellopterin and todalenone showed the most potent with IC_{50} less than 100 µM. Structure–activity relationship analysis indicated that the lipophilicity has impacts on inhibitory activity. Coumarins which possessed log P less than 2, similar to fraxinol (logP = 1.51) and toddalolactone (logP = 1.84), provided unfavorable effect, which displayed inhibitory activity with IC_{50} values higher than 200 µM. However, the balance between hydrophilic and lipophilic properties should be concerned. We found that the substitution with higher lipophilic group at position 6 or 8 led to declined inhibitory potency; for instances, compared among the coumarins bearing different substituents at position 8, toddalenone (log P = 2.30) showed higher inhibitory activity than artanin (log P = 3.03) and toddacoumaquinone (log P = 3.3), respectively. Our results also demonstrated that the furan substitution of phellopterin (IC_{50} = 95 µM) at position 6-7 exhibited higher inhibitory activity than the corresponding OCH_3-substituted artanin (IC_{50} = 124 µM). The furan ring might increase the binding affinity by electron delocalization.

3.4. Binding Interaction Study by Molecular Docking

3.4.1. Binding Interaction with AChE

To clearly understand the mechanism of action between our test compounds and AChE, a molecular modeling technique was performed to determine the binding orientation. The binding orientations of nine coumarins in AChE are shown in Figure 2. The docking results revealed that the coumarin ring of all derivatives was bound to the catalytic anionic site (CAS) of AChE. The coumarin moiety had a planar structure, which is inserted into the CAS of AChE. Therefore, our results suggested that the coumarin moiety is the important structure for AChE inhibitory action by interfering with ACh hydrolysis at the CAS binding site. Some studies showed that the coumarin moiety binds preferably to interact at the PAS of AChE, and they are mostly modified the long chain substituents at positions 3 or 4 of coumarin ring [12,37], but Fellarero et al. [29] demonstrated that coumarin could interact with Ser200 at CAS and have π–π stacking interaction with Phe330. Thus, our data seem to support that substitutions of the alkyl chain at position 6 or 8 forced coumarin ring locating at CAS. Therefore, the coumarin moiety could interact with both the CAS and PAS of AChE depending on the substituents.

In the case of toddalenone (Figure 2H) and toddacoumaquinone (Figure 2I), their binding orientations were quite different from other coumarins. In the middle gorge, the coumarin ring of toddalenone had π–π stacking and π–sigma interactions against Phe330 and Trp432, respectively, and the methoxy group at position 5 formed hydrogen bonds with Tyr442 and Trp84. Moreover, the carbonyl group on alkyl chain at position 8 could also form hydrogen bonds with Ser200, Gly118, and Gly119. Similarly, toddacoumaquinone could form π–π stacking interactions with Phe330 and Tyr121. Interestingly, the naphthoquinone ring, which was substituted on position 8, could interact with Tyr121 and the indole ring of Trp84 to form hydrogen bonds and π–π interactions, respectively. Moreover, the methyl group on the naphthoquinone ring also formed two π–sigma interactions with Tyr334 and Trp432 in the PAS. The result indicated that the naphthoquinone ring at position 8 located in PAS binding site.

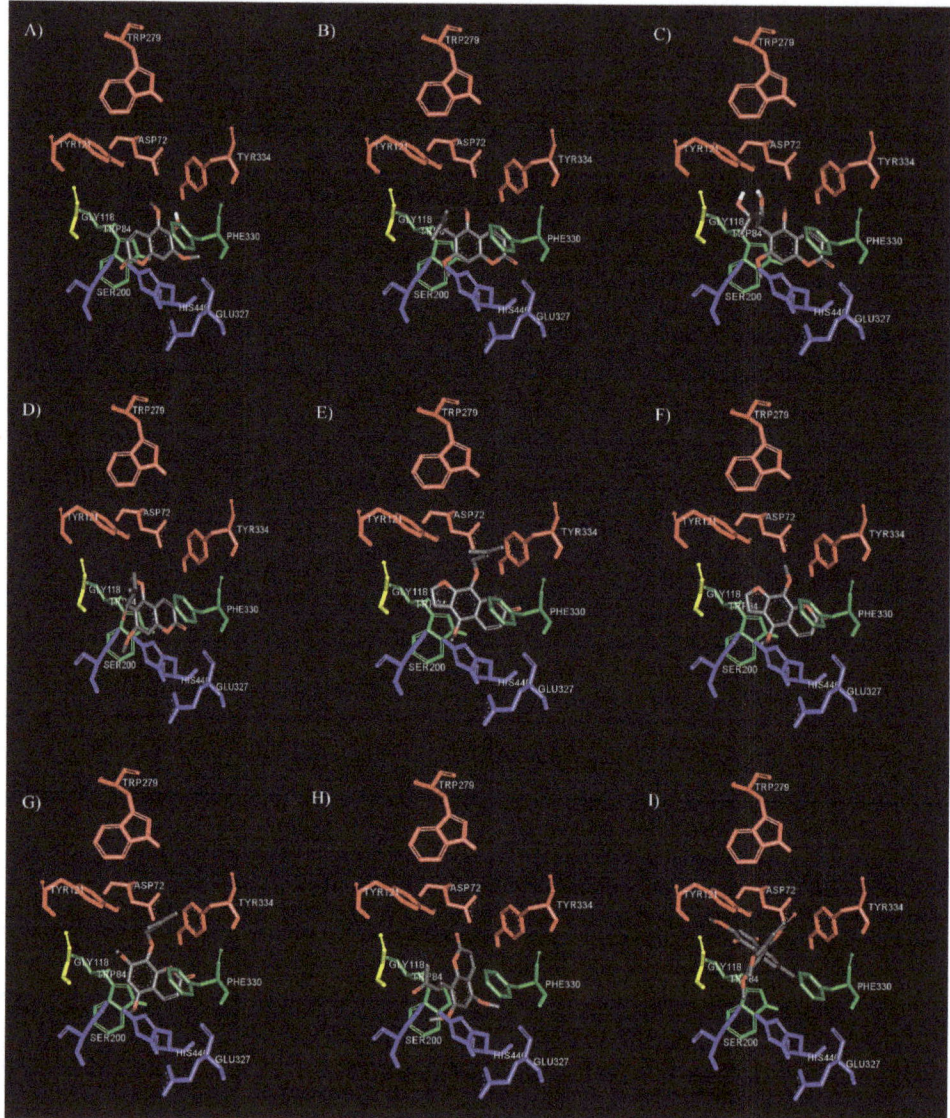

Figure 2. Binding mode of coumarin derivatives fraxinol (**A**), toddaculin (**B**), toddalolactone (**C**), toddanone (**D**), phellopterin (**E**), isopimpinellin (**F**), artanin (**G**), toddalenone (**H**), and toddacoumaquinone (**I**) at the binding site of AChE predicted by molecular docking. The active sites are coded with different colors (CAS; blue, AS; green, oxyanion hole; yellow, and PAS; red).

With regard to the substituent at the 6th position of the coumarin ring, substitution of bulky groups or long side chains affected AChE inhibitory activity. The docking study showed that fraxinol (4.28 Å, a distance between oxygen atom at position 1 on coumarin ring and carboxylic group of His440) could enter the active site CAS closer than toddaculin (4.90 Å), toddanone (5.22 Å), or toddalolactone (4.92 Å), which had bulky substitution groups (Figure 2A). The substitution of bulky moieties might generate the steric effect and related to the decrease of binding affinity between coumarins and

CAS. Then, this might cause the decrease of AChE inhibitory activity. Interestingly, the long alkyl chain at position 6 could interact with Tyr121, which is a key residue of PAS. The alkyl side chain of toddaculin (Figure 2B) and toddanone (Figure 2D) established π–alkyl interaction with Tyr121, while toddalolactone (Figure 2C) interacted with Tyr121 via hydrogen bonds. Therefore, these compounds exhibited a multi-target profile encompassing inhibitory activities toward AChE and Aβ aggregation induced by AChE, resulting from their dual site to CAS and PAS, as predicted by the docking study.

Additionally, the influence of a furan ring and the length of side chain at position 8 on the inhibitory potency was examined with phellopterin (Figure 2E), artanin (Figure 2G), and isopimpinellin (Figure 2F). The addition of a furan ring of phellopterin compared to artanin revealed that the furan ring seemed to increase the affinity because it could form π–π stacking against the indole ring of Trp84. Moreover, the longer alkyl chain established π–alkyl interactions with peripheral anionic site residues, including Tyr121, Phe330, and Tyr334. Likewise, the alkyl chain of artanin formed π–alkyl interactions with Tyr121, Phe330, and Tyr334.

Thus, our data suggested that coumarins exhibited the inhibitory activity of AChE by binding to CAS and AS. Moreover, the presence of long alkyl side chains at positions 6 or 8 allowed for additional interaction with the PAS, thereby enabling a dual-site interaction. Previous studies revealed that AChE could induce Aβ fibril formation by forming AChE–Aβ complexes throughout the PAS of AChE [12,37]. Our docking results were also relevant to our AChE-induced Aβ aggregation inhibitory activity results. The test inhibitors with the alkyl chain interacting with amino acid residues of the PAS exhibited the inhibition of AChE-induced Aβ aggregation. Therefore, these data supported that coumarins with the long alkyl chain were able to enhance cholinergic tone by reducing the hydrolytic activity of AChE and prevent the deposition of Aβ fibrils as dual action inhibitors.

3.4.2. Binding Interaction with Aβ

In order to get further insight into the binding mode, we performed a docking study to generate the binding mode for coumarins on $A\beta_{1-42}$ (Protein Data Bank (PDB) ID: 2BEG). The assemblies of Aβ are composed of monomers, soluble oligomers, and insoluble fibrils. The soluble oligomers have different sizes which are ranging from dimers, trimers, tetramers, pentamers, and dodecamers [38]. The folded monomers are self-associates to form nucleus for fibril elongation, which derived a paranucleus [39]. After that, the paranuclei self-associate to form protofibrils and sequentially become fibrils. The Aβ monomers could bind with the hydrophobic stretch of residues 17–21 at the tip of the protofibrils [40], which Ile41 was essential for mediating paranucleus formation and Ala42 was required for self-association of paranuclei [41]. Based on previous studies [36,41,42], $A\beta_{1-42}$ fibrils have parallel and in-register β-sheets, of which they have inter-sheet interactions to stabilize conformation between two β-strands. The two strands composed of residues 12–24 and 30–42 are connected by a turn at residue 25–29. In addition, to stabilize the structure and connect the two β strands, there are inter-sheet contacts which are formed by hydrophobic interactions between Phe19 and Gly38, and Ala21 and Val36, as well as a salt bridge between Asp23 and Lys28.

Considering the results, the coumarin ring of all test inhibitors could interact with $A\beta_{1-42}$ at the inter-sheet against Phe19 and Val40 via π–π and π–sigma interactions, respectively (Figure 3). According to the significance role of Phe19 on amyloid aggregation, Cukalevasi et al. [43] reported that the substitution of Phe19 with leucine dramatically has a slower aggregation rate than the wild type. Moreover, Phe19 also formed the inter-sheet contact to stabilize the Aβ structure as above. Therefore, these data supported that the coumarin ring could interfere with Aβ destabilization through the π–π interaction with Phe19. In the case of fraxinol (Figure 3A), it was found that its hydroxyl group at position 6 and carbonyl group at position 2 could form hydrogen bonds with Leu17 and Val39, respectively. With regard to the substituents at the 6th position of the coumarin ring, the docking results revealed that the alkyl chain with two hydroxyl groups at position 6 of toddalolactone (Figure 3C) could bind to the residue Val39 with hydrogen bonds. However, the carbonyl group on alkyl chain of toddanone (Figure 3D) and the vinyl group on alkyl chain of toddaculin (Figure 3B) could form a hydrogen bond and a van der Waals interaction, respectively, with Ile41 which it is the crucial residue for promoting the initial oligomerization of Aβ$_{42}$ [41]. Therefore, they possessed a higher activity than fraxinol and toddalolactone.

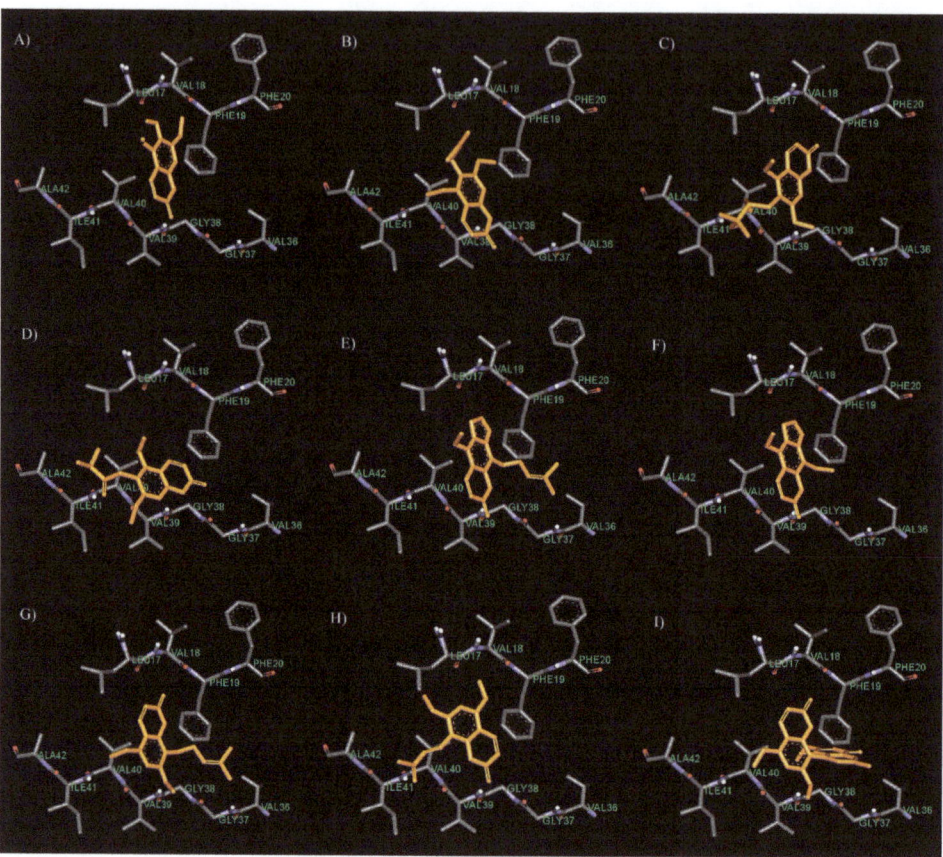

Figure 3. Binding mode for interactions of fraxinol (**A**), toddaculin (**B**), toddalolactone (**C**), toddanone (**D**), phellopterin (**E**), isopimpinellin (**F**), artanin (**G**), toddalenone (**H**), and toddacoumaquinone (**I**) docked into Aβ$_{1-42}$ fibrils.

For the comparison between the furan ring and methoxy group at position 6–7, the results showed that phellopterin with furan ring (Figure 3E) exhibited better activity than artanin, which contains a methoxy group (Figure 3G). The docking results indicated that the furan ring which has high electron delocalization could form π–π interaction with the aromatic ring of Phe19 and Val40. The furan ring of isopimpinellin (Figure 3F) is also stacked against the aromatic ring of Phe19 through the π–π interaction. The results suggested that the addition of the furan ring seemed to afford the binding affinity between the coumarins and Aβ.

Additionally, the substitution at position 8 showed that the length of the substituents affected the inhibitory activity. Compared to isopimpinellin, phellopterin bearing longer alkyl chain at position 8 possessed higher activity than isopimpinellin. The docking result showed that the long alkyl chain at position 8 of phellopterin is expanded to bind with residues Ala21 and Val36 via π–alkyl interactions (Figure 3E). Similarly, the long alkyl chain of artanin (Figure 3G) could interact with residues Ala21 and Val36, which could indicate that the presence of long alkyl side chain at position 8 allowed to gain additional interaction with Aβ, thereby increasing the binding affinity.

3.5. Neuroprotective Activity against H_2O_2 and $A\beta_{1-42}$-Induced Neuronal Cell Death

For neuroprotective evaluation, we selected phellopterin as the most potent compound which possessed the multimode-action of anti-AChE, AChE- and self-induced Aβ aggregation inhibition. To evaluate the cytotoxicity of phellopterin in human neuroblastoma SH-SY5Y cells, the MTT assays revealed that there was no significant change in the viability of SH-SY5Y cells after treatment with the phellopterin at concentration of 0.1 to 10 μM for 24 h (Figure 4). Thus, this data indicates that phellopterin at those concentrations are non-toxic for use in further neuroprotective effects investigations.

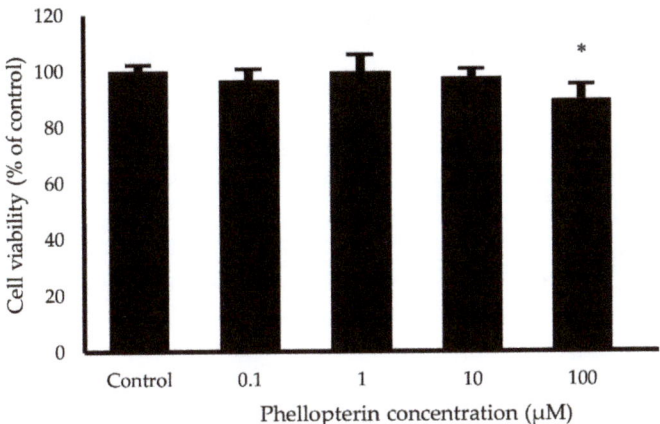

Figure 4. Effects of phellopterin on cell viability of SH-SY5Y cells. The values are reported as mean ± SD ($n = 4$), Paired t-test was used to compare between control and test inhibitors, * $p < 0.05$.

Oxidative stress has been widely implicated in neuronal cell death, which has been considered as the pathogenic mechanism underlying neurodegenerative disorders including AD [44]. Oxidative stress is characterized by the imbalance in the production of reactive oxygen species (ROS) and antioxidative defense systems which are responsible for the removal of ROS. ROS are able to initiate cell death. H_2O_2 is commonly used as an exogenous source of ROS and neuronal cells exposed to H_2O_2 undergo cell death with oxidative stress [45]. Several studies reported that H_2O_2 could induce oxidative stress in neuronal cell by several pathways such as free radical generation, oxidative enzyme induction, intracellular signaling pathway activation, etc [46–49]. Therefore, an H_2O_2-induced cytotoxicity model is considered suitable for the study of neurodegeneration induced by oxidative stress.

The neuroprotective effect of phellopterin against oxidative stress was determined by colorimetric MTT assay in SH-SY5Y cells. Hydrogen peroxide at concentration 100 μM was used to induce oxidative damage. SH-SY5Y cells were pretreated with phellopterin at a concentration of 0.1 to 10 μM for 24 h prior to exposure to H_2O_2 for 2 h. The H_2O_2 treatment decreased the cell viability to 60.61%; however, pre-incubation with 10 μM of phellopterin significantly attenuated the H_2O_2-induced cell damage compared to the H_2O_2 treated group (Figure 5). Thus, these findings indicated that phellopterin exhibited potential protective effects against oxidative stress induced by H_2O_2 in SH-SY5Y cells.

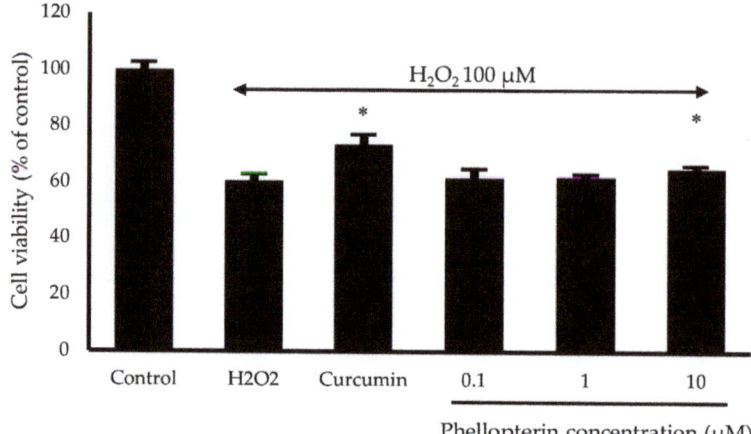

Figure 5. Effects of phellopterin on H_2O_2-induced cell damage in SH-SY5Y cells. Curcumin at 10 μM was used as a reference standard. The values are reported as mean ± SD (n = 3). Paired t-test, * $p < 0.05$ versus H_2O_2 treated group.

Aβ has been implicated in the pathogenesis of AD. Several evidences demonstrated that Aβ protein-induced neurotoxicity is a major pathological mechanism of AD and leads to neuronal cell death [13,50,51]. Therefore, the neuroprotective effect against $Aβ_{1-42}$ toxicity of phellopterin was also determined in SH-SY5Y cells. $Aβ_{1-42}$ at concentration 25 μM was treated with cells in the presence or absence of phellopterin at a concentration 0.1 to 10 μM for 24 h, and then the cell viability was determined by MTT assay. Our results showed that phellopterin could significantly increase cell viability compared to only the $Aβ_{1-42}$-induced group in SH-SY5Y, as shown in Figure 6. Several studies indicated that Aβ could induce neuronal cell damage by evoking a cascade of oxidative damage to neurons [52,53]. The neuroprotective effect of the coumarins might partly come from anti-oxidative stress action. Taken together, these findings suggested that phellopterin significantly protected H_2O_2 and Aβ-induced cell damage in SH-SY5Y cells.

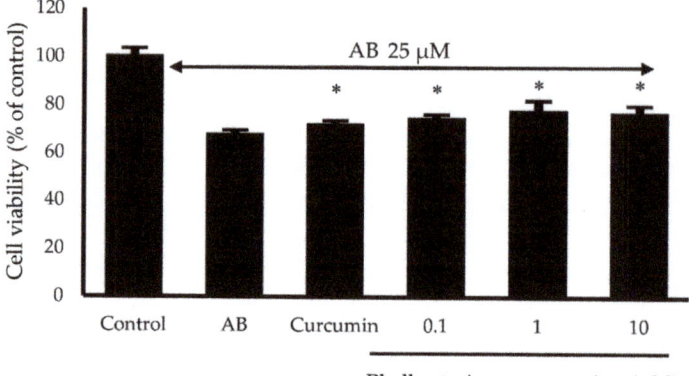

Figure 6. Effects of phellopterin at the concentration of 0.1 to 10 μM on $Aβ_{1-42}$-induced cell damage in SH-SY5Y cells. Curcumin at 10 μM was used as a reference standard. The values are reported as mean ± SD (n = 3). Paired t-test, * $p < 0.05$ compared to $Aβ_{1-42}$ treated group.

4. Conclusions

In summary, nine coumarins from *Toddalia asiatica* root were evaluated for activities related to the pathogenesis of Alzheimer's disease, including anti-AChE function, AChE- and self-induced Aβ aggregation. Seven out of nine coumarins were identified as multifunctional compounds inhibiting the pathogenesis of AD. The most potent multifunctional coumarin, phellopterin showed an ability to protect neuronal cell damage induced by H_2O_2 and $A\beta_{1-42}$. The structure–activity relationship and molecular docking studies suggested that the substituents on position 6, 7, and 8 of coumarin ring influenced anti-AChE function and anti-Aβ aggregation. The structure–activity relationship information obtained from this study might be useful in the development of new anti-AD drugs.

Author Contributions: Conceptualization, C.B., P.W., C.Y., P.T., B.S., R.L., P.K., and P.R.; methodology, P.T., P.W., and C.B.; formal analysis, P.T., and C.B.; investigation, P.T., and C.B.; resources, C.Y., and C.B.; writing—original draft preparation, P.T., and C.B.; writing—review and editing, P.W., and C.B.; project administration, C.B. All authors have read and agreed to the published version of the manuscript.

Funding: This research was funded by Khon Kaen University, grant number 601H108, Thailand Research Fund, grant number DBG6080006 and the Center for Research and Development of Herbal Health Products, Khon Kaen University, Thailand.

Conflicts of Interest: The authors declare no conflict of interest. The funders had no role in the design of the study; in the collection, analyses, or interpretation of data; in the writing of the manuscript, or in the decision to publish the results.

Abbreviations

AD	Alzheimer's disease
Aβ	amyloid beta
AChE	acetylcholinesterase
ACh	acetylcholine
CAS	catalytic anionic site
PAS	peripheral anionic site
APP	amyloid precursor protein
MTDLs	multi-target directed ligands
ThT	Thioflavin T
SAR	the structure–activity relationship
H_2O_2	hydrogen peroxide
MTT	3-(4,5-dimethyl-2-thiazolyl)-2,5-diphenyl-2H-tetrazolium bromide
DTNB	5,5′-dithiobis(2-nitrobenzoic acid)
DMSO	dimethyl sulfoxide

References

1. Jahn, H. Memory loss in Alzheimer's disease. *Dialogues Clin. Neurosci.* **2013**, *15*, 445–454. [PubMed]
2. Tarawneh, R.; Holtzman, D.M. The clinical problem of symptomatic Alzheimer disease and mild cognitive impairment. *Cold Spring Harb. Perspect. Med.* **2012**, *2*, 1–16. [CrossRef]
3. Ferreira-Vieira, T.H.; Guimaraes, I.M.; Silva, F.R.; Ribeiro, F.M. Alzheimer's disease: Targeting the cholinergic system. *Curr. Neuropharmacol.* **2016**, *14*, 101–115. [CrossRef] [PubMed]
4. Murphy, M.P.; LeVine, H. Alzheimer's Disease and the Amyloid-β Peptide. *J. Alzheimer's Dis.* **2010**, *19*, 311–323. [CrossRef] [PubMed]
5. Querfurth, H.W.; LaFerla, F.M. Alzheimer's Disease. *N. Engl. J. Med.* **2010**, *362*, 329–344. [CrossRef] [PubMed]
6. Madeo, J. The role of oxidative stress in Alzheimer's Disease. *J. Alzheimer's Dis. Park.* **2013**, *03*. [CrossRef]
7. Hasselmo, M.E. The role of acetylcholine in learning and memory. *Curr. Opin. Neurobiol.* **2006**, *16*, 710–715. [CrossRef] [PubMed]
8. Colovic, M.B.; Krstic, D.Z.; Lazarevic-Pasti, T.D.; Bondzic, A.M.; Vasic, V.M. Acetylcholinesterase inhibitors: Pharmacology and toxicology. *Curr. Neuropharmacol.* **2013**, *11*, 315–335. [CrossRef]

9. Pinho, B.R.; Ferreres, F.; Valentão, P.; Andrade, P.B. Nature as a source of metabolites with cholinesterase-inhibitory activity: An approach to Alzheimer's disease treatment. *J. Pharm. Pharmacol.* **2013**, *65*, 1681–1700. [CrossRef]
10. De Ferrari, G.V.; Canales, M.A.; Shin, I.; Weiner, L.M.; Silman, I.; Inestrosa, N.C. A structural motif of acetylcholinesterase that promotes amyloid β-peptide fibril formation. *Biochemistry* **2001**, *40*, 10447–10457. [CrossRef]
11. Kwon, Y.E.; Park, J.Y.; No, K.T.; Shin, J.H.; Lee, S.K.; Eun, J.S.; Yang, J.H.; Shin, T.Y.; Kim, D.K.; Chae, B.S.; et al. Synthesis, *in vitro* assay, and molecular modeling of new piperidine derivatives having dual inhibitory potency against acetylcholinesterase and Abeta1-42 aggregation for Alzheimer's disease therapeutics. *Bioorg. Med. Chem.* **2007**, *15*, 6596–6607. [CrossRef] [PubMed]
12. Inestrosa, N.C.; Alvarez, A.; Pérez, C.A.; Moreno, R.D.; Vicente, M.; Linker, C.; Casanueva, O.I.; Soto, C.; Garrido, J. Acetylcholinesterase accelerates assembly of amyloid-beta-peptides into Alzheimer's fibrils: Possible role of the peripheral site of the enzyme. *Neuron* **1996**, *16*, 881–891. [CrossRef]
13. Hardy, J.; Selkoe, D.J. The amyloid hypothesis of Alzheimer's disease: Progress and problems on the road to therapeutics. *Science* **2002**, *297*, 353–356. [CrossRef]
14. Madav, Y.; Wairkar, S.; Prabhakar, B. Recent therapeutic strategies targeting beta amyloid and tauopathies in Alzheimer's disease. *Brain Res. Bull.* **2019**, *146*, 171–184. [CrossRef] [PubMed]
15. Anand, P.; Singh, B.; Singh, N. A review on coumarins as acetylcholinesterase inhibitors for Alzheimer's disease. *Bioorg. Med. Chem.* **2012**, *20*, 1175–1180. [CrossRef] [PubMed]
16. Ali, M.Y.; Jannat, S.; Jung, H.A.; Choi, R.J.; Roy, A.; Choi, J.S. Anti-Alzheimer's disease potential of coumarins from *Angelica decursiva* and *Artemisia capillaris* and structure-activity analysis. *Asian Pac. J. Trop. Med.* **2016**, *9*, 103–111. [CrossRef]
17. Thiratmatrakul, S.; Yenjai, C.; Waiwut, P.; Vajragupta, O.; Reubroycharoen, P.; Tohda, M.; Boonyarat, C. Synthesis, biological evaluation and molecular modeling study of novel tacrine-carbazole hybrids as potential multifunctional agents for the treatment of Alzheimer's disease. *Eur. J. Med. Chem.* **2014**, *75*, 21–30. [CrossRef]
18. Zhao, Q.; Brett, M.; Van Osselaer, N.; Huang, F.; Raoult, A.; Van Peer, A.; Verhaeghe, T.; Hust, R. Galantamine pharmacokinetics, safety, and tolerability profiles are similar in healthy Caucasian and Japanese subjects. *J. Clin. Pharmacol.* **2002**, *42*, 1002–1010. [CrossRef]
19. Ji, H.; Zhang, H. Multipotent natural agents to combat Alzheimer's disease. Functional spectrum and structural features. *Acta Pharmacol. Sin.* **2008**, *29*, 143–151. [CrossRef]
20. Rajkumar, M.; Chandra, R.H.; Asres, K.; Veeresham, C. *Toddalia asiatica* (Linn.) Lam.—A Comprehensive Review. *Pharmacogn. Rev.* **2008**, *2*, 386–397.
21. Orwa, J.A.; Jondiko, I.J.O.; Minja, R.J.A.; Bekunda, M. The use of *Toddalia asiatica* (L) Lam. (Rutaceae) in traditional medicine practice in East Africa. *J. Ethnopharmacol.* **2008**, *115*, 257–262. [CrossRef] [PubMed]
22. Orwa, J.A.; Ngeny, L.; Mwikwabe, N.M.; Ondicho, J.; Jondiko, I.J.O. Antimalarial and safety evaluation of extracts from *Toddalia asiatica* (L) Lam. (Rutaceae). *J. Ethnopharmacol.* **2013**, *145*, 587–590. [CrossRef] [PubMed]
23. Piller, N.B. A comparison of the effectiveness of some anti-inflammatory drugs on thermal oedema. *Br. J. Exp. Pathol.* **1975**, *56*, 554–560.
24. Kumagai, M.; Watanabe, A.; Yoshida, I.; Mishima, T.; Nakamura, M.; Nishikawa, K.; Morimoto, Y. Evaluation of aculeatin and toddaculin isolated from *Toddalia asiatica* as anti-inflammatory agents in LPS-stimulated RAW264 macrophages. *Biol. Pharm. Bull.* **2018**, *41*, 132–137. [CrossRef] [PubMed]
25. Vázquez, R.; Riveiro, M.E.; Vermeulen, M.; Mondillo, C.; Coombes, P.H.; Crouch, N.R.; Ismail, F.; Mulholland, D.A.; Baldi, A.; Shayo, C.; et al. Toddaculin, a natural coumarin from *Toddalia asiatica*, induces differentiation and apoptosis in U-937 leukemic cells. *Phytomedicine* **2012**, *19*, 737–746. [CrossRef] [PubMed]
26. Kaneko, T.; Tahara, S.; Takabayashi, F. Suppression of lipid hydroperoxide-induced oxidative damage to cellular DNA by esculetin. *Biol. Pharm. Bull.* **2003**, *26*, 840–844. [CrossRef] [PubMed]
27. Mayer, G.A.; Connell, W.F. Effect of bishydroxycoumarin (dicumarol) on clotting time of whole blood. *J. Am. Med. Assoc.* **1956**, *161*, 806. [CrossRef]
28. Basile, A.; Sorbo, S.; Spadaro, V.; Bruno, M.; Maggio, A.; Faraone, N.; Rosselli, S. Antimicrobial and antioxidant activities of coumarins from the roots of *Ferulago campestris* (Apiaceae). *Molecules* **2009**, *14*, 939–952. [CrossRef]

29. Abu-Aisheh, M.N.; Al-Aboudi, A.; Mustafa, M.S.; El-Abadelah, M.M.; Ali, S.Y.; Ul-Haq, Z.; Mubarak, M.S. Coumarin derivatives as acetyl- and butyrylcholinestrase inhibitors: An *in vitro*, molecular docking, and molecular dynamics simulations study. *Heliyon* **2019**, *5*, e01552. [CrossRef]
30. Sukieum, S.; Sang-aroon, W.; Yenjai, C. Coumarins and alkaloids from the roots of *Toddalia asiatica*. *Nat. Prod. Res.* **2018**, *32*, 944–952. [CrossRef]
31. Hirunwong, C.; Sukieum, S.; Phatchana, R.; Yenjai, C. Cytotoxic and antimalarial constituents from the roots of *Toddalia asiatica*. *Phytochem. Lett.* **2016**, *17*, 242–246. [CrossRef]
32. Ellman, G.L.; Courtney, K.D.; Andres, V.; Featherstone, R.M. A new and rapid colorimetric determination of acetylcholinesterase activity. *Biochem. Pharmacol.* **1961**, *7*, 88–95. [CrossRef]
33. Bartolini, M.; Bertucci, C.; Cavrini, V.; Andrisano, V. β-Amyloid aggregation induced by human acetylcholinesterase: Inhibition studies. *Biochem. Pharmacol.* **2003**, *65*, 407–416. [CrossRef]
34. LeVine, H. Quantification of beta-sheet amyloid fibril structures with thioflavin T. *Methods Enzymol.* **1999**, *309*, 274–284.
35. Kang, S.Y.; Lee, K.Y.; Sung, S.H.; Park, M.J.; Kim, Y.C. Coumarins isolated from *Angelica gigas* inhibit Acetylcholinesterase: Structure–Activity Relationships. *J. Nat. Prod.* **2001**, *64*, 683–685. [CrossRef]
36. Fallarero, A.; Oinonen, P.; Gupta, S.; Blom, P.; Galkin, A.; Mohan, C.G.; Vuorela, P.M. Inhibition of acetylcholinesterase by coumarins: The case of coumarin 106. *Pharmacol. Res.* **2008**, *58*, 215–221. [CrossRef]
37. Muñoz, F.J.; Inestrosa, N.C. Neurotoxicity of acetylcholinesterase amyloid β-peptide aggregates is dependent on the type of Aβ peptide and the AChE concentration present in the complexes. *FEBS Lett.* **1999**, *450*, 205–209. [CrossRef]
38. Sengupta, U.; Nilson, A.N.; Kayed, R. The Role of Amyloid-β Oligomers in Toxicity, Propagation, and Immunotherapy. *EBioMedicine* **2016**, *6*, 42–49. [CrossRef]
39. Roychaudhuri, R.; Yang, M.; Hoshi, M.M.; Teplow, D.B. Amyloid β-protein assembly and Alzheimer disease. *J. Biol. Chem.* **2009**, *284*, 4749–4753. [CrossRef]
40. Luhrs, T.; Ritter, C.; Adrian, M.; Riek-Loher, D.; Bohrmann, B.; Dobeli, H.; Schubert, D.; Riek, R. 3D structure of Alzheimer's amyloid- (1-42) fibrils. *Proc. Natl. Acad. Sci. USA* **2005**, *102*, 17342–17347. [CrossRef]
41. Bitan, G.; Kirkitadze, M.D.; Lomakin, A.; Vollers, S.S.; Benedek, G.B.; Teplow, D.B. Amyloid beta -protein (Abeta) assembly: Abeta 40 and Abeta 42 oligomerize through distinct pathways. *Proc. Natl. Acad. Sci. USA* **2003**, *100*, 330–335. [CrossRef] [PubMed]
42. Petkova, A.T.; Ishii, Y.; Balbach, J.J.; Antzutkin, O.N.; Leapman, R.D.; Delaglio, F.; Tycko, R. A structural model for Alzheimer's β-amyloid fibrils based on experimental constraints from solid state NMR. *Proc. Natl. Acad. Sci. USA* **2002**, *99*, 16742–16747. [CrossRef] [PubMed]
43. Cukalevski, R.; Boland, B.; Frohm, B.; Thulin, E.; Walsh, D.; Linse, S. Role of aromatic side chains in amyloid β-protein aggregation. *ACS Chem. Neurosci.* **2012**, *3*, 1008–1016. [CrossRef] [PubMed]
44. Alexi, T.; Borlongan, C.V.; Faull, R.L.; Williams, C.E.; Clark, R.G.; Gluckman, P.D.; Hughes, P.E. Neuroprotective strategies for basal ganglia degeneration: Parkinson's and Huntington's diseases. *Prog. Neurobiol.* **2000**, *60*, 409–470. [CrossRef]
45. Hampton, M.B.; Orrenius, S. Dual regulation of caspase activity by hydrogen peroxide: Implications for apoptosis. *FEBS Lett.* **1997**, *414*, 552–556. [CrossRef]
46. Chen, L.; Liu, L.; Yin, J.; Luo, Y.; Huang, S. Hydrogen peroxide-induced neuronal apoptosis is associated with inhibition of protein phosphatase 2A and 5, leading to activation of MAPK pathway. *Int. J. Biochem. Cell Biol.* **2009**, *41*, 1284–1295. [CrossRef]
47. Sanvicens, N.; Gomez-Vicente, V.; Messeguer, A.; Cotter, T.G. The radical scavenger CR-6 protects SH-SY5Y neuroblastoma cells from oxidative stress-induced apoptosis: Effect on survival pathways. *J. Neurochem.* **2006**, *98*, 735–747. [CrossRef]
48. Yu, Y.; Du, J.-R.; Wang, C.-Y.; Qian, Z.-M. Protection against hydrogen peroxide-induced injury by Z-ligustilide in PC12 cells. *Exp. Brain Res.* **2008**, *184*, 307–312. [CrossRef]
49. Nakajima, Y.; Inokuchi, Y.; Nishi, M.; Shimazawa, M.; Otsubo, K.; Hara, H. Coenzyme Q10 protects retinal cells against oxidative stress *in vitro* and *in vivo*. *Brain Res.* **2008**, *1226*, 226–233. [CrossRef]
50. Sadigh-Eteghad, S.; Sabermarouf, B.; Majdi, A.; Talebi, M.; Farhoudi, M.; Mahmoudi, J. Amyloid-Beta: A crucial factor in Alzheimer's Disease. *Med. Princ. Pract.* **2015**, *24*, 1–10. [CrossRef] [PubMed]
51. Mohamed, T.; Shakeri, A.; Rao, P.P.N. Amyloid cascade in Alzheimer's disease: Recent advances in medicinal chemistry. *Eur. J. Med. Chem.* **2016**, *113*, 258–272. [CrossRef] [PubMed]

52. Carrillo-Mora, P.; Luna, R.; Colín-Barenque, L. Amyloid beta: Multiple mechanisms of toxicity and only some protective effects? *Oxid. Med. Cell. Longev.* **2014**, *2014*, 795375. [CrossRef] [PubMed]
53. Wang, H.; Xu, Y.; Yan, J.; Zhao, X.; Sun, X.; Zhang, Y.; Guo, J.; Zhu, C. Acteoside protects human neuroblastoma SH-SY5Y cells against β-amyloid-induced cell injury. *Brain Res.* **2009**, *1283*, 139–147. [CrossRef] [PubMed]

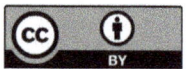

© 2020 by the authors. Licensee MDPI, Basel, Switzerland. This article is an open access article distributed under the terms and conditions of the Creative Commons Attribution (CC BY) license (http://creativecommons.org/licenses/by/4.0/).

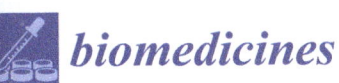

Article

Insights into the Interaction Mechanism of DTP3 with MKK7 by Using STD-NMR and Computational Approaches

Annamaria Sandomenico [1,†], Lorenzo Di Rienzo [2,†], Luisa Calvanese [3], Emanuela Iaccarino [1], Gabriella D'Auria [1,4], Lucia Falcigno [1,4], Angela Chambery [5], Rosita Russo [5], Guido Franzoso [6], Laura Tornatore [6], Marco D'Abramo [7], Menotti Ruvo [1], Edoardo Milanetti [2,8,*] and Domenico Raimondo [9,*]

1. Institute of Biostructures and Bioimaging (IBB)-CNR, Via Mezzocannone 16, 80134 Naples, Italy; annamaria.sandomenico@gmail.com (A.S.); emanuela.iaccarino@unicampania.it (E.I.); gabriella.dauria@unina.it (G.D.); falcigno@unina.it (L.F.); menotti.ruvo@unina.it (M.R.)
2. Center for Life Nano Science@Sapienza, Italian Institute of Technology, Viale Regina Elena 291, 00161 Rome, Italy; lorenzo.dirienzo@uniroma1.it
3. CIRPeB, University of Naples Federico II, 80134 Naples, Italy; luisa.calvanese@unina.it
4. Department of Pharmacy, University of Naples "Federico II", Via Mezzocannone 16, 80134 Naples, Italy
5. Department of Environmental, Biological and Pharmaceutical Sciences and Technologies, University of Campania Luigi Vanvitelli, 81100 Caserta, Italy; angela.chambery@unicampania.it (A.C.); rosita.russo@unicampania.it (R.R.)
6. Centre for Molecular Immunology and Inflammation, Department of Immunology and Inflammation, Imperial College London, London W12 0NN, UK; g.franzoso@imperial.ac.uk (G.F.); la.tornatore@gmail.com (L.T.)
7. Department of Chemistry, Sapienza University of Rome, Piazzale Aldo Moro 5, 00185 Rome, Italy; marco.dabramo@uniroma1.it
8. Department of Physics, Sapienza University of Rome, Piazzale Aldo Moro 5, 00185 Rome, Italy
9. Department of Molecular Medicine, Sapienza University of Rome, Viale Regina Elena 291, 00161 Rome, Italy
* Correspondence: edoardo.milanetti@uniroma1.it (E.M.); domenico.raimondo@uniroma1.it (D.R.)
† These authors contributed equally to this work.

Abstract: GADD45β/MKK7 complex is a non-redundant, cancer cell-restricted survival module downstream of the NF-κB survival pathway, and it has a pathogenically critical role in multiple myeloma, an incurable malignancy of plasma cells. The first-in-class GADD45β/MKK7 inhibitor DTP3 effectively kills MM cells expressing its molecular target, both in vitro and in vivo, by inducing MKK7/JNK-dependent apoptosis with no apparent toxicity to normal cells. DTP3 combines favorable drug-like properties, with on-target-specific pharmacology, resulting in a safe and cancer-selective therapeutic effect; however, its mode of action is only partially understood. In this work, we have investigated the molecular determinants underlying the MKK7 interaction with DTP3 by combining computational, NMR, and spectroscopic methods. Data gathered by fluorescence quenching and computational approaches consistently indicate that the N-terminal region of MKK7 is the optimal binding site explored by DTP3. These findings further the understanding of the selective mode of action of GADD45β/MKK7 inhibitors and inform potential mechanisms of drug resistance. Notably, upon validation of the safety and efficacy of DTP3 in human trials, our results could also facilitate the development of novel DTP3-like therapeutics with improved bioavailability or the capacity to bypass drug resistance.

Keywords: GADD45β; MKK7; multiple myeloma; protein-ligand interaction; STD-NMR

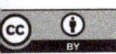

1. Introduction

Mitogen-activated protein (MAP) kinases are evolutionarily conserved serine–threonine protein kinases that are activated in response to a wide variety of extracellular or intracellular stimuli. They play a key role in a number of intracellular networks where they transduce and integrate cellular signals into complex cytoplasmatic and nuclear processes, including proliferation, differentiation, and apoptosis [1,2]. These MAP kinases are activated by dual phosphorylation events on threonine and tyrosine residues within a Thr-Xaa-Tyr motif, which are systematically mediated by three-tiered cascades consisting of a MAP kinase (MAPK), a MAP kinase kinase (MAPKK, MEK, or MKK), and a MAP kinase kinase kinase (MAPKKK, MEKK, or MKKK). Ultimately, this signaling cascade results in the activation of the three major MAPKs pathways: the c-Jun N-terminal kinase (JNK) pathway, the p38 MAP kinase pathway, and the extracellular signal-regulated kinase (ERK) pathway [1,2]. Among MAPKKs, MKK7 is one of two the essential regulators of the JNK signaling and has been recently suggested to represent an emerging therapeutic target in cancer [3]. MKK7 consists of three domains: the D (docking) domain (residues 37–57), which contains a conserved docking site and is required for the binding to MAPK substrates; the kinase domain; and the DVD (domain for versatile docking) domain [2]. The MKK7 N-terminal D domain is involved in the binding to, and activation of, JNK. The central kinase domain (residues 120–380) contains a Ser–Xaa–Ala–Lys–Thr (S–X–A–K–T) kinase motif that is phosphorylated by upstream MKKKs. The C-terminal DVD domain, located at residues 377–400, plays an important role in the docking of upstream MAP3Ks such as MLKs, ASKs, TAKs, and LZK.

The activity of MKK7 is also regulated by direct physical interactions with several scaffold proteins (i.e., JIP proteins) and other partners (i.e., GADD45β and TIPRL), which play a crucial role in controlling the binding duration and signal intensity of MAP3K/MAP2K/MAPK complexes in the MAPK pathway [1–4]. We have recently identified the interaction between the NF-κB-regulated antiapoptotic factor, GADD45β, and the JNK kinase, MKK7, as a therapeutic target in multiple myeloma (MM), an incurable plasma cell malignancy accounting for about 2% of all cancer deaths and representing a paradigm for NF-κB-driven cancers [2,5]. GADD45β is upregulated in MM cells by NF-κB, associates with poor outcome in patients, and promotes myeloma cell survival by suppressing proapoptotic MKK7/JNK signaling [5].

GADD45β mediates this activity by interacting directly with MKK7 and blocking its enzymatic activity by engaging the enzyme catalytic pocket, thereby preventing the access of ATP (See Figure 1a) [6,7]. DTP3 is a D-tripeptide of sequence Ac-D-Tyr-D-Arg-D-Phe-NH2 that has been identified through the screening of a combinatorial library of synthetic peptides targeting the GADD45β/MKK7 complex (See Figure 1b) [5,8–10]. By undertaking a drug discovery approach, we developed DTP3, which disrupts the GADD45β/MKK7 interaction and kills MM cells effectively by inducing MKK7/JNK-dependent apoptosis, without overt toxicity to normal tissues [5]. Preclinical studies demonstrated that the first-in-class GADD45β/MKK7 inhibitor DTP3 is a promising candidate therapeutic agent with a novel mode of action that selectively targets the NF-κB survival axis and has significant clinical potential for development in oncology [8]. The safety, tolerability, pharmacokinetics, and pharmacodynamics of DTP3 were recently evaluated in a pilot clinical study in patients with relapsed or refractory MM (first-in-human phase-I/IIa trial, EudraCT: 2015-003459-23), with encouraging initial clinical results [8,9].

Mass spectrometry (MS)-based footprinting and chemical cross-linking (CX-MS) analyses and modeling studies of the GADD45β–MKK7 and MKK7–DTP3 complexes have established that DTP3 interacts with two spatially adjacent MKK7 outer regions, which form a shallow pocket located proximally to the ATP pocket, and that the interactions of GADD45β and DTP3 with MKK7 are mutually exclusive. These data also suggested that the DTP3 binding to MKK7 induces a conformational rearrangement, which contributes to the dissociation of GADD45β from MKK7 [5,11]. GADD45β recognizes the MKK7 catalytic pocket through a flexible acidic loop encompassing residues 103–117. While the 3D crystallographic structure of the kinase domain has been solved [6,12], no structural data are so far available for GADD45β or the complexes GADD45β/MKK7 and DTP3/MKK7 complexes.

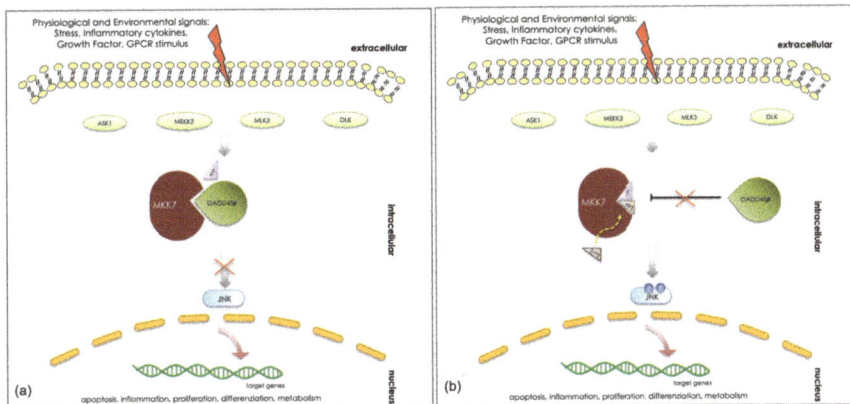

Figure 1. The GADD45β-regulated MKK7 signaling cascade in absence (**a**) and in presence (**b**) of the DTP3 peptide inhibitor. DTP3 interaction with MKK7 restores its kinase activity and the JNK-mediated apoptotic signal by preventing the GADD45β inhibition.

In an attempt to further refine at the atomic level the interaction between DTP3 and MKK7 and to shed light on the molecular mechanisms underpinning the effects of DTP3 on the GADD45β/MKK7 interaction, we have investigated the peptide groups that are more directly involved in the binding to MKK7 by using STD-NMR. These analysis were complemented by an extensive computational examination of the interaction mechanisms that could guide future studies aimed at designing novel DTP3-like chemical entities with improved bioavailability and/or drug-like characteristics.

2. Materials and Methods

2.1. Synthesis and Purification of FITC-βAla$_2$-DTP3 and FITC-βAla$_2$-SCRB Peptides

DTP3 (Ac-D-Tyr-D-Arg-D-Phe-NH2) and the related scramble (SCRB) peptide (Ac-D-Arg-D-Phe-D-Tyr-NH2) were prepared as previously reported [10]. The fluoresceine isothiocyanate (FITC)-labeled variants (FITC-βAla$_2$-DTP3 and FITC-βAla$_2$-SCRB) were similarly assembled on the solid phase introducing on the N-terminus two additional β-alanines and then FITC at the N-terminus via direct overnight coupling (room temperature) to the resin. FITC was dissolved in DMF and used at 5-fold excess at slightly basic pH. After removal from the solid support by treatment with a TFA/H$_2$O/tri-isopropylsilane(TIS) mixture at 90:5:5 ($v/v/v$) (RT, 3 h, 1.0 mL mixture/100 mg resin) and lyophilization, peptides were purified by reversed-phase HPLC using an X-Bridge Prep C18 Column (19 × 150 mm ID) by applying a linear gradient of solvent B (0.1% TFA in CH$_3$CN) over solvent A (0.1% TFA in H$_2$O) from 5% to 70% in 15 min (flow rate 15 mL/min) using a Waters HPLC preparative system. Products purity and identity were assessed by ESI-TOF-MS analyses. The recombinant kinase domain of MKK7 (MKK7-KD), residues 101–405, was prepared as reported elsewhere [5,10].

2.2. Fluorescence Quenching Ligand Binding Assay

Fluorescence quenching binding analyses were performed by titrating FITC-βAla$_2$-DTP3 and FITC-βAla$_2$-SCRB, both at 10 nM, with soluble MKK7-KD at increasing concentrations ranging between 0 and 1000 nM. Experiments were performed in 96-well black plates using 200 μL volume samples in quadruplicates. Excitation was set at 488 nm, while emission spectra were collected between 500 nm and 600 nm. Maximum emission values at 517 nm were averaged and the blank subtracted. K_Ds Δfluorescence value were obtained by subtracting the fluorescence signal of the peptide alone plotted against the kinase concentration and then fitted using a nonlinear one-site total algorithm implemented in GraphPad Prism version 5.00 for Windows (GraphPad Software, San Diego, CA, USA). Experiments were repeated at least twice in triplicate. The concentrations of the labeled peptides were determined according to the Lambert–Beer law by using the molar absorptivity of FITC at 488 nm (73,000 cm^{-1}M^{-1}). The very strong emission of FITC prevented the exploration of the wider concentration intervals required to assess the non-specific interaction of the control peptide with the kinase at concentrations above those shown. Experiments were therefore performed by monitoring the tryptophan fluorescence quenching as a function of the concentration of the added peptides. MKK7-KD was used at 1.25 µM in phosphate buffer pH 7.5 together with both DTP3 or SCRB in the concentration range between 10 nM and 140 µM, as previously reported [5]. Experiments were performed at least twice, and data were averaged and plotted against the change in fluorescence emission at 334 nm (ΔFluorescence 334 nm) as a function of the peptide concentrations. To estimate the KD values, data were fitted using GraphPad with a nonlinear algorithm (log[inhibitor] vs. response—Variable slope) to account for the entire concentration range.

2.3. NMR Analyses

2.3.1. NMR Spectroscopy of Free Molecules

All NMR experiments were performed at T = 301 K by using a Varian Inova spectrometer located at the "Istituto di Biostrutture e Bioimmagini (IBB) of CNR, Napoli", operating at a proton frequency of 600 MHz, and equipped with a 5 mm inverse-detection cryoprobe and z-gradient. The free MKK7-KD protein was measured by NMR at 10 µM concentration in 600 µL of deuterated TRIS buffer 20 mM/D2O (100%) at pH 7.5, with NaCl 50 mM and TCEP (Tris(2 carboxyethyl)phosphine) 0.5 mM.

One-dimensional and STD spectra of the free MKK7-KD protein were obtained to test the integrity of the protein and to determine appropriate saturation frequencies, respectively. The frequency of −3045 Hz (0 ppm) was chosen as the best one for the magnetization transfer from protein to the peptide binder. Analogously, STD spectra were acquired for each peptide, DTP3, SCRB, and a unrelated control peptide (1 mM in D2O), to verify that they were not excited by the pulse at the frequency chosen for protein saturation. In such a way, the saturation frequency at 0 ppm could be confirmed as the best also for the peptides. The concentration of the unlabelled peptides and protein were spectrophotometrically determined according to the Lambert–Beer law using ϵ_{275nm} = 1420 cm^{-1}M^{-1} and ϵ_{280nm} = 31,400 cm^{-1}M^{-1}, respectively.

2.3.2. NMR Spectroscopy of Tripeptide–Protein Interactions

STD NMR experiments were performed at T = 301 K by adding increasing amounts of peptide to the protein samples at 10 µM in 600 µL of buffered D2O (solvent composition specified above) in order to achieve peptide/protein molar ratios, R, ranging from 10 (R10) to 100 (R100). The excitation sculpting pulse sequences were used to suppress the water signals in the spectra. The protein was irradiated at δ H 0 ppm (on-resonance) and δ H 27 ppm (off-resonance) with a train of Gaussian shaped pulses (50 ms). The broad resonances of the protein were suppressed with a 50 ms spin-lock pulse. The setup of the STD NMR experiments was optimized by a series of experiments using ligand-only samples to ensure that the irradiation at the selected frequency for on-resonance scan did not affect the ligand, as reported above. The saturation time used in the STD experiments was 2 s. Following the method of Mayer and Meyer [13] we also performed a Group Epitope Mapping (GEM) study to identify the binding surfaces on the ligand using STD methods. This approach was based on the comparison of the STD response for different protons within a ligand. This was done by normalizing all the measured STD signals against the one most intense in the spectrum, which is arbitrarily assumed to be the 100% value. The set of resulting STD percentages qualitatively delineates the chemical moieties that are critical for the molecular interaction, as they are intimately recognized by the protein (STD values close to 100%), and the regions of the ligand situated far from the receptor binding site. The proton resonances of the peptides detected in the presence of the protein, assigned at the peptide/protein ratio equal to R100, are reported in Tables S1 and S2 (Supplementary Material).

2.4. Computational Studies

2.4.1. Molecular Dynamics Simulations

We used the PDB files of the MKK7 and the .mol2 file of the peptides DTP3 and SCRB that were employed in our previous work [5]. SwissParam software was used to generate the topologies and parameters based on the Merck molecular force field, in a functional form that is compatible with the CHARMM force field [14]. After solvation using the SPC water model [15] and minimization procedure performed by the steepest descent algorithm, a 100 ps long NVT and a 100 ps long NPT equilibration runs were performed for each system. Finally, production runs lasting 15 ns for both the peptides and 500 ns for the protein, with a time step of 2 fs, was performed. The Verlet cut-off scheme was adopted and the particle–mesh Ewald method was utilized to treat long-range electrostatic interactions. The temperature was kept constant by means of the velocity rescale algorithm (300 K) [16]. The simulations were executed using Gromacs Software version 2019.4 [17].

2.4.2. Zernike Descriptors

First, we calculated the electrostatic potential by assigning to each atom of the system a partial charge as obtained using the PDB2PQR algorithm [18,19]. Given a function $f(r,\theta,\phi)$ describing the molecular surface shape or electrostatics, the Zernike formalism relies on a series expansion in an orthonormal sequence of polynomials:

$$f(r,\theta,\phi) = \sum_{n=0}^{\infty} \sum_{l=0}^{n} \sum_{m=-l}^{l} C_{nlm} Z_{nl}^{m}(r,\theta,\phi)$$

where C_{nlm} are the Zernike moments and Z_{nl}^{m} are the Zernike polynomials. The order N at which the sum over n is truncated selects the level of representation details. In this work, we chose N = 20. The invariant 3D Zernike descriptors are defined as

$$D_{nl} = ||C_{nlm}|| = \sqrt{\sum_{m=-l}^{l} (C_{nlm})^2}$$

Selecting N = 20, we deal with 121 descriptors D_{nl}. A detailed mathematical treatment is reported in Venkatraman et al. [20].

In order to characterize the binding properties of the interfaces between two interacting molecules, we considered both their shape and electrostatic complementarity. As both binding regions can be correctly described with a set of Zernike descriptors, we were able to quantify the degree of complementarity (DOC) between the two interfaces measuring the distance between the two vectors of Zernike descriptors. In particular, the higher was the shape complementarity between the two interacting regions, the shorter was the distance between the corresponding Zernike descriptors (i.e., similar surfaces have similar descriptors). In order to analyze the role of the electrostatics in the binding process, we compare, in terms of the Zernike descriptors, the surface corresponding to the positive electrostatic potential with the surface of the negative electrostatic potential (and vice versa). This approach is justified since the positive potential descriptors of one region has to be similar to the negative potential descriptors of the interacting region (and vice versa). Therefore, the complementarity between regions A and B is defined as

$$[A-B]_{shape} = D(X^A_{shape}, X^B_{shape})$$

$$[A-B]_{elec} = \frac{(D(X^A_{elec,+}, X^B_{elec,-}) + (D(X^A_{elec,-}, X^B_{elec,+}))}{2}$$

where X_{shape}, $X_{elec,+}$, and $X_{elec,-}$ are the shape, the electrostatic positive, and the electrostatic negative descriptors, respectively. D represents the cosine distance. Note that high complementarity is achieved when these distances are small.

2.4.3. Binding Sites Detection and Molecular Docking

DTP3 binding sites on MKK7 protein were predicted by using the P2Rank approach, a template-free, machine learning-based method for ligand binding site prediction which uses a random forest model to predict "ligandability" scores for each point on a protein's surface [21]. Cluster points with high scores into resulting pocket scores are used to rank the putative pockets. AutoDock Vina (version 1.1.2) was used in this study to perform docking experiments [22]. We used the same PDB files of the MKK7 (receptor) and the .mol2 file of the peptides DTP3 and SCRB (ligands) that were used in our previous work [5]. The parameters were set employing AutoDock Tools [22], and the protein structural files were translated to PDBQT (Protein Data Bank, Partial Charge (Q), and Atom Type (T)) format by adding polar hydrogens and Kollman charges in the same software. All rotatable bonds within the peptides (ligands) were allowed to rotate freely. One of the critical parameters for ligand docking is the size of a search space used to identify low-energy binding poses of ligand candidates. The docking search space was defined according to the procedure for calculating the optimal docking box size that maximizes the accuracy of binding pose prediction described by Feinstein et al. [23]. Autodock Vina software provides a parameter called "Exhaustiveness" to change the amount of computational effort used during a docking experiment. The default exhaustiveness value is 8, but we increased the exhaustiveness of search parameter to the value of 256 (the number of final binding modes produced by Vina was set to 20) in order to give a more consistent docking result. All other docking parameters were set to the default values. Subsequently, each of the conformation was visualized on UCSF Chimera, and the best docked orientation was selected based on docking score and binding interactions with the protein. The hydrogen bond (HB) and hydrophobic (HP) contacts between ligand and receptor were estimated using the protein-ligand interaction profiler LigPlot+ [24].

3. Results

3.1. Peptide Synthesis

DTP3, SCRB, and the FITC-peptides were obtained with average yields of 90% and after RP-HPLC purification homogeneous products were isolated. Experimental molecular masses were consistent with the expected values (DTP3 and SCRB: MWtheor 526.20 amu/MWexp 526.18 amu. FITC-βAla_2-DTP3 and FITC-βAla_2-SCRB: MWtheor 944.16 amu/MWexp 943.37 amu).

3.2. Fluorescence Quenching Ligand Binding Assay

According to previously reported results, obtained by similar experiments [5], the binding affinity of DTP3 (tested as FITC-βAla_2-DTP3) to MKK7-KD was in the nanomolar range (KD = 123.2 ± 35.3 nM). DTP3/MKK7-KD binding was assessed evaluating the fluorescence quenching of the FITC molecule, covalently bound to the DTP3 N-terminus, that we obtain as the peptide is located in proximity to the kinase. In a parallel experiment performed with the control peptide FITC-βAla_2-SCRB, no such quenching was observed, indicating that the binding was due to the tripeptide and not the N-terminal FITC molecule (See Figure 2a). The fluorescence quenching binding curves obtained by titrating DTP3 and SCRB in the range of concentrations between 10 nM and 140 μM with the kinase domain of MKK7 are reported in Figure 2b. Under these conditions, DTP3 bound to MKK7-KD with a KD of 0.240 ± 0.070 μM in substantial agreement with the previous experiment using an alternative methodology. Titration of the SCRB peptide with MKK7-KD instead only showed some binding at concentrations above 10 μM (with a ΔFluorescence at 334 nm of about 4 units) and was not saturated up to 140 μM. Fitting of the SCRB data with the same algorithm provided a KD of around 41 μM.

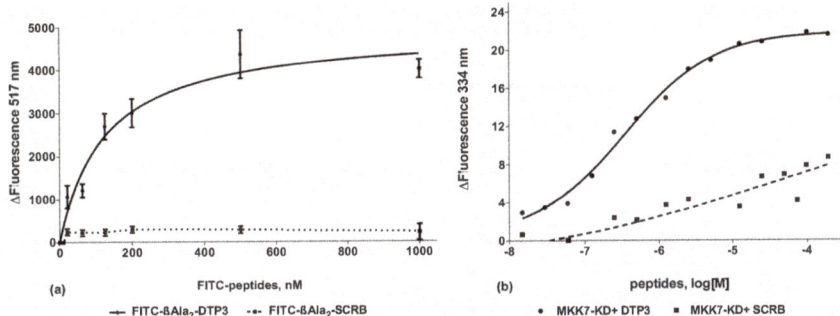

Figure 2. Fluorescence quenching binding analysis of N-terminally fluoresceinated DTP3 to MKK7-KD. (**a**) ΔFluorescence values at 517 nm of FITC-βAla_2-DTP3 and FITC-βAla_2-SCRB (10 nM) plotted against the concentration of MKK7-KD (0.05 ÷ 1000 nM) are reported. Values denote means ± SD (n = 4). (**b**) Fluorescence quenching binding analysis of DTP3 and SCRB to MKK7-KD as obtained by monitoring the ΔFluorescence at 334 nm. ΔFluorescence values plotted against the concentration of peptides (10 nM ÷ 140 µM) are reported. Values denote means ± SE (n = 2).

3.3. Interaction studies of DTP3 and SCRB with MKK7-KD by STD-NMR

Using a STD-NMR technique, we investigated the interaction of MKK7-KD with DTP3, SCRB, and other unrelated peptides. For each peptide, a series of STD spectra was acquired by using a fixed protein concentration of 10 µM and increasing peptide/protein R ratios. The full STD spectra together with expansions of the aromatic region, obtained for DTP3/MKK7-KD at ratio values from 5 to 100, are shown in Figure 3a,b. While for R = 5 no signals were visible, STD signals from D-Tyr^1 and D-Phe^3 aromatic protons appear starting from R = 10. Signals due to βCH and βCH2 protons of D-Arg^2 and acetyl group were observed only starting from R = 50. A comparison of the 1D and STD spectra is shown in Figure S1 (Supplementary material). At each R value, different nuclei are more or less affected by magnetization transfer in reason of their closeness to the enzyme surface during the contact events. A picture of the binding epitope of the ligand can be obtained by Group Epitope Mapping (GEM) [13], that is by comparing the STD effects of the protons once normalized with respect to the highest STD response. The set of normalized STD values qualitatively describes the portions of the ligand that are most involved in the interaction with the target protein. The GEM analysis performed for DTP3 (at R = 100) shows that the aromatic side chains are the most important for the interaction with MKK7-KD (Figure 3c). Taken together with the lower effects measured for the central residue, this result suggests that the most productive DTP3 conformation for MKK7 binding requires an iso-orientation of D-Tyr^1 and D-Phe^3 aromatic rings and an opposite localization of the D-Arg^2 side chain.

A GEM analysis of the binding surface of SCRB evaluated at R = 100 shows that, as for DTP3, the aromatic side chains are the moieties most involved in the MKK7-KD interaction (Figure 4c). A comparison of 1D and STD spectra is reported in Figure S2 in the Supplementary Material. At the concentrations used for STD analysis, DTP3 and SCRB peptides are both able to interact with the enzyme even though with different affinities (Figure 4). Indeed, the STD comparison demonstrates that the presence and the arrangement of the two aromatic residues do matter, with the distanced arrangement (i and i + 2 positions) that are more effective than the sequential one (i and i + 1). The saturation transfer effect also observed with the SCRB peptide likely derives from the high concentrations of the peptide necessarily required for the NMR STD experiments. However, it is apparent from the comparison spectra shown in Figure S3 that the STD effect observed with DTP3 can be recorded, yet at R20, it is almost absent in the parallel experiment with SCRB. Moreover, the STD intensities recorded in the parallel experiments conducted at grater concentration ratios are higher for DTP3 than for SCRB, suggesting a stronger interaction of MKK7 with DTP3 than with SCRB. Potentially owing to the structure similarity of the two isomeric tripeptides, at concentrations above 10 µM, the SCRB peptide also showed some binding with the kinase, consistent with results from the fluorescence quenching experiments (see Figure 2b). However, experiments performed at more biologically relevant concentrations demonstrated that DTP3, but not SCRB was capable of binding to MKK7 (See Figure 2, see also Tornatore et al. [5] and Rega et al. [11]). To confirm the specificity of DTP3 for MKK7-KD, we investigated the potential interactions with additional peptides having a similar size but no aromatic side chains. The set of STD spectra acquired under similar conditions with one of these control peptides [25] is reported in Figure S4 (Supplementary Material), which shows no binding to MKK7-KD at any of the concentrations tested.

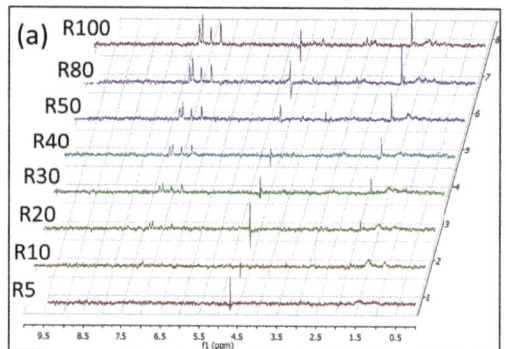
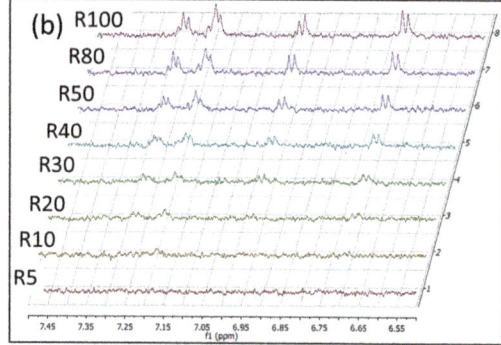
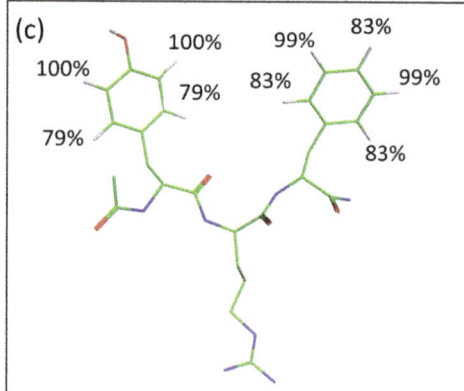

Figure 3. (a) STD spectra acquired at 10 µM of MKK7-KD and DTP3/MKK7-KD ratio values in the range 5 ÷ 100; (b) Zoom-in of the aromatic region; (c) Molecular model of DTP3 reporting the group epitope mapping (GEM) at R100.

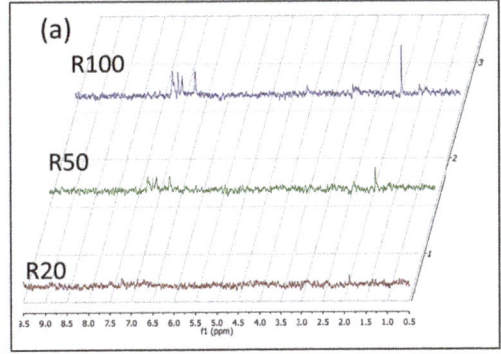
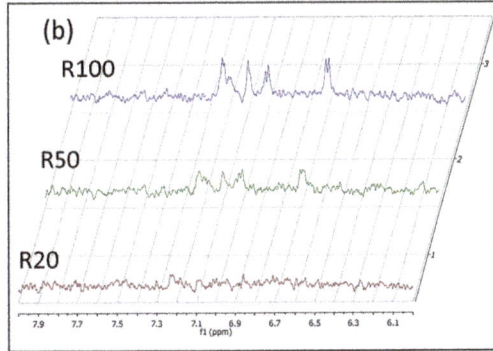
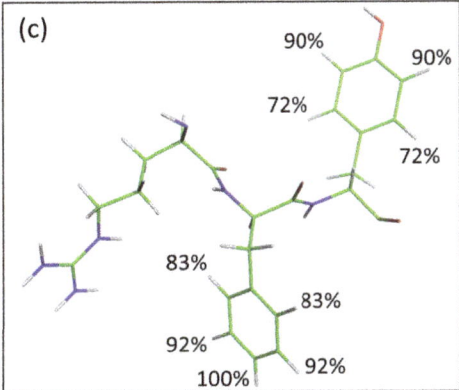

Figure 4. (a) STD spectra acquired at 10 μM of MKK7-KD and SCRB/MKK7-KD ratio values in the range 5 ÷ 100; (b) Zoom-in of the aromatic region; (c) Molecular model of SCRB reporting the group epitope mapping (GEM) at R100.

3.4. Identification of the DTP3 Binding Sites on MKK7-KD Surface and Their Characterization by Using Zernike Polynomials

While we previously identified the petide segments of MKK7-KD involved in the interaction with DTP3 (Y113-K136 and L259-K274, according to UNIPROT numbering) [11], the molecular details of the 3D kinase binding site and modality of the DTP3-dependent interaction remain unknown.

To identify the DTP3 binding sites of MKK7, we first used the P2Rank software. P2Rank scanned the surface and identified four top ranked binding pockets, hereafter defined as BP1, BP2, BP3, and BP4, that are potentially involved in the interaction with the DTP3 peptide. BP3 and BP4 pockets (Figure 5) were selected for further evaluation because they are in complete agreement with previous predictions [5] and experimental data [11]. In particular, several residues of BP3 and BP4 were previously identified as being involved in the interaction with DTP3 [11] (depicted as red ribbons in Figure 5). Of note, BP1 corresponds to the ATP binding site, which was previously reported not to be involved in the DTP3 interaction [11]. BP3 lies within the N-lobe of the MKK7-KD, while BP4 is located in the cleft between the N- and C-terminal lobes. BP3 and BP4 are defined by the residues 119, 120, 139, 142, 144, 146, 183, 186, and 195, and 162, 165, 166, 169, 239, 262, 263, 264, 265, 266, and 267, respectively (Figure 5).

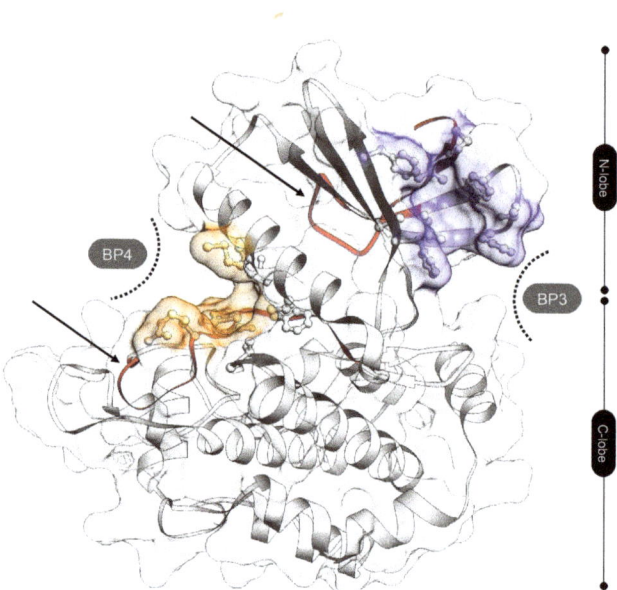

Figure 5. BP3 (in blue) and BP4 (in orange) binding sites on the kinase domain surface of MKK7, potentially occupable by DTP3. MKK-KD is shown in cartoon and surface representations. The residues defining the binding site are depicted in ball and stick representation. MKK7 linear peptides involved in the interaction with DTP3 [11] are reported as red ribbons (black arrows, residues 113–136 and 259–274).

We subsequently investigated the interaction between DTP3 with both BP3 and BP4 by using a method dealing with series expansion of the function that represents the protein molecular surface based on the Zernike polynomials. The norm of the expansion coefficients provides a local description of the shape and the electrostatic configuration of the regions involved in the interaction [20,26,27]. Once the molecular surfaces are described with the Zernike descriptors, complementarity metrics for both the shape and the electrostatics can be easily defined using a pairwise distance (we adopted the Cosine distance). It results that the lower the distance between their Zernike descriptors, the higher the complementarity between the two potentially interacting molecular regions (See Experimental Section) [28,29]. By such an approach, we can quantitatively assess the complementarity between two molecular regions, belonging to different molecular partners, that are supposed to interact. To let the peptides and the protein explore their own conformational spaces at equilibrium and to obtain a more statistically robust result, we performed Molecular Dynamics (MD) simulations to get representative snapshots of the structures of the molecules. In particular, we matched, by means of Zernike descriptors, the 60 conformations of both DTP3 and SCRB, obtained using a 15 ns long MD simulation performed in water for each peptide, with the 500 BP3 and BP4 conformations obtained from 500 ns long MD simulation of MKK7-KD in water. Before going further, MKK7 stability and its conformational behavior were investigated. We studied the backbone RMSD and gyration radius evolution over the MD trajectory, revealing how the initial 30 ns are required for MKK7 equilibration. Then, a reliable structural stability was reached and the protein does not destabilize the global conformation during the simulation (Supplementary Figures S5 and S6a). We also evaluated the local conformational mobility of the regions potentially interacting with DTP3, BP3, and BP4, by means of studying RMSF parameter and how the volume of BPs changes during the MD simulation. Results of this analysis, reported in Figure S7, showed that the BP4 pocket residues do not display great displacement since the corresponding RMSF values are low for each residue. The BP3 cavity is characterized by higher atomic mobility during molecular dynamics (especially residues 119 and 142), but it is not the region of the protein with the greatest structural variation. Moreover, BP3 is partially composed by the last N-terminal region of MKK7 and this may explain its higher mobility. In fact, even BP3 volume variation analysis did not display any marked variation during MD simulation (Figure S7b) Then, we evaluated the shape and electrostatic complementarity between the peptides and the two pockets on the MKK7-KD surface.

The Zernike descriptors of shape and electrostatics complementarity, obtained as results of this analysis, are depicted in Figure 6a–d. It is worth noting that shape complementarity is a distinguishing feature of the binding properties of DTP3 and SCRB, and likely drives the specific interaction of DTP3, but not SCRB, with both BP3 and BP4 (Figure 6a,c, respectively). The density distribution difference of the Zernike distances is statistically significant (KS-test p-value is less than 2.2×10^{-16}). In particular, DTP3 has a lower Zernike shape distance than SCRB in both the BP3 and BP4 pockets, suggesting a higher shape complementarity. On the other hand, the electrostatic interactions do not seem to play a role in the selective binding of DTP3 relative to SCRB to BPs. Indeed, the DTP3 and SCRB Zernike electrostatic distance density distributions are substantially overlapped. (Figure 6b,d).

The shape analysis also reveals that the Zernike distances estimated for the BP3 cavity, positioned at the N-terminus of MKK7, are lower compared to that exhibited by BP4 (Figure 6c) regardless of the peptide involved. These findings suggests an overall better predisposition of BP3, in terms of shape complementarity, to the interaction with these peptides in all their possible conformations.

Starting from the STD data and considering the atomic structures DTP3 and SCRB, we also investigated, through the procedure based on the Zernike formalism, the changes in the complementarities between the binding site of the protein and the corresponding interacting peptide. In particular, we analyzed, comparatively for the two peptides, the distribution of the spatial distances between the centroids of the side chain (geometric center of the heavy atoms) of the aromatic residues during the thermal motion in water as calculated by Molecular Dynamics (MD) simulations. This measure allows us to characterize the different conformations of the peptides, recognizing more open conformations from more compact ones.

We also evaluated the correlation between the explored distances with shape complementarity, measured for the putative binding pockets (BP3 and BP4). From these analyses, we found that the aromatic residues of DTP3 (position i and i + 2) explore a very wide range of distances (Figure 7a, blue line), while the distance between the aromatic rings of SCRB (i and i + 1) is on average lower than that observed with DTP3 (Figure 7a, red line). A relevant result for clarifying the molecular mechanisms of the DTP3 binding to MKK7, is the anticorrelation between the aromatic ring distances of the DTP3 peptide with the Zernike shape distance (Figure 7b,c, blue dots). Aromatic distances have a Pearson correlation coefficient value of -0.64 and -0.58 with BS4 and BS3, respectively (p-value less than 10^{-5}). SCRB peptide aromatic distances demonstrate instead no correlation with the Zernike shape distance (Figure 7b,c, red dots). These results clearly demonstrate that the complementarity of DTP3 with BP3 and BP4 is mainly mediated by the possibility of this molecule to increase the distance between the two aromatic rings. In particular, we found that the further the aromatic residues are, the higher the complementary of the peptides with the pockets is. On the other hand, having an almost fixed "aromatic distance", the SCRB peptide cannot achieve the same complementarity for BP3 and BP4 as DTP3.

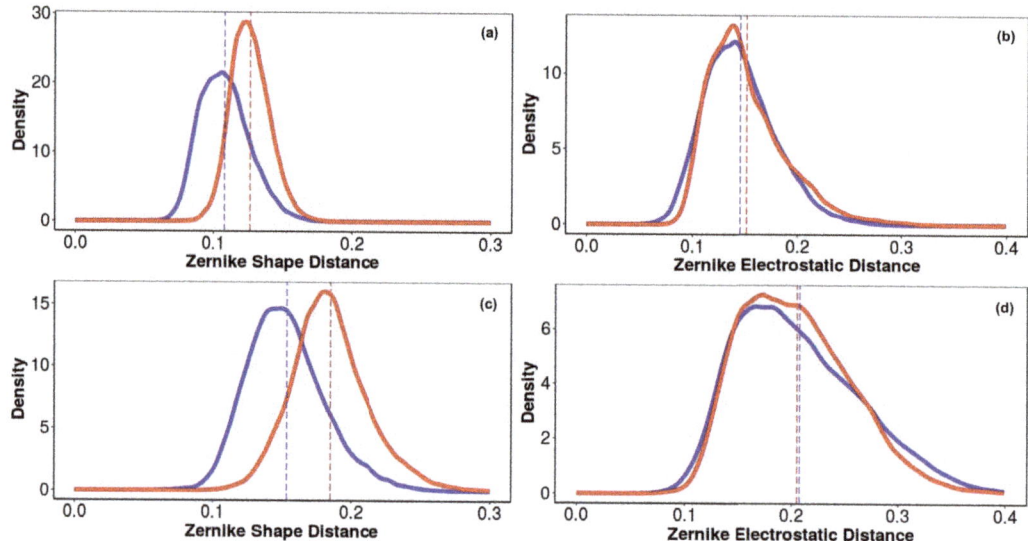

Figure 6. Density distribution of Zernike descriptors calculated for DTP3 and SCRB are reported. Shape and electrostatic complementarity between DTP3 (blue lines) and SCRB (red lines) peptides with BP3 (**a,b**) and BP4 (**c,d**) pockets of the MKK7 surface.

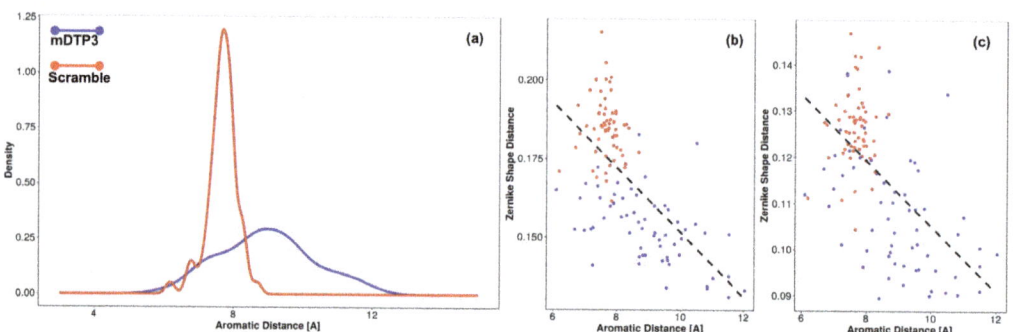

Figure 7. (**a**) Distribution of spatial distances between side chain heavy atoms geometrical center of aromatic residues of DTP3 and SCRB peptides. (**b,c**) Correlation of the distances explored by the peptides with shape complementarity to the binding pockets BP3 and BP4, respectively.

3.5. MKK7-DTP3 Molecular Docking Studies

Subsequently, we obtained a more accurate picture of the binding modalities of DTP3 with BP3 and BP4 by means of a focused molecular docking study. These two cavities were defined in the docking experiment using the residues identified in the previous section, and the docking analyses were performed using the Autodock Vina program. Hydrogen bond (HB) and hydrophobic (HP) contacts between DTP3 and MKK7-KD were estimated using LigPlot+ software [24].

Figure 8a shows the best docked conformation (top-ranked pose) of DTP3 with the BP3 cavity of MKK7-KD ($\Delta G = -11.47$ kcal/mol). The 2D ligand interaction diagram of DTP3 is shown in Figure 8b.

This top-ranked pose suggests a positioning of the tripeptide that is able to make contacts with several protein residues and to adopt an iso-orientation of the D-Tyr[1] and D-

Phe³ aromatic rings and an opposite localization of the D-Arg³ side chain. This is consistent with results from the NMR-STD experiments, although the NMR data were not used as restraints in the docking run. These results are also consistent with Zernike analysis which confirms that the conformation and the relative orientations adopted by D-Tyr¹ and D-Phe³ residues are crucial for the interaction of DTP3 with the MKK7 protein. The residues of the kinase domain involved in hydrogen bonds and hydrophobic interactions with a specific portion of DTP3 are shown in Figure 8b.

In particular, D-Tyr¹ formed two H-bonds with Arg140. The phenyl group of D-Phe³ appears to be embedded in a cavity formed primarily by residues Phe139, Phe183, and Phe186. In this conformation, D-Phe³ may form a potential π-stacking with the β2 Phe139. D-Arg² appears to form two H-bonds with the Ile187 backbone oxygen, while the DTP3 backbone is involved in two H-bonds with Asn118 and Asp119. Taken together, the experimental and computational data point toward the presence of a well-defined and previously unknown binding site in the N-terminal region of MKK7 that is explored by DTP3 molecule. This site, which was found to exhibit allosteric dynamics [5,11], is likely involved in the modulation of the protein-protein interactions with GADD45β [11]. The presence of DTP3 around this N-terminal allosteric site is also consistent with the FITC-tripeptide fluorescence quenching effect induced by the β2 Trp135 side chain [11] located in proximity of the putative DTP3 binding site (Figure 7a).

We also subjected DTP3 to molecular docking at the BP4 site of MKK7 that is located between the αC helix, the activation loop and the D-F-G motif (see Figure 5). The generated docked complexes were examined based on binding affinity values (Kcal/mol) and bonding interaction patterns. The best pose (ΔG = −9.22 kcal/mol according to Autodock Vina program), is reported in Figure 9a. Considering the results, the DTP3/BP4 interface is stabilized by several van der Waals interactions and by a series of intermolecular hydrogen bonds (Figure 9b). Of particular note was the binding mode of DTP3 where the moiety protruded into a hydrophobic pocket in proximity to the αC helix, formed by residues Met 49, Val 123, Ile 148, and Ala 157. This conformation assumed by DTP3 in proximity to the MKK7 surface could destabilize the D–F–G protein motif thus resulting in a MKK conformation alteration.

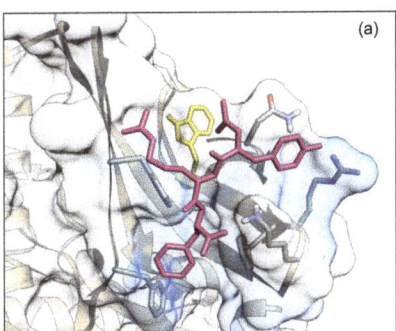 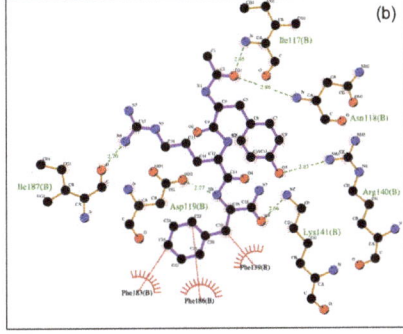

Figure 8. (**a**) Surface model of DTP3 docked to BP3 (cyan) where the protein molecule is shown as surface and DTP3 is shown in stick (magenta). Trp135 located in proximity of the DTP3 binding site is depicted as yellow sticks; (**b**) Interactions of the MKK-KD residues with DTP3 interactions of the MKK-KD residues with DTP3 are displayed in a two dimensional model. The main interactions between the protein and the ligands are shown as dotted lines, hydrogen bonds are in green, while the hydrophobic interactions are shown in red.

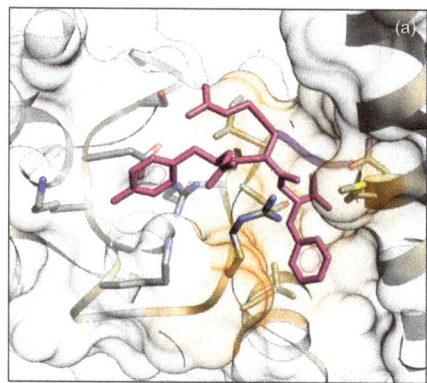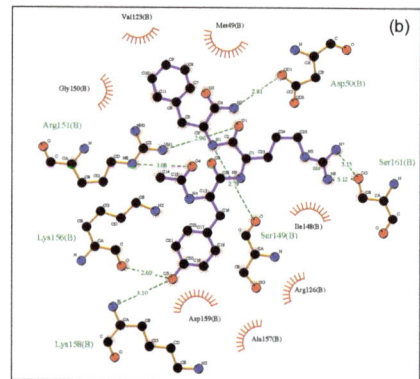

Figure 9. (a) Surface model of DTP3 docked to BP4 cavity (orange) where the protein molecule is shown as surface and DTP3 is shown in stick (magenta); (b) Interactions of the MKK-KD residues with DTP3 are displayed in a two dimensional model. The main interactions between the protein and the ligands are shown as dotted lines, hydrogen bonds are in green, while the hydrophobic interactions are shown in red.

4. Discussion

We have investigated the interaction of DTP3 with the kinase domain of MKK7, the therapeutic target, which is relieved from GADD45β-mediated inhibition upon binding to DTP3, with activation of JNK-dependent apoptosis. Our NMR binding data support the view that DTP3 predominantly interacts with the protein kinase domain via its aromatic side chains and that its arginine residue has a less relevant role in the binding to MKK7. A detailed computational investigation performed by molecular dynamics, prediction of binding sites and molecular docking studies has further elucidated the localization of the best putative MKK7-KD binding site of DPT3 and provided an atomistic view of the interactions established with the protein. A Zernicke analysis has also clarified the nature of the MKK7/DTP3 interactions and provided a basis for the selectivity of DTP3 as compared to the control scrambled (SCRB) peptide. The NMR-STD study has provided information about the peptide surface involved in the interaction with MKK7. Parallel experiments suggested that high, non-biologically relevant concentrations of the SCRB peptide can also force an interaction with MKK7. However, this interaction is lost at concentrations in the therapeutic nanomolar range. Consistently, the STD technique works with dimensionally different molecule pairs that interact with KD values in the millimolar to low micromolar range (10^{-3}–10^{-8} M), ensuring a proper exchange between the bound and free ligand states that originate the STD signal. Thus, given the NMR technique experimental limitations, it is possible that these experiments only provide a partial view of the molecular MKK7/DTP3 complex and the peptide interacting atoms. Similarly, on the basis of previous data with other control D-tripeptides [5], it is possible that the central arginine also plays a role in the interaction, contributing to the higher affinity measured by fluorescence. The STD intensities of the DTP3 protons demonstrate that the aromatic side chains of D-Tyr[1] and D-Phe[3] come into contact with the MKK7 surface closer to the side chain of the central residue D-Arg[2]. The Zernike analysis further suggests that the distance between the two aromatic side chains is critical for an efficient recognition. Thus, altogether, the data suggest that the hydrophobic interactions mediated by the phenylalanine and tyrosine rings play a main role in the docking of DTP3 to MKK7 and possibly in the allosteric effect leading to the dissociation of GADD45β from MKK7.

5. Conclusions

The molecular complex formed by MKK7 and GADD45β has been identified as a key therapeutic target downstream of NF-κB in MM. DTP3 effectively blocks the GADD45β/MKK7 interaction, thereby restoring MKK7 kinase activity, and as such is a promising candidate therapeutic for clinical development in oncology. Here, we investigated the interaction of DTP3 with the kinase domain of MKK7 and further elucidated the main molecular determinants underpinning this interaction. We have identified the key hydrophobic groups involved in the MKK7/DTP3 binding and clarified the peptide geometries and main kinase binding pockets, thus advancing the understanding of the mechanism of recognition. Together, the experimental data from our NMR, fluorescence, and computational studies point toward an interaction of the tripeptide with the protein N-terminal region, in agreement with previous observations, and corroborate the hypothesis of a dynamic interaction that ultimately leads to dissociation of the GADD45β/MKK7 complex. These findings improve the understanding of the interactions between these molecules and provide further molecular details for the generation of novel MKK7/GADD45β inhibitors.

Supplementary Materials: The following are available online at https://www.mdpi.com/2227-9059/9/1/20/s1. Figure S1: Comparison of 1D spectrum of DTP3 with STD of DTP3/MKK7-KD. Figure S2: Comparison of 1D spectrum of SCRB peptide with STD of SCRB/MKK7-KD. Figure S3: Comparison of STD full spectra acquired at R20 of DTP3 and SCRB vs MKK7-KD. Figure S4: STD spectra at different peptide/protein R ratios of peptide used as negative control. Figure S5: Evolution of MKK7 gyration radius over the MD trajectory. Figure S6: (a) Root Mean Square Deviation (RMSD) values assumed by the 500 structures of MKK7 selected from the MD simulation (b) Principal Component Analysis of the 500 MKK7 frames employing protein alpha carbon atoms. Figure S7: (a) Analysis of local conformational mobility of the BP3 and BP4. Root Mean Square Fluctuation (RMSF) values are reported. (b) BP3 cavity volume evolution during the simulation. Table S1: Chemical shifts of DTP3 at peptide/KD R100 molar ratio. Table S2: Chemical shifts of SCRB at peptide/KD R100 molar ratio.

Author Contributions: Methodology—protein and peptide preparation, binding experiments, A.S. and E.I.; methodology—NMR experiments, L.C., L.F., and G.D.; methodology—computational experiments, L.D.R., E.M., and D.R.; Data analysis A.S., M.R., L.F., G.D., L.T., M.D., G.F., R.R., and A.C. Writing—original draft preparation A.S., M.R., L.F., G.D., E.M, and D.R. Writing-review and editing M.R., D.R., L.F., G.D., and G.F. Conceptualization: M.R., A.S., M.D., E.M., and D.R.; All authors have read and agreed to the published version of the manuscript.

Funding: This research was funded by Sapienza University of Rome, Regione Campania for the projects: (i) Development of novel therapeutic approaches for treatment-resistant neoplastic diseases (SATIN); (ii) Fighting Cancer resistance: Multidisciplinary integrated Platform for a technological Innovative Approach to Oncotherapies (Campania Oncotherapies); (iii) NANOCAN, NANOfotonica per la lotta al CANcro. This work was supported in part by an NIHR Imperial Biomedical Research Centre (BRC) Push for Impact award to G.F. Infrastructure support for this research was provided in part by the NIHR Imperial BRC.

Institutional Review Board Statement: Not applicable.

Informed Consent Statement: Not applicable.

Data Availability Statement: The data presented in this study are available on request from the corresponding author.

Acknowledgments: We wish to acknowledge Leopoldo Zona and Maurizio Amendola for their support in this paper.

Conflicts of Interest: M.R., G.F., and L.T. are listed as inventors in patents describing the use of DTP3 as a therapeutic agent against multiple myeloma.

References

1. Chang, L.; Karin, M. Mammalian MAP kinase signalling cascades. *Nature* **2001**, *410*, 37–40. [CrossRef] [PubMed]
2. Cuevas, B.D.; Abell, A.N.; Johnson, G.L. Role of mitogen-activated protein kinase kinase kinases in signal integration. *Oncogene* **2007**, *26*, 3159–3171. [CrossRef] [PubMed]
3. Park, J.G.; Aziz, N.; Cho, J.Y. MKK7, the essential regulator of JNK signaling involved in cancer cell survival: A newly emerging anticancer therapeutic target. *Ther. Adv. Med. Oncol.* **2019**, *11*, 1758835919875574. [CrossRef] [PubMed]

4. Haeusgen, W.; Herdegen, T.; Waetzig, V. The bottleneck of JNK signaling: Molecular and functional characteristics of MKK4 and MKK7. *Eur. J. Cell Biol.* **2011**, *90*, 536–544. [CrossRef] [PubMed]
5. Tornatore, L.; Sandomenico, A.; Raimondo, D.; Low, C.; Rocci, A.; Tralau-Stewart, C.; Capece, D.; D'Andrea, D.; Bua, M.; Boyle, E.; et al. Cancer-Selective Targeting of the Nf-KB Survival Pathway With Gadd45B/Mkk7 Inhibitors. *Cancer Cell* **2014**, *26*, 495–508. [CrossRef]
6. Shraga, A.; Olshvang, E.; Davidzohn, N.; Khoshkenar, P.; Germain, N.; Shurrush, K.; Carvalho, S.; Avram, L.; Albeck, S.; Unger, T.; et al. Covalent Docking Identifies a Potent and Selective MKK7 Inhibitor. *Cell Chem. Biol.* **2019**, *26*, 98–108.e5. [CrossRef]
7. Pettersen, E.F.; Goddard, T.D.; Huang, C.C.; Couch, G.S.; Greenblatt, D.M.; Meng, E.C.; Ferrin, T.E. UCSF Chimera—A visualization system for exploratory research and analysis. *J. Comput. Chem.* **2004**, *25*, 1605–1612. [CrossRef]
8. Tornatore, L.; Capece, D.; D'Andrea, D.; Begalli, F.; Verzella, D.; Bennett, J.; Acton, G.; Campbell, E.A.; Kelly, J.; Tarbit, M.; et al. Preclinical toxicology and safety pharmacology of the first-in-class GADD45β/MKK7 inhibitor and clinical candidate, DTP3. *Toxicol. Rep.* **2019**, *6*, 369–379. [CrossRef]
9. Tornatore, L.; Capece, D.; D'Andrea, D.; Begalli, F.; Verzella, D.; Bennett, J.; Acton, G.; Campbell, E.A.; Kelly, J.; Tarbit, M.; et al. Clinical proof of concept for a safe and effective NF-κB-targeting strategy in multiple myeloma. *Br. J. Haematol.* **2019**, *185*, 588. [CrossRef]
10. Tornatore, L.; Marasco, D.; Dathan, N.; Vitale, R.M.; Benedetti, E.; Papa, S.; Franzoso, G.; Ruvo, M.; Monti, S.M. Gadd45β forms a Homodimeric Complex that Binds Tightly to MKK7. *J. Mol. Biol.* **2008**, *378*, 97–111. [CrossRef]
11. Rega, C.; Russo, R.; Focà, A.; Sandomenico, A.; Iaccarino, E.; Raimondo, D.; Milanetti, E.; Tornatore, L.; Franzoso, G.; Pedone, P.V.; et al. Probing the interaction interface of the GADD45β/MKK7 and MKK7/DTP3 complexes by chemical cross-linking mass spectrometry. *Int. J. Biol. Macromol.* **2018**, *114*, 114–123. [CrossRef] [PubMed]
12. Schröder, M.; Tan, L.; Wang, J.; Liang, Y.; Gray, N.S.; Knapp, S.; Chaikuad, A. Catalytic Domain Plasticity of MKK7 Reveals Structural Mechanisms of Allosteric Activation and Diverse Targeting Opportunities. *Cell Chem. Biol.* **2020**, *27*, 1285–1295. [CrossRef] [PubMed]
13. Mayer, M.; Meyer, B. Group epitope mapping by saturation transfer difference NMR to identify segments of a ligand in direct contact with a protein receptor. *J. Am. Chem. Soc.* **2001**, *123*, 6108–6117. [CrossRef] [PubMed]
14. Zoete, V.; Cuendet, M.A.; Grosdidier, A.; Michielin, O. SwissParam: A fast force field generation tool for small organic molecules. *J. Comput. Chem.* **2011**, *32*, 2359–2368. [CrossRef] [PubMed]
15. Mark, P.; Nilsson, L. Structure and dynamics of the TIP3P, SPC, and SPC/E water models at 298 K. *J. Phys. Chem. A* **2001**, *105*, 9954–9960. [CrossRef]
16. Bussi, G.; Donadio, D.; Parrinello, M. Canonical sampling through velocity rescaling. *J. Chem. Phys.* **2007**, *126*, 014101. [CrossRef]
17. Abraham, M.J.; Murtola, T.; Schulz, R.; Páll, S.; Smith, J.C.; Hess, B.; Lindah, E. Gromacs: High performance molecular simulations through multi-level parallelism from laptops to supercomputers. *SoftwareX* **2015**, *1–2*, 19–25. [CrossRef]
18. Fogolari, F.; Corazza, A.; Yarra, V.; Jalaru, A.; Viglino, P.; Esposito, G. Bluues: A program for the analysis of the electrostatic properties of proteins based on generalized Born radii. *BMC Bioinform.* **2012**, *13*, S18. [CrossRef]
19. Dolinsky, T.J.; Nielsen, J.E.; McCammon, J.A.; Baker, N.A. PDB2PQR: An automated pipeline for the setup of Poisson-Boltzmann electrostatics calculations. *Nucleic Acids Res.* **2004**, *32*, W665. [CrossRef]
20. Venkatraman, V.; Sael, L.; Kihara, D. Potential for protein surface shape analysis using spherical harmonics and 3d zernike descriptors. *Cell Biochem. Biophys.* **2009**, *54*, 23–32. [CrossRef]
21. Krivák, R.; Hoksza, D. P2Rank: Machine learning based tool for rapid and accurate prediction of ligand binding sites from protein structure. *J. Cheminform.* **2018**, *10*, 39. [CrossRef] [PubMed]
22. Trott, O.; Olson, A.J. AutoDock Vina: Improving the speed and accuracy of docking with a new scoring function, efficient optimization, and multithreading. *J. Comput. Chem.* **2009**, *31*, 455–461. [CrossRef] [PubMed]
23. Feinstein, W.P.; Brylinski, M. Calculating an optimal box size for ligand docking and virtual screening against experimental and predicted binding pockets. *J. Cheminform.* **2015**, *7*, 18. [CrossRef]
24. Laskowski, R.A.; Swindells, M.B. LigPlot+: Multiple ligand-protein interaction diagrams for drug discovery. *J. Chem. Inf. Model.* **2011**, *51*, 2778–2786. [CrossRef]
25. Sandomenico, A.; Russo, A.; Palmieri, G.; Bergamo, P.; Gogliettino, M.; Falcigno, L.; Ruvo, M. Small peptide inhibitors of acetyl-peptide hydrolase having an uncommon mechanism of inhibition and a stable bent conformation. *J. Med. Chem.* **2012**, *55*, 2102–2111. [CrossRef] [PubMed]
26. Di Rienzo, L.; Milanetti, E.; Lepore, R.; Olimpieri, P.P.; Tramontano, A. Superposition-free comparison and clustering of antibody binding sites: Implications for the prediction of the nature of their antigen. *Sci. Rep.* **2017**, *7*, 1–10. [CrossRef]
27. Kihara, D.; Sael, L.; Chikhi, R.; Esquivel-Rodriguez, J. Molecular Surface Representation Using 3D Zernike Descriptors for Protein Shape Comparison and Docking. *Curr. Protein Pept. Sci.* **2011**, *12*, 520–530. [CrossRef]
28. Di Rienzo, L.; Milanetti, E.; Alba, J.; D'Abramo, M. Quantitative Characterization of Binding Pockets and Binding Complementarity by Means of Zernike Descriptors. *J. Chem. Inf. Model.* **2020**, *2020*, 1390–1398. [CrossRef]
29. Daberdaku, S.; Ferrari, C. Exploring the potential of 3D Zernike descriptors and SVM for protein-protein interface prediction. *BMC Bioinform.* **2018**, *19*, 35. [CrossRef]

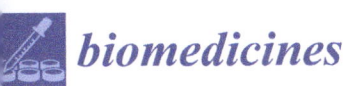

Article

UV-B Filter Octylmethoxycinnamate Alters the Vascular Contractility Patterns in Pregnant Women with Hypothyroidism

Margarida Lorigo [1,2,3], Carla Quintaneiro [4], Luiza Breitenfeld [1,2] and Elisa Cairrao [1,2,3,*]

1. CICS-UBI, Health Sciences Research Centre, University of Beira Interior, 6200-506 Covilhã, Portugal; margarida.lorigo@gmail.com (M.L.); luiza@fcsaude.ubi.pt (L.B.)
2. FCS-UBI, Faculty of Health Sciences, University of Beira Interior, 6200-506 Covilhã, Portugal
3. C4-UBI, Cloud Computing Competence Centre, University of Beira Interior, 6200-501 Covilhã, Portugal
4. Centre for Environmental and Marine Studies (CESAM), Department of Biology, University of Aveiro, 3810-193 Aveiro, Portugal; cquintaneiro@ua.pt
* Correspondence: ecairrao@fcsaude.ubi.pt; Tel.: +351-275-329049

Citation: Lorigo, M.; Quintaneiro, C.; Breitenfeld, L.; Cairrao, E. UV-B Filter Octylmethoxycinnamate Alters the Vascular Contractility Patterns in Pregnant Women with Hypothyroidism. *Biomedicines* **2021**, *9*, 115. https://doi.org/10.3390/biomedicines9020115

Academic Editor: Fabio Altieri
Received: 22 December 2020
Accepted: 22 January 2021
Published: 26 January 2021

Publisher's Note: MDPI stays neutral with regard to jurisdictional claims in published maps and institutional affiliations.

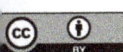

Copyright: © 2021 by the authors. Licensee MDPI, Basel, Switzerland. This article is an open access article distributed under the terms and conditions of the Creative Commons Attribution (CC BY) license (https://creativecommons.org/licenses/by/4.0/).

Abstract: Increasing evidence relating the exposure and/or bioaccumulation of endocrine-disrupting compounds (EDCs) with cardiovascular system are arising. Octylmethoxycinnamate (OMC) is the most widely used UV-B filter and as EDC interacts with TH receptors. However, their effects on thyroid diseases during pregnancy remain unknown. The purpose of this work was to assess the short- and long-term effects of OMC on arterial tonus of pregnant women with hypothyroidism. To elucidate this, human umbilical artery (HUA) rings without endothelium were used to explore the vascular effects of OMC by arterial and cellular experiments. The binding energy and the modes of interaction of the OMC into the active center of the TSHR and THRα were analyzed by molecular docking studies. Our results indicated that OMC altered the contractility patterns of HUA contracted with serotonin, histamine and KCl, possibly due to an interference with serotonin and histamine receptors or an involvement of the Ca^{2+} channels. The molecular docking analysis show that OMC compete with T_3 for the binding center of THRα. Taken together, these findings pointed out to alterations in HUA reactivity as result of OMC-exposure, which may be involved in the development and increased risk of cardiovascular diseases.

Keywords: thyroid diseases; endocrine disruptor compound; human umbilical artery; vascular homeostasis

1. Introduction

The use of personal care products (PCPs) containing UV filters is a common practice in the population [1,2]. Recently, their safety has been questioned since several UV filters are classified as endocrine-disrupting compounds (EDCs). Among the main endocrine disruptive activities of EDCs the modulation of thyroid activity is highlighted [1], with studies reporting that EDCs exposure may be correlated with the incidence of thyroid diseases [3,4]. This is particularly relevant on populations more susceptible to endocrine disruption, such as pregnant women and developing fetuses [1,5–8].

The EDCs can disrupt maternal thyroid hormones (TH) production [9–11] inducing hypo- and hyperthyroidism. People with these pathologies have higher risk of developing cardiovascular diseases (CVDs), since small changes in TH levels can modulate vascular homeostasis [12,13]. However, the fact that the effects of UV filters acting as EDCs of the human thyroid system (and their consequences at the vascular level) during pregnancy remain unknown is a major concern.

Octylmethoxycinnamate (OMC) is probably the world's most widely used UV-B filter [14] in the cosmetics industry [15]. In addition to its presence in hair products, lipsticks, makeup, perfumes and skin care products [16–19], the OMC is also widely found in powder samples [20], pool, tap and drinking water [21–23], increasing human exposure to this UV filter. Due to its high lipophilic character, low molecular weight and poor degradability, OMC is an emerging contaminant that can be bioaccumulated in several organisms [15]. Recently, this UV-B filter was banned in Hawaii owing to its toxic effects on marine ecosystems [2,24]. The toxic effects to other species have alarmed the general public about its potential to have impacts on human health when applied in human skin [2,25,26]. Indeed, the OMC can penetrate through the epidermis and dermis, and reach the systemic circulation. Consequently, OMC has been detected in urine, plasma [27], breast milk samples [19,28] and placenta [29], which raises concerns about its adverse consequences on fetal development. Several studies pointed OMC as an EDC, which have an endocrine disrupting potential by interaction with TH receptors [30,31]. In rats, it was reported that OMC-induced changes on iodine intake, on 3,5,3'Triiodothyronine (T_3), thyroxine (T_4) and thyroid-stimulating hormone (TSH) levels, on iodothyronine deiodinase 1 (DIO1) activity, on TSHR expression levels and on thyroid weight (see review [25]). Regarding human studies, OMC can modulate thyroid hormone receptor (THR) in human hepatocarcinoma cell lines (HepG2) [30] and is a deiodinase-disrupting chemical since it alters the expression of related genes (e.g., type II iodothyronine deiodinase (DIO2)) as reported by Song, et al. in human neuroblastoma cells [31]. However, other authors suggested that the amount of OMC absorbed by the skin after topical application does not interfere with TH homeostasis in human adults [32]. Although not entirely consensual, these results pointed an interference of OMC in the human thyroid system. However, to our knowledge no studies were performed to explore the effects of OMC in the human vasculature of pregnant women with thyroid diseases.

In this context, the purpose of the current study was to analyze the short- and long-term effects of the UV-filter OMC on arterial tonus of pregnant women with hypothyroidism. To elucidate this, human umbilical artery (HUA) rings were used in ex vivo organ bath experiments to analyze the effect and the mode of action (MOA) of OMC on the vascular contractility. Furthermore, the HUA were also used to perform cultures of vascular smooth muscle cells (SMC), which were used to evaluate cellular contractility by the planar cell surface area (PCSA) experiments to support data from organ bath. Moreover, the binding energy and the modes of interaction of the OMC into the active centre of the thyroid stimulating hormone receptor (TSHR) and thyroid hormone receptor alpha (THRα) were analyzed by molecular docking studies.

2. Materials and Methods

Experimental studies were performed in Health Sciences Research Centre (CICS-UBI, University of Beira Interior, Covilhã, Portugal). This work was approved by the local ethic committees (CHUCB, No.33/2018, 18 July 2018, Centro Hospitalar Universitário da Cova da Beira E.P.E., Covilhã, Portugal) and (ULS-Guarda, No.02324/2019, 27 February 2019, Unidade Local de Saúde da Guarda, Guarda, Portugal). Pregnant women gave written informed consent in accordance with the principles of the Declaration of Helsinki.

2.1. Sample Collection

Human umbilical cord (UC) samples were collected (n = 33) from normal full-term pregnancies after vaginal delivery. All donor mothers were under medication with folic acid during the first trimester of gestation or iron supplementation during the last trimester of gestation. There were two groups of pregnant women: (1) healthy donor mothers (control group) and (2) donor mothers with hypothyroidism (hypothyroidism group) treated with oral levothyroxine (Euthyrox, 2.5 µg) in generic tablets formulation, according to the standard therapy for patients with hypothyroidism [33]. Sample collection was performed after signing their written informed consent. Samples were resected from the proximal half of the UC (20 cm) and collected within 10–20 min after delivery. The tissue was immediately stored in cold (4 °C) for 4–24 h in sterile physiological saline (PSS) solution supplemented with antibiotics (penicillin, 5 U/mL, streptomycin, 5 µg/mL and amphotericin B, 12.5 ng/mL) and antiproteases (leupeptin, 0.45 mg/L; benzamidine,

26 mg/L and trypsin inhibitor, 10 mg/L) to avoid contamination and tissue degradation, respectively.

2.2. Preparation of HUA Rings for Vascular Reactivity Studies

Short- and long-term effects of OMC on vascular contractility patterns in pregnant women with and without hypothyroidism were investigated. The short-term effects were analyzed in HUA rings that were not incubated. To analyze the long-term effects of OMC, the HUA were preincubated 24 h with OMC at 50 µmol/L. Then, rings were used to perform vascular reactivity studies, more specifically, the arterial contractility experiments using the organ bath technique.

Human umbilical vessels were dissected as described by Cairrao, et al. [34]. Briefly, HUA were dissected free from Wharton's jelly and cut into rings of 3–5 mm. Vascular endothelium was mechanically removed by gentle rubbing of arterial lumen with a cotton bud. The rings were mounted throughout two stainless steel wire hooks inserted through the lumen. HUA rings were suspended in the organ bath chambers LE01.004 (Letica, Madrid, Spain) filled with 20 mL of Krebs-bicarbonate solution maintained at a 37 °C and aerated with 95% O_2 and 5% CO_2 (pH = 7.4). Changes in isometric tension were measured in millinewton (mN) with isometric force transducers (model TRI201, Panlab SA, Madrid, Spain) coupled to an ML118/D Quad Bridge amplifier (AD Instruments, Oxford, UK) and an interface Power Lab/4SP ML750 (ADInstruments, Oxford, UK). Chart5 Power Lab software program (ADInstruments, Oxford, UK) was used to chart recording and to data acquisition. Baseline load of 20–25 mN was initially placed on the HUA rings. The rings were allowed to equilibrate for 45 min (during which the Krebs solution was replaced every 15 min) in order for the rings stretch to an optical resting tension (basal tension) of 20–25 mN.

2.3. Arterial Contractility Experiments

The tension recordings of HUA were performed according to our previous work [35]. Following the equilibration period and before starting the experiments, rings were transiently challenged with a supramaximal concentration of 5-HT (1 µmol/L) to assess the functional state of each vessel. Rings with a maximum contraction of <10 mN were not used [34]. Afterward, responses were stopped by washing rings with fresh Krebs solution. Vascular rings recuperated for at least 45 min, during which Krebs solution was replaced every 15 min.

In the first series of experiments, HUA rings were exposed to cumulative doses of OMC (0.001–50 µmol/L), in six steps, to evaluate their effect on basal tension of the arteries. Then, rings were contracted with 1 µmol/L of serotonin (5-HT) and the produced response was analyzed.

The next step was the analysis of OMC short-term effects. Each ring was precontracted using 5-HT (1 µmol/L), histamine (His, 10 µmol/L) or potassium chloride (KCl, 60 mmol/L). Cumulative pharmacologic concentrations (0.001–50 µmol/L) were used according to the previous studies [35,36]. Control experiments were performed using solvent (ethanol) at same % used to dissolve the OMC.

The long-term effects of 50 µmol/L of OMC were also analyzed, to observe if there is an alteration of the contractility patterns induced by exposure to OMC. In this sense, the same procedures described above to short-term effects were repeated. To avoid photodegradation of OMC [37,38] all the arterial contractility experiments were carried out with no UV light exposure.

2.4. Primary Cultures of HUA Smooth Muscle Cells (HUASMCs)

Cultures of HUA smooth muscle cells (HUASMCs) were obtained through explants of the umbilical artery, as previously described [35]. The SMC were grown at 37 °C in a 5% CO_2 atmosphere in culture medium DMEM-F12 supplemented with bovine serum albumin (BSA, 0.5%), heat-inactivated fetal bovine serum (FBS, 5%), epidermal growth factor (EGF,

5 µg/mL), fibroblast growth factor (FGF, 0.5 ng/mL), heparin (2 µg/mL), insulin (5 µg/mL), penicillin (5 U/mL), streptomycin (5 µg/mL) and amphotericin B (12.5 ng/mL). The culture medium was changed three times a week. When cell growth reached a confluent culture, a trypsinization with commercial trypsin-EDTA solution (0.025%) was performed. Each culture was used until P4. HUASMC from the different passages were used to perform cellular contractility experiments (see below). Before experiments, HUASMC were placed 24 h in culture medium without FBS (FBS-free culture medium), at 37 °C in a 5% CO_2 atmosphere, to express the required contractile phenotype [39,40].

2.5. Preparation of HUASMC for Vascular Reactivity Studies

Short- and long-term effects of OMC on vascular contractility patterns in pregnant women with and without hypothyroidism were investigated. Short-term effects were analyzed with non-incubated HUASMC. Long-term effects of OMC were analyzed using HUASMC that were preincubated 24 h with OMC at 50 µmol/L. Then, cells were used to perform vascular reactivity studies, namely, to evaluate cellular contractility using planar cell surface area (PCSA) technique.

HUASMC were prepared as described by our group [35,41], with some modifications as described above. Briefly, the cells were trypsinized and planted in specific Petri dishes, at 37 °C in a 5% CO_2 atmosphere for 2 h. Then, the cells were washed with a specific saline solution (PCSA solution) and placed in an inverted fluorescence microscope (Zeiss Axio Observer Z1, Jena, Germany) with an incubation system (maintained at 37 °C) and a high-speed monochrome digital camera Axio Cam Hsm (Zeiss, Jena, Germany). Changes in the cellular area were determined in micrometres^2 (μm^2) by measuring the area along time through serial photographs taken before and after all experimental additions. Axion vision 4.8 software (Zeiss, Jena, Germany) was used to determine PCSA data. Measurements of the actual area were calculated using supplementary "Automatic Measurement program" (Zeiss). For data treatment 4–8 cells/photograph were chosen and a suitable sharp margin for its planimetric analysis was always considered.

2.6. Cellular Contractility Experiments

In the first series of experiments, the effect of 50 µmol/L of OMC on basal tension of HUASMC was evaluated. Then, SMC were contracted with 5-HT (1 µmol/L) and the produced effect was analyzed.

The next step was to analyze the short-term effect of OMC (50 µmol/L) on the contractile force of precontracted HUASMC, which were contracted using 5-HT (1 µmol/L) or His (10 µmol/L). After 20 min, a steady contraction was achieved, and 50 µmol/L of OMC was added to the PCSA medium to record the vascular effect.

The long-term effect of OMC 50 µmol/L was also analyzed, to observe if there is an alteration of the contractility patterns induced by exposure to OMC. In this sense, similar methodology described for short-term effects was used to evaluate the long-term effects of OMC.

The chosen concentration of OMC was 50 µmol/L since it is the concentration where the maximum effect was achieved according to organ bath data. Control experiments were always performed using solvent (ethanol) at same % used to dissolve OMC. Cellular contractility experiments were carried out with no UV light exposure to avoid OMC photodegradation.

2.7. Drugs, Chemicals, and Solutions

The umbilical cords samples were stored in PSS solution (pH = 7.4) with the composition: EDTA (0.50 mmol/L), KCl (5 mmol/L), HEPES (10 mmol/L), $MgCl_2$ (2 mmol/L), $NaHCO_3$ (10 mmol/L), KH_2PO_4 (0.5 mmol/L), NaH_2PO_4 (0.5 mmol/L), glucose (10 mmol/L), NaCl (110 mmol/L) and $CaCl_2$ (0.16 mmol/L).

The composition of the Krebs' modified solution (used in organ bath experiments) was: KCl (5.0 mmol/L), EDTA (0.03 mmol/L), $MgSO_4 \cdot 7H_2O$ (1.2 mmol/L), KH_2PO_4

(1.2 mmol/L), ascorbic acid (0.6 mmol/L), NaCl (119 mmol/L), CaCl$_2$ (0.5 mmol/L), glucose (11 mmol/L) and NaHCO$_3$ (25 mmol/L) with a pH of 7.4.

The composition of the PCSA solution (used in PCSA experiments) was: NaCl (124.0 mmol/L), HEPES (5.0 mmol/L), tetraethylammonium sodium salt (TEA, 10.0 mmol/L), glucose (6.0 mmol/L), CaCl$_2$ (5.0 mmol/L) and KCl (4.5 mmol/L) with a pH of 7.4.

All drugs and chemicals were purchased from Sigma-Aldrich Química (Sintra, Portugal). Stock solutions were prepared by dissolving OMC in absolute ethanol and by dissolving all the other drugs in distilled water. All of the stock solutions were stored at −20 °C. Final solutions of OMC and ethanol control were prepared daily by dilution with Krebs solution or FBS-free culture medium (according to each experiment). The final concentration of solvent never exceeded 0.05%.

2.8. Statistical Analysis

In arterial contractility experiments, the tension was expressed in millinewton (mN) of force elicited by HUA-rings in the presence of 5-HT, His or KCl 60 mmol/L. The relaxant responses induced by OMC were expressed as a % of reduction of the maximal contraction induced by vasoconstriction drugs. Results were expressed as mean ± standard error of the mean (S.E.M) of the number of HUA used (n).

Concerning cellular contractility experiments, the area achieved by HUASMC in the presence of 5-HT or His was expressed in micrometres^2 (μm^2). The relaxant responses induced by OMC were expressed as a % of reduction of the maximal area induced by vasoconstriction drugs. Results were expressed as mean ± standard error of the mean (S.E.M) of the number of the HUA used to obtain smooth muscle cells (n).

All statistical analysis was performed using SigmaStat Statistical Analysis System version 3.5 (2006) for a significance level of 0.05 and the graphic design was performed in the Software Origin 8.5.1. To analyze differences on the tension and areas induced by the contractile agents or in the % of relaxation of HUA and HUASMC, the two-way ANOVA followed by the Holm-Sidak (parametric) post-hoc test was used. This procedure was performed to compare the interactions between factors (pathological conditions and incubation with OMC) and to identify the significantly differences. When necessary, data sets were log$_{10}$ transformed to achieve normal distribution. These criteria were checked by the Levene's mean test and the Kolmogorov–Smirnov for homoscedasticity and normality, respectively.

2.9. Molecular Docking Studies

The Autodock4 program (http://autodock.scripps.edu/) was chosen to calculate the binding energy and the modes of interaction of the OMC into the active centre of the TSHR and TRHα. The 3D structural coordinates for selected target proteins TSHR and TRHα were obtained from the Protein Data Bank (https://www.rcsb.org/) and OMC was obtained from the Database of Endocrine Disrupting Chemicals and Their Toxicity profiles (DEDuCT) (https://cb.imsc.res.in/deduct/). The crystal structure of TSHR (PDB ID: 2XWT) at 1.90 Å co-complexed with its natural ligand, 2-acetamido-2-deoxy-beta-D-glucopyranose (NAG) was retrieved. Similarity, the crystal structure of TRHα (PDB ID: 2H79) at 1.87 Å co-complexed with its natural ligand, 3,5,3′Triiodothyronine (T3) was downloaded.

The Autodock Tools 1.5.6 and Quimera 1.15 software's were used to prepare the proteins and ligands, respectively (removing water molecules, merging non-polar hydrogens atoms and adding Gasteiger partial charges) [42]. The structures of the ligands were designed in 2D using the ChemBioDraw 18.2 software and their PubChem compound identities (CIDs) and Chemical Abstracts Service Registry Number (CASRN) are presented in Table 1. To obtain 3D structures, hydrogen atoms were added, and energy minimization and geometry optimization were performed by the MMFF94 force field using the ChemBio3D 13.0 software. For the docking simulations all the structure files were saved in PDBQT format.

Table 1. Nomenclature, commonly used abbreviations, PubChem IDs and the Chemical Abstracts Service Registry Number (CASRN) of ligands for molecular docking studies with the thyroid stimulating hormone receptor (TSHR) and thyroid hormone receptor alpha (TRHα).

S. No	Name	Abbreviation	PubChem ID	CASRN
1	3,5,3′Triiodothyronine	T_3	5920	6893-02-3
2	2-acetamido-2-deoxy-beta-D-glucopyranose	NAG	24139	7512-17-6
3	octylmethoxycinnamate	OMC	5355130	5466-77-3

The Autogrid 4 was used to perform the calculations of the grid map based on the coordinates of each crystal protein structure active centre. The grid boxes with the dimensions size of 14 × 26 × 16 Å and 30 × 24 × 32 Å (along x, y, and z) with grid spacing of 0.375 Å was constructed around the active site of TSHR and TRHα, respectively.

The validation of molecular docking was achieved by RMSD values less than 2 Å and the results were subsequently confirmed using Autodock Vina. The Lamarkian genetic algorithm by Autodock 4 was used to perform all docking calculations and the remaining docking parameters were maintained as default. Finally, a total of 10 hybrid runs were obtained for each simulation and the dominating configuration of the binding complex with minimum binding energy (ΔG) was analyzed. The interactions between OMC and the selected target proteins within their active centers were visualized using the Quimera 1.15 software.

3. Results

3.1. Contractility Experiments in HUA

Direct application of different concentrations of OMC (0.001–50 µmol/L) on the control group (pregnant without pathology) and in the hypothyroidism group (pregnant with hypothyroidism) did not change their basal tension. Moreover, the incubation of 50 µmol/L of OMC did not change their basal tension. The solvent used (ethanol 0.05%) in control and hypothyroidism groups did not have an effect on the basal tension (data not shown).

3.1.1. Tension Measurements of Arteries Contracted with 5-HT, His and KCl

The tension produced by 5-HT contraction in the two groups are present in Figure 1A. The results show a statistically interaction between the pathological conditions and the preincubation with OMC ($p = 0.026$). The incubation with 50 µmol/L of OMC induced a significantly higher contraction of 5-HT in the hypothyroidism group.

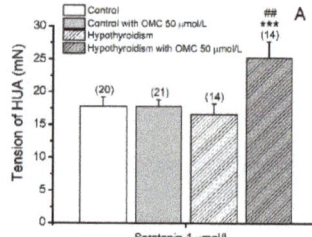
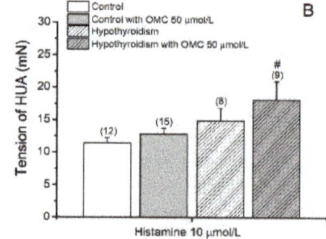
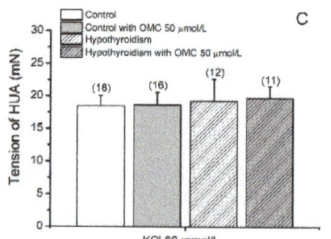

Figure 1. Tension (mN) (at time 15 min) of the human umbilical artery (HUA) rings without (control) and with hypothyroidism incubated with octylmethoxycinnamate (OMC, 0 and 50 µmol/L) and contracted by (**A**) serotonin (5-HT; 1 µmol/L), (**B**) histamine (His; 10 µmol/L) and (**C**) potassium chloride (KCl; 60 mmol/L). Each bar represents the mean, vertical lines the S.E.M. and the number within brackets the n. Asterisk * represents a significant difference versus incubation: *** $p < 0.001$, and hashtag # represents a significant difference versus hypothyroidism: # $p < 0.05$ and ## $p < 0.01$; two-way ANOVA method followed by Holm–Sidak post-hoc tests.

The contraction with His produced stables contractions only in arteries from control groups (Figure 2). For this reason, the tensions present in Figure 1B were attained at

15 min. The HUA from the hypothyroidism group incubated with 50 µmol/L of OMC produced a higher contraction with His (18.13 ± 2.80 mN, p = 0.018) when compared with the control group.

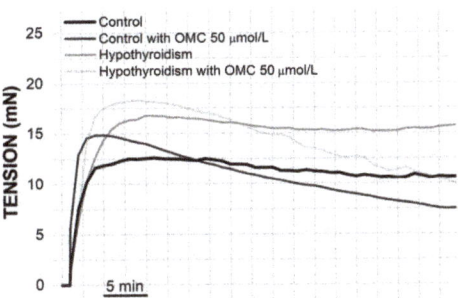

Figure 2. Real tension (mN) of the human umbilical artery (HUA)-rings without (control) and with hypothyroidism incubated with octylmethoxycinnamate (OMC, 0 and 50 µmol/L) and contracted by histamine (His; 10 µmol/L).

The tension produced by KCl contraction in the two groups are present in Figure 1C. The results show that the tensions produced by KCl were similar in the two groups ($p > 0.05$).

3.1.2. Effects of OMC on Arteries Contracted with 5-HT

In Figure 3 the effects of OMC on arteries contracted with 5-HT is present. The results show a statistically significant interaction between the pathological conditions in HUA without incubation ($p \leq 0.001$) and preincubated with 50 µmol/L of OMC ($p = 0.001$). Contrarily to the vasorelaxant effect observed for the control group, the exposure of cumulative concentrations of OMC (Figure 3A) induced a contraction effect in the hypothyroidism group. Concerning the effects of the incubation for 24 h with 50 µmol/L of OMC (Figure 3B), the results show that OMC induce a similar contractile response in the two groups, except for the highest one (OMC, 50 µmol/L) that OMC induced a small relaxation (8.03% ± 5.78%) in the hypothyroidism group, contrarily to the contraction effect observed for the control group.

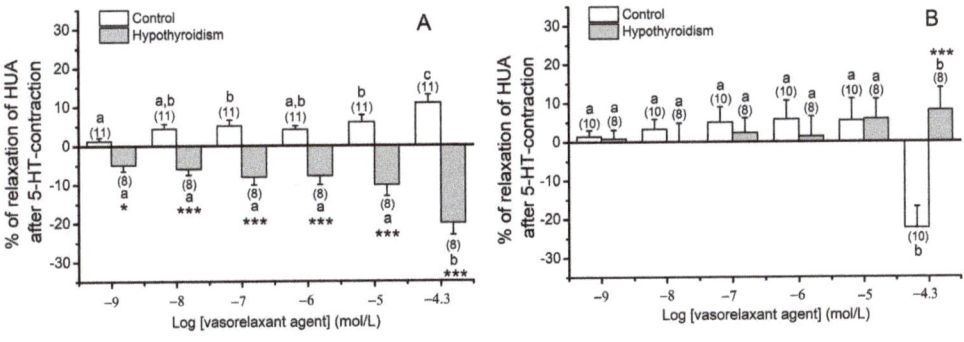

Figure 3. Percentage of relaxation of human umbilical artery (HUA) rings without (control) and with hypothyroidism incubated with (**A**) 0 µmol/L and (**B**) 50 µmol/L of octylmethoxycinnamate (OMC) and contracted by serotonin (5-HT; 1 µmol/L). Each bar represents the mean, vertical lines the S.E.M. and the number within brackets the n. Asterisk * represents a significant difference versus hypothyroidism: * $p < 0.05$ and *** $p < 0.001$, and the different letters represents significant differences between OMC concentrations ($p < 0.05$); two-way ANOVA method followed by Holm–Sidak post-hoc tests.

3.1.3. Effects of OMC on Arteries Contracted with His

Concerning the effects of OMC on arteries non-incubated contracted with His (Figure 4), the results show a statistically significant interaction between the pathological condition and the different concentrations of OMC of exposure ($p \leq 0.001$). The exposure of cumulative concentrations of OMC induced a higher relaxation in the hypothyroidism group. The long-term effects of OMC on HUA contracted with His could not be assessed since stable contractions were not obtained.

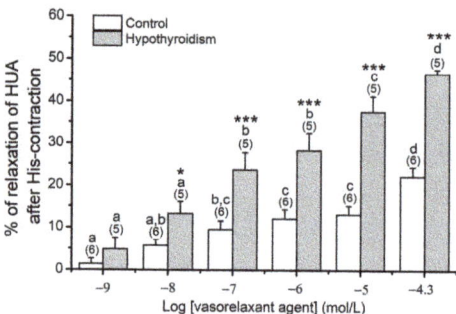

Figure 4. Percentage of relaxation of human umbilical artery (HUA) rings without (control) and with hypothyroidism non-incubated with octylmethoxycinnamate (OMC, 0 μmol/L) and contracted by histamine (His; 10 μmol/L). Each bar represents the mean, vertical lines the S.E.M. and the number within brackets the n. Asterisk * represents a significant difference versus hypothyroidism: * $p < 0.05$ and *** $p < 0.001$, and the different letters represents significant differences between OMC concentrations ($p < 0.05$); two-way ANOVA method followed by Holm–Sidak post-hoc tests.

3.1.4. Effects of OMC on Arteries Contracted with KCl

In Figure 5 the effects of OMC on arteries contracted with KCl is present. The results show a statistically significant interaction between the pathological conditions in the preincubation with 50 μmol/L of OMC ($p \leq 0.001$). The exposure of cumulative concentrations of OMC (Figure 5A) induced a similar contractile response (relaxation) in the two groups, except for the highest concentration (OMC, 50 μmol/L) in the hypothyroidism group that induces a smaller relaxing effect. Concerning the effects of the incubation for 24 h with 50 μmol/L OMC (Figure 5B), the results show that the exposure of OMC induced a relaxation in the hypothyroidism group contrary to the observed for the control group.

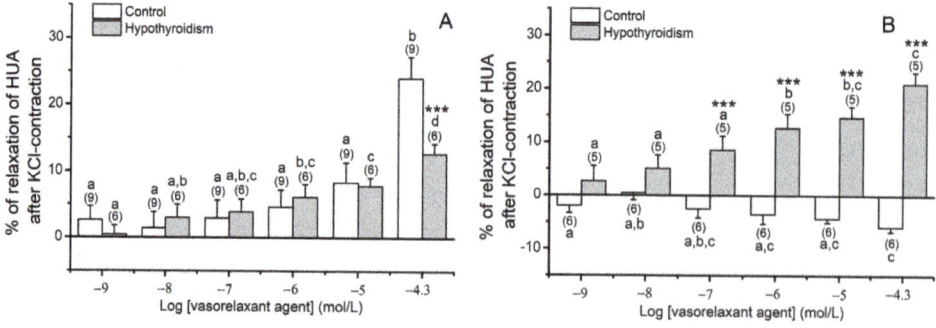

Figure 5. Percentage of relaxation of human umbilical artery (HUA) rings without (control) and with hypothyroidism incubated with (**A**) 0 μmol/L and (**B**) 50 μmol/L of octylmethoxycinnamate (OMC) and contracted by potassium chloride (KCl; 60 mmol/L). Each bar represents the mean, vertical lines the S.E.M. and the number within brackets the n. Asterisk * represents a significant difference versus hypothyroidism: *** $p < 0.001$, and the different letters represents significant differences between OMC concentrations ($p < 0.05$); two-way ANOVA method followed by Holm–Sidak post-hoc tests.

3.2. Contractility Experiments in HUASMC

Direct application of OMC at 50 µmol/L on the control group (pregnant without pathology) and in the hypothyroidism group (pregnant with hypothyroidism) did not change their basal area. Moreover, the incubation of 50 µmol/L of OMC did not change their basal area. The solvent used (ethanol 0.05%) in control and hypothyroidism groups did not have an effect on the basal area (data not shown).

In Figure 6 the effects of OMC on cells contracted with 5-HT is present. The results show that OMC induced a vasoconstriction effect in the hypothyroidism group, contrary to the observed in the control group (Figure 6C).

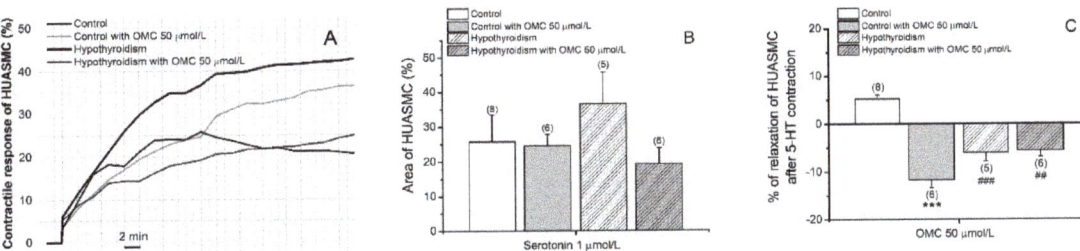

Figure 6. Effects of OMC on the human umbilical artery smooth muscle cells (HUASMCs) without (control) and with hypothyroidism incubated with octylmethoxycinnamate (OMC, 0 and 50 µmol/L) and contracted by serotonin (5-HT; 1 µmol/L). (**A**) Contractile response of HUASMC (%) during 40 min; (**B**) area (%) (at time 20 min) of the HUASMC and (**C**) percentage of relaxation of HUASMC after 5-HT contraction. Each bar represents the mean, vertical lines the S.E.M. and the number within brackets the n. Asterisk * represents a significant difference versus incubation: *** $p < 0.001$, and Hashtag # represents a significant difference versus hypothyroidism: ## $p < 0.01$ and ### $p < 0.001$; two-way ANOVA method followed by Holm–Sidak post-hoc tests.

The effects of OMC on cells contracted with His are present in Figure 7. The contraction with His produced stables contractions only in HUASMC from control groups (Figure 7A). The results show that OMC in the short-term produced a vasorelaxation effect in the hypothyroidism group similarly to the control group (Figure 7C).

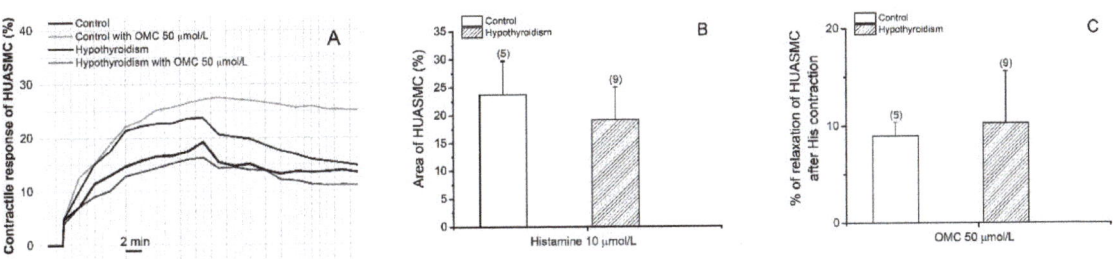

Figure 7. Effects of OMC on the human umbilical artery smooth muscle cells (HUASMCs) without (control) and with hypothyroidism incubated with octylmethoxycinnamate (OMC, 0 and 50 µmol/L) and contracted by histamine (His; 10 µmol/L). (**A**) Contractile response of HUASMC (%) during 40 min; (**B**) area (%) (at time 20 min) of the HUASMC and (**C**) percentage of relaxation of HUASMC after His contraction. Each bar represents the mean, vertical lines the S.E.M. and the number within brackets the n.

3.3. Molecular Docking Simulations

Rigid docking of OMC was carried out in the active site of the THRα and TSHR. The molecular docking results are present in Table 2 and the docking views are shown in Figures 8 and 9. The molecular docking of natural ligand T_3 with THRα shown that T_3 is in a hydrophobic environment involving an interaction with the amino acid residues

Met 259, Ser 277 and Leu 276. As shown in Figure 8A,C, T$_3$ formed two H-bonds with residues Ala 180 in distances of 4.399 Å and 4.351 Å. Concerning the molecular docking of OMC with THRα, the results show that OMC is in a hydrophobic environment involving an interaction with the amino acid residues Met 259, Ser 277 and Leu 276 likewise T$_3$, but also act by a hydrophobic interaction with the amino acid residues Ala 261, Ala 263, Phe 218 and Ile 222. The docking analyses show that OMC bound to the active centre of THRα with binding energy of −7.69 kcal/mol and no H-bonds were formed (Figure 8B,D).

Table 2. Binding energies of ligands T3, NAG and OMC (1–10) calculated from molecular docking studies.

Compound	TRHα	TSH
T$_3$	−10.80	-
NAG	-	−1.61
OMC_1	−7.69	0.68
OMC_2	−7.67	0.69
OMC_3	−7.65	0.73
OMC_4	−7.63	0.96
OMC_5	−7.60	1.08
OMC_6	−7.56	1.16
OMC_7	−6.92	1.01
OMC_8	−7.35	1.11
OMC_9	−7.16	1.30
OMC_10	−6.71	1.23

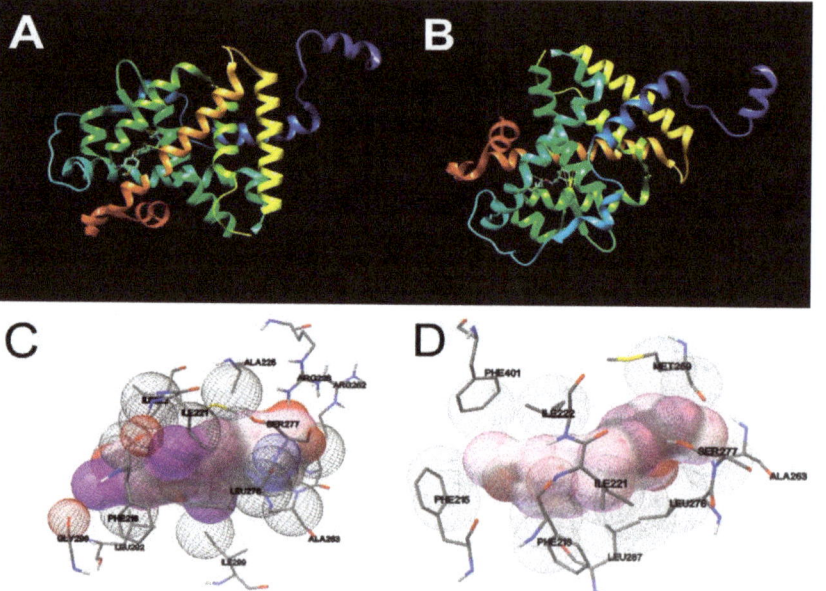

Figure 8. Docking views of the complex between the ligands with THRα using Quimera 1.15 software. (**A,B**) show the 3D representations of the interactions and preferred conformation between natural 3,5,3'Triiodothyronine (T3) and octylmethoxycinnamate (OMC), respectively, within THRα active centre. (**C,D**) show the interactions between natural ligand 3,5,3'Triiodothyronine (T3) and octylmethoxycinnamate (OMC), respectively, to the amino acid residues in the THRα active centre.

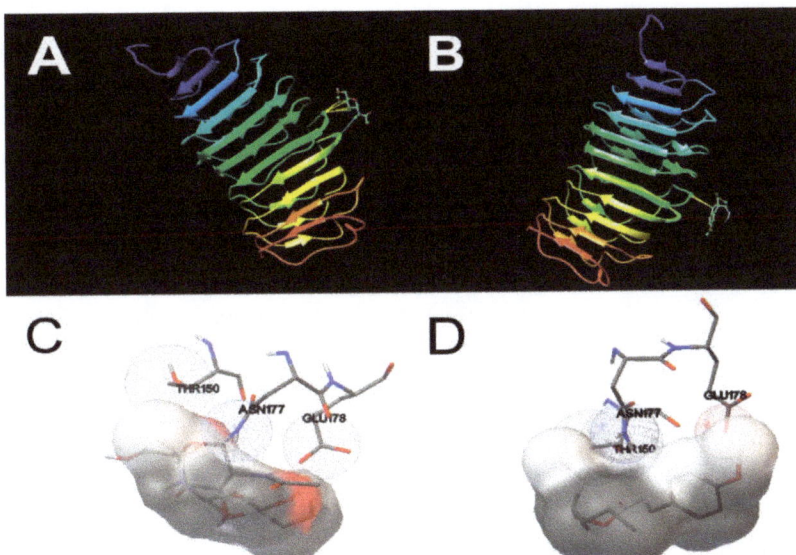

Figure 9. Docking views of the complex between the ligands with TSHR using Quimera 1.15 software. (**A,B**) show the 3D representations of the interactions and preferred conformation between natural ligand 2-acetamido-2-deoxy-beta-D-glucopyranose (NAG) and octylmethoxycinnamate (OMC), respectively, within TSHR active centre. (**C,D**) show the interactions between natural ligand 2-acetamido-2-deoxy-beta-D-glucopyranose (NAG) and octylmethoxycinnamate (OMC), respectively, to the amino acid residues in the TSHR active centre.

Concerning the molecular docking results of natural ligand NAG with TSHR, the results shown that NAG is in a hydrophilic environment involving five interactions with the amino acid residue Thr 150. Moreover, NAG formed H-bonds with residue Asn 177 in a distance of 4.725 Å (see Figure 9A,C). Similarly, the molecular docking results of OMC with TSHR shown that OMC was in a hydrophilic environment, however these binding complex involved only two interactions with the amino acid residue Thr 150, and it was observed only at a greater distance (−1.5 Å). The docking analyses show that OMC bound to the active centre of TSHR with binding energy of 0.68 kcal/mol and no H-bonds were formed (Figure 9B,D).

4. Discussion

The proposed aim of this work was to understand how the exposure of the UV filter OMC affects the arterial tonus of pregnant women with hypothyroidism. According to Benvenga, et al. hypothyroidism is a common disorder that has a prevalence of approximately 5% and an incidence of approximately 250/100,000 per year in the adult population [43]. Oral administration of levothyroxine is the standard treatment for patients with hypothyroidism [33]. During pregnancy, supplementation with iron and folic acid is widely used and recommended in Portugal. However, several evidences indicated an interaction between iron and levothyroxine [44–46], which is dependent on the formulation of levothyroxine [43]. In our research, all donor mothers were under medication with folic acid during the first trimester of gestation or iron supplementation during the last trimester of gestation. Donor mothers with hypothyroidism were treated with oral levothyroxine (Euthyrox, 2.5 µg) in generic tablets formulation, according to the standard therapy for patients with hypothyroidism [33]. However, the absorption of levothyroxine appears to be reduced when the iron is present, probably due to the formation of an insoluble complex between them [46]. The simultaneous intake of levothyroxine with the oral formulation of iron leads to the need to adjust the levothyroxine dose to achieve the same levels of TH. Regarding the liquid formulation of levothyroxine, Benvenga, et al. demonstrated that it is more resistant to sequestration by calcium bicarbonate or ferrous sulphate [43] than the tablet formulation (used in this work). Thus, it would be interesting to know the levels of TH during pregnancy. Ideally, all women with hypothyroidism should be educated about the potential interaction between iron pills and levothyroxine and should be advised to avoid simultaneous intake of both [46].

Pregnant women without pathology after exposure to the UV filter OMC presented a rapid vasodilatation of HUA [35] and long-term exposure impair the vascular homeostasis of these arteries. It is known that effects of UV filters acting as EDCs of the human thyroid system (and their consequences at the vascular level) during pregnancy is a major concern as it remains unknown. Using the organ bath technique, firstly the direct effect of OMC on the basal tension of the arteries was studied. The results showed that the exposure of cumulative concentrations of OMC or the incubation of 50 μmol/L OMC did not affect the basal tension of the HUA from hypothyroidism group.

In the next step, the rapid/short and long-term effects (incubation for 24 h with 50 μmol/L) of OMC on endothelium-denuded HUA from hypothyroidism group was evaluated. The results show that OMC in the short-term induced vasoconstriction while in the long-term induced vasorelaxation of the HUA from hypothyroidism group that were precontracted with 5-HT. Nevertheless, in HUA from the control groups, OMC produced a relaxation response, which is in accordance to work demonstrated by our research group [35]. Furthermore, it was observed that the incubation with 50 μmol/L of OMC induced a significantly higher contraction of 5-HT in the hypothyroidism group. These results can be explained by the interaction observed between the pathological conditions and the preincubation with OMC but also by the vascular MOA of 5-HT as the contractile agent. Serotonin (5-HT) is the most potent vasoactive agent to contract the HUA [47] and induce vascular contraction by activation of the $5-HT_{2A}$, $5-HT_{1B}/5-HT_{1D}$ and $5-HT_7$ receptors [34,48,49]. The activation of $5-HT_{2A}$ receptors stimulates the PLC/IP_3 pathway and the $5-HT_{1B}/5-HT_{1D}$ activation leads to an inhibition of adenyl cyclase. On the other hand, the activation of $5-HT_7$ receptors (Gs-protein coupled) promotes vasorelaxation by activation of adenyl [48–50].

The contractility experiments in HUASMC contracted with 5-HT and exposed to OMC were in accordance with the obtained in organ bath experiments, where OMC at short-term increases the area (relax) of HUASMC from the control group and decreases these areas (contraction) in HUASMC preincubated with 50 μmol/L of OMC. In relation to the experiments on HUASMC from the hypothyroidism group, OMC induced a decrease in the cell areas (relaxation), according to the organ bath data. In summary, our results suggested for the first time that the OMC could modulate the vascular homeostasis of HUA from pregnant women with hypothyroidism probably by an interference with 5-HT receptors.

In relation to the experiments regarding the effects of OMC on the vascular tone of HUA contracted with His, the results show that in the hypothyroidism group OMC in the short-term induced pronounced vasorelaxation of the HUA. In arteries from the control group, OMC also relaxes HUA according to that previously demonstrated [35]. Furthermore, it was observed that the incubation with 50 μmol/L of OMC induced a significantly higher contraction of His in the hypothyroidism group. These results can be explained by the interaction observed between the pathological conditions and the different concentrations of OMC of exposure. Concerning the long-term effects of OMC on the vascular tone of HUA contracted with His, we did not expose the HUA to the OMC since a sustained contraction of the arteries was only achieved for the control group. The fact that HUA incubated with OMC did not achieve a stable contraction with His suggests a strong interference from OMC with histamine receptors. Moreover, the pathological conditions did not alter this effect. These results might be explained by the vascular MOA of His as the contractile agent. Some authors reported that their contractile effects are due to activation of the H_1 receptor (coupled to the Gq protein), which is present in HUA [34,49].

The His promotes vasoconstriction through the H_1 receptor acts by PLC/IP_3 signaling cascade and increasing $[Ca^{2+}]_i$ [49,51,52]. On the other hand, vasorelaxation was promoted through activation of the H_2 receptor (Gs-protein coupled) which will activate the adenyl cyclase and decreases $[Ca^{2+}]_I$ [34,49,52]. Furthermore, the contractility experiments in HUASMC contracted with His and exposed to OMC were in accordance with the obtained in organ bath experiments, the HUASMC preincubated with 50 μmol/L of OMC, also did not promote a sustained contraction. Taken together, our results suggested for the first time that the OMC could modulate the vascular homeostasis of HUA from pregnant women with hypothyroidism probably by an interference with His receptors.

Concerning the experiments regarding the effects of OMC on the vascular tone of HUA contracted with KCl, the results show that OMC in the short-term induces less vasorelaxation of HUA from the hypothyroidism group than HUA from the control group. With respect to the long-term effects of OMC on vasculature of HUA, OMC induces relaxation of HUA from the hypothyroidism group contrary to that observed for the control group. These results can be explained by the interaction observed between the pathological conditions and the preincubation with OMC but also by the vascular MOA of KCl as the contractile agent. As described by our research group in previous studies, KCl contracts HUA by an influx of extracellular Ca^{2+}, leading to depolarization and L-Type VOCC opening [50,53]. The contractility experiments in HUASMC for this contractile agent were not evaluated since it was impossible to perform the depolarization with isosmotic KCl (60 mmol/L) solution. Therefore, and taking into account that $[Ca^{2+}]_i$ is key for the contractile responses of HUA [40], our results suggest that OMC also modulates vascular homeostasis of HUA from pregnant women with hypothyroidism probably by an interference with Ca^{2+} channels. According to the literature, the dysregulation of the normal functioning of the Ca^{2+} channels (namely an increase in activity) has been associated with hypertension (HT) and other cardiovascular (CV) complications [54].

Several authors have observed an association between the CV system and the thyroid diseases, but few studies have assessed the correlation between hypothyroidism and cardiac pathologies, with the exception of atrial fibrillation and tachyarrhythmias [55–58]. The SMC, as modulators of vascular tone, are a fundamental target for the action of TH [59]. Tian, et al. suggested that TSH may have a direct vascular effect on SMC [60]. Moreover, Makino, et al. demonstrated that SMC predominantly expresses the TRHα, playing a key role in the regulation of the vascular tone [61]. According to the literature, the TH (mainly T_3) may act directly in the vascular smooth muscle cells inducing relaxation [62–64]. Ojamaa, et al. demonstrated that this vasorelaxation occurs within 10 min after T_3 is bound to specific binding sites in the SMC. The authors were unable to detect increases in cGMP levels in endothelial cells (EC) after T_3 stimulation, which is suggestive that NO was not produced in these cells. Therefore, these results suggested that T_3 acts by a non-genomic mechanism and endothelium-independent [65]. Moreover, Fukuyama, et al. suggested that the mechanism for this vasorelaxant effect may be due to decreasing the expression of angiotensin II type 1 receptors by T_3, and thereby reduces the contractile response to angiotensin II [66]. According to these authors, Carrillo-Sepulveda, et al. also demonstrated that T_3 causes nitric oxide (NO)-dependent rapid relaxation of vascular SMC by activation of PI3K/Akt-mediated endothelial nitric oxide synthase signaling pathway [67]. Consequently, recent epidemiological studies have shown that patients with hypothyroidism or with subclinical hypothyroidism may develop increased diastolic blood pressure, probably via decreased endothelium-mediated relaxation and vascular compliance [55,62,68]. In this sense, some studies suggested that this vasodilation is a result of the T_3 effects on the PI3K/Akt pathway mediated by non-genomic and genomic actions [69,70]. Interesting, Napoli, et al. reported that TSH (thyroid stimulating hormone) can promote endothelial mediated vasodilation of conduit arteries, independent of systemic hemodynamic changes [71]. Moreover, Zwaveling, et al. suggested that relaxation induced by TH may be the result of a joint effect between EC and SMC. Briefly, TH can act directly on SMC and EC, and these last cells can induce indirect effects on SMC [72]. Taken together, these data indicate that TH exerts vasorelaxant effects at the vascular level.

The TH plays a fundamental role in CV homeostasis and vascular remodeling [12,73]; myocardial and vascular endothelial tissues have thyroid receptors and even subtle changes in circulating TH concentrations can adversely influence the CV system [12]. However, specific links and mechanisms between an altered thyroid metabolism and CV diseases, during the progression of disease from organ specific to systemic disorder, are not known and need to be established. Furthermore, current human exposure to ubiquitous chemicals (from cosmetics to environment), which might act as thyroid disrupting chemicals by disrupting thyroid homeostasis can contribute to the development and increased risk of CV diseases [74].

Organic UV filters are emerging contaminants present ubiquitously in the environment. Human exposure to these EDCs is a global concern due to their adverse effects on human hormone systems [75,76] and an important target for thyroid disruption [76] namely in vulnerable populations such as pregnant women [1,5–9].

The EDCs affect the normal functioning of TH at a molecular level by different mechanisms, including hormone receptor proteins. The THR is the nuclear receptor responsible for thyroid signaling [76] and TSHR is the primary regulator of thyrocyte function that regulates the levels of circulating T_3 and T_4 hormones [77]. Therefore, both TRHα and TSHR are proteins involved in thyroid physiology that can be potential targets for EDCs.

One of the main research difficulties is to clarify whether the mode of action of EDCs with receptors is due to an endocrine hormone mimicking action or an interference with the signal transduction process [78]. In this way, molecular docking analysis helped us by providing some information on structure–activity relationships for thyroid receptors by OMC. The results of our study revealed that OMC successfully binds to the active centre of TRHα, but the same was not observed for TSHR. Interactions of the OMC with more amino acid residues were found with TRHα, when compared with the native ligand, the hormone T_3. Comparing with the natural TSHR ligand (NAG ligand), the OMC binding involved fewer interactions with amino acid residues, and a greater distance was required for these interactions to be observed. Therefore, our results indicate that OMC has a higher binding affinity for TRHα than for TSHR, which is also confirmed by the binding energies. Typically, lower binding energies indicate a higher possibility of stable binding [75], and the OMC binding energy value for the TRHα receptor (-7.69 kcal/mol) has a more negative value than for the TSHR (0.68 kcal/mol). Moreover, the OMC is a hydrophobic compound [79], so it is not surprising that its binding to the TRHα receptor occurred in the internal hydrophobic cavity. Contrary, the OMC binding to TSHR in a hydrophilic environment, which supports the weak affinity of this UV filter to TSHR. Thus, our results seem to indicate that OMC has the potential to interfere with the binding of T_3 to TRHα. One of the reasons for the greater potential of OMC binding to the TRHα receptor compared to TSHR may be due to the structural similarity shared between OMC and T_3 (both have a double ring chemical structure). Therefore, it is expected that OMC will imitate T_3 and compete for the active centre of TRHα. Although molecular docking simulation cannot provide an absolute or precise mode of action of OMC, our results suggested that OMC seems to disrupt TH signaling pathways, which have implications at the genomic and non-genomic level, supporting the contractility data obtained.

According to Couderq, et al. [80] assessing the effects of a compound's endocrine disruption is a challenge due to (i) the existence of non-monotonic responses, which leads to questioning where the "safe" threshold doses are determined; (ii) the endocrine system is an integrative and complex system that may involve different hormonal pathways; (iii) the existence of critical stages of development such as pregnancy, which are more vulnerable to exposure to EDC and (iv) the effects of exposure may occur at a later stage of development or even extend to future generations. This concept was introduced by the Developmental Origins of Health and Disease theory (DOHaD), which highlights the importance that EDCs can play in fetal programming [81]. Fetal programming is understood as the "result of epigenetic changes that occurs in response to various stimuli that come from the environment that can affect the life and health of the baby even in adulthood" [82]. According to previous studies, the placenta is not fully effective against these chemical compounds, and even its exposure in pregnant women has been associated with the entry of these compounds into fetal circulation [83–85]. Regarding the OMC, it is described that this UV-B filter can penetrate through the epidermis and dermis and reach the systemic circulation. Consequently, OMC has been detected in urine, plasma [27], breast milk samples [19,28] and placenta [29]. Thus, our results may indicate that the OMC effects may be remarkable in the future generation, since the developing fetus is more sensitive to EDCs than a human adult [81]. Based on the fetal programming hypothesis, pregnancies affected by diseases such as gestational diabetes appear to be associated with endothelial dysfunction of the human umbilical vein (HUV) [86]. Moreover, in HUVEC from women's with pre-eclampsia presented functional abnormalities of calcium handling and NO production [87]. More recently, sex differences in HUVEC have also been reported. However, this sex difference was not observed in HUASMC [82]. Therefore, taken together, our findings suggested that alterations in maternal reactivity vasculature as a result of OMC exposure might reflect long-term "programming" of the fetal cardiovascular system. According to this concept, the exposure to OMC in the prenatal stage may be involved in the development and increased risk of cardiovascular diseases.

In summary, our results suggested that OMC alters the vascular contractility patterns in pregnant women with hypothyroidism. Pronounced vasorelaxation or vasoconstriction as the ones obtained in this study as a response to OMC might be harmful to the CV system of pregnant women. However, further studies are needed to unravel the vascular MOA of OMC, which may also be related with 5-HT and His receptors or the Ca^{2+} and/or K^+ channels. The activation of ion channels could also be an explanation for the exaggerated relaxation observed in HUA from the hypothyroidism group contracted with His and explain the non-sustained contractions obtained. According to Gokina and Bevan working with rabbit cerebral arteries, sustained contractions of His may be due to an increase in Ca^{2+} currents through VOCC, sensitization of the contractile apparatus and the non-selective cationic channels [88]. Therefore, these results are in accordance with other investigations reporting that long-term exposure to EDCs can be the inductor of CV complications [1,11,89–91] and are extremely important at a physiological and pharmacological level to improve thyroid and CV maternofetal health.

5. Conclusions

To the best of our knowledge, this study is the first report to rapid- and long-term effects of the UV filter octylmethoxycinnamate (OMC) on vasculature from pregnant women with hypothyroidism. Our results indicated that OMC altered the contractility patterns of HUA contracted with serotonin, histamine and KCl, possibly due to interference with serotonin and histamine receptors or an involvement of the Ca^{2+} channels. The molecular docking analysis show that OMC compete with T_3 for the binding centre of THRα. Taken together, these findings pointed out alterations in HUA reactivity as a result of OMC-exposure, which may be involved in the development and increased risk of cardiovascular diseases.

In conclusion, this work represents a new and promising research field that remains practically unexplored, and therefore requires further investigations. Given the ubiquity of this UV filter in the environment and its potentially adverse effects on human health, studying human exposure to OMC may lead to a better understanding of the role of this EDC in cardiovascular diseases. Furthermore, due to the close relationship between the CV and thyroid systems, it highlights the need to identify the molecular pathways involved in the effects of EDCs for better prevention and treatment of CVD in pregnant women with hypothyroidism.

Author Contributions: M.L.: Methodology; Formal analysis; Investigation; Writing—Original Draft; Visualization. C.Q.: Conceptualization; Formal Analysis; Validation; Writing—Review and Editing; Supervision; Funding acquisition. L.B.: Conceptualization; Writing—Review and Editing; Supervision; Funding acquisition. E.C.: Conceptualization; Methodology; Investigation; Software; Validation; Formal analysis; Resources; Data Curation; Writing—Review and Editing; Supervision; Project administration; Funding acquisition. All authors have read and agreed to the published version of the manuscript.

Funding: This research was supported by FEDER funds through the POCI-COMPETE 2020—Operational Program Competitiveness and Internationalisation in Axis I-Strengthening research, technological development and innovation (Project POCI-01-0145-FEDER007491) and National Funds by FCT—Foundation for Science and Technology (Project UID/Multi/00709/2019). This work was also supported by the European Regional Development Fund through the "Programa Operacional Regional do Centro (Centro 2020)—Sistema de Apoio à Investigação Científica e Tecnológica—Programas Integrados de IC&DT" (Project Centro-01-0145-FEDER-000019—C4—Centro de Competências em Cloud Computing). M.L. acknowledges the PhD fellowship from FCT (Reference: 2020.06616.BD). The work of C.Q. is funded by national funds (OE), through FCT—Fundação para a Ciência e a Tecnologia, I.P., in the scope of the framework contract foreseen in the numbers 4, 5 and 6 of the article 23, of the Decree-Law 57/2016, of August 29, changed by Law 57/2017, of July 19. Thanks are due to FCT/MCTES for the financial support to CESAM (UIDB/50017/2020 + UIDP/50017/2020), through national funds.

Institutional Review Board Statement: The study was conducted according to the guidelines of the Declaration of Helsinki, and approved by the Institutional Review Board (or Ethics Committee) of CHUCB (No.33/2018, 18 July 2018, Centro Hospitalar Universitário da Cova da Beira E.P.E., Covilhã, Portugal) and ULS-Guarda (No. 02324/2019, 27 February 2019, Unidade Local de Saúde da Guarda, Guarda, Portugal).

Informed Consent Statement: Informed consent was obtained from all subjects involved in the study.

Data Availability Statement: Data is contained within the article.

Acknowledgments: The authors would like to thank all donors' mothers who agreed to participate in this study and all the technical staff from Gynaecology–Obstetrics Department staff of "Centro Hospitalar Universitário da Cova da Beira E.P.E." (CHUCB, Covilhã, Portugal) and from maternity of "Unidade de Saúde Local da Guarda" (ULS, Guarda, Portugal), particularly to all medical, nurses and health technicians for their disinterested collaboration. The authors also thanks to Nelson Oliveira, Fernando Pimenta, Cremilde Sousa, Maria Inês Fonseca, Manuel Pouso, Carolina Mangana and Rui Rodrigues for their contribution in this research.

Conflicts of Interest: The authors declare no conflict of interest.

References

1. Kelley, A.S.; Banker, M.; Goodrich, J.M.; Dolinoy, D.C.; Burant, C.; Domino, S.E.; Smith, Y.R.; Song, P.X.K.; Padmanabhan, V. Early pregnancy exposure to endocrine disrupting chemical mixtures are associated with inflammatory changes in maternal and neonatal circulation. *Sci. Rep.* **2019**, *9*, 5422. [CrossRef]
2. Suh, S.; Pham, C.; Smith, J.; Mesinkovska, N.A. The banned sunscreen ingredients and their impact on human health: A systematic review. *Int. J. Dermatol.* **2020**. [CrossRef]
3. Gore, A.C.; Chappell, V.A.; Fenton, S.E.; Flaws, J.A.; Nadal, A.; Prins, G.S.; Toppari, J.; Zoeller, R.T. EDC-2: The Endocrine Society's Second Scientific Statement on Endocrine-Disrupting Chemicals. *Endocr. Rev.* **2015**, *36*, E1–E150. [CrossRef]
4. Jugan, M.-L.; Levi, Y.; Blondeau, J.-P. Endocrine disruptors and thyroid hormone physiology. *Biochem. Pharmacol.* **2010**, *79*, 939–947. [CrossRef]
5. Padula, A.M.; Monk, C.; Brennan, P.A.; Borders, A.; Barrett, E.S.; McEvoy, C.T.; Foss, S.; Desai, P.; Alshawabkeh, A.; Wurth, R. A review of maternal prenatal exposures to environmental chemicals and psychosocial stressors—Implications for research on perinatal outcomes in the ECHO program. *J. Perinatol.* **2020**, *40*, 10–24. [CrossRef]
6. Rager, J.E.; Bangma, J.; Carberry, C.; Chao, A.; Grossman, J.; Lu, K.; Manuck, T.A.; Sobus, J.R.; Szilagyi, J.; Fry, R.C. Review of the environmental prenatal exposome and its relationship to maternal and fetal health. *Reprod. Toxicol.* **2020**, *98*, 1–12. [CrossRef]
7. Marie-Pierre, S.-R.; Cabut, S.; Vendittelli, F.; Sauvant-Rochat, M.-P. Changes in Cosmetics Use during Pregnancy and Risk Perception by Women. *Int. J. Environ. Res. Public Health* **2016**, *13*, 383. [CrossRef] [PubMed]
8. Tanner, E.M.; Hallerbäck, M.U.; Wikström, S.; Lindh, C.; Kiviranta, H.; Gennings, C.; Bornehag, C.-G. Early prenatal exposure to suspected endocrine disruptor mixtures is associated with lower IQ at age seven. *Environ. Int.* **2020**, *134*, 105185. [CrossRef]

9. Ghassabian, A.; Trasande, L. Disruption in Thyroid Signaling Pathway: A Mechanism for the Effect of Endocrine-Disrupting Chemicals on Child Neurodevelopment. *Front. Endocrinol.* **2018**, *9*, 204. [CrossRef]
10. Vancamp, P.; Houbrechts, A.M.; Darras, V.M. Insights from zebrafish deficiency models to understand the impact of local thyroid hormone regulator action on early development. *Gen. Comp. Endocrinol.* **2019**, *279*, 45–52. [CrossRef]
11. Street, M.E.; Bernasconi, S. Endocrine-Disrupting Chemicals in Human Fetal Growth. *Int. J. Mol. Sci.* **2020**, *21*, 1430. [CrossRef]
12. Jabbar, A.; Pingitore, A.; Pearce, S.H.S.; Zaman, A.J.A.; Iervasi, A.P.G.; Razvi, A.J.S.H.S.P.A.Z.S. Thyroid hormones and cardiovascular disease. *Nat. Rev. Cardiol.* **2017**, *14*, 39–55. [CrossRef]
13. Razvi, S.; Jabbar, A.; Pingitore, A.; Danzi, S.; Biondi, B.; Klein, I.; Peeters, R.; Zaman, A.; Iervasi, G. Thyroid Hormones and Cardiovascular Function and Diseases. *J. Am. Coll. Cardiol.* **2018**, *71*, 1781–1796. [CrossRef]
14. Lorigo, M.; Cairrao, E. Antioxidants as stabilizers of UV filters: An example for the UV-B filter octylmethoxycinnamate. *Biomed. Dermatol.* **2019**, *3*, 1–9. [CrossRef]
15. Ferraris, F.K.; Garcia, E.B.; Chaves, A.D.S.; De Brito, T.M.; Doro, L.H.; Da Silva, N.M.F.; Alves, A.S.; Pádua, T.A.; Henriques, M.D.G.M.O.; Machado, T.S.C.; et al. Exposure to the UV Filter Octyl Methoxy Cinnamate in the Postnatal Period Induces Thyroid Dysregulation and Perturbs the Immune System of Mice. *Front. Endocrinol.* **2020**, *10*. [CrossRef]
16. Benson, H.A.E.; Sarveiya, V.; Risk, S.; Roberts, M.S. Influence of anatomical site and topical formulation on skin penetration of sunscreens. *Ther. Clin. Risk Manag.* **2005**, *1*, 209–218.
17. Krause, M.; Klit, A.; Jensen, M.B.; Søeborg, T.; Frederiksen, H.; Schlumpf, M.; Lichtensteiger, W.; Skakkebaek, N.E.; Drzewiecki, K.T. Sunscreens: Are they beneficial for health? An overview of endocrine disrupting properties of UV-filters. *Int. J. Androl.* **2012**, *35*, 424–436. [CrossRef]
18. Kunz, P.Y.; Fent, K. Multiple hormonal activities of UV filters and comparison of in vivo and in vitro estrogenic activity of ethyl-4-aminobenzoate in fish. *Aquat. Toxicol.* **2006**, *79*, 305–324. [CrossRef]
19. Schlumpf, M.; Kypke, K.; Wittassek, M.; Angerer, J.; Mascher, H.; Mascher, D.; Vökt, C.; Birchler, M.; Lichtensteiger, W. Exposure patterns of UV filters, fragrances, parabens, phthalates, organochlor pesticides, PBDEs, and PCBs in human milk: Correlation of UV filters with use of cosmetics. *Chemosphere* **2010**, *81*, 1171–1183. [CrossRef]
20. Negreira, N.; Rodríguez, I.; Rubí, E.; Cela, R. Determination of selected UV filters in indoor dust by matrix solid-phase dispersion and gas chromatography–tandem mass spectrometry. *J. Chromatogr. A* **2009**, *1216*, 5895–5902. [CrossRef]
21. Zwiener, C.; Ichardson, S.D.R.; Arini, D.M.D.E.M.; Grummt, T.; Launer, T.G.; Rimmel, F.R.H.F. Drowning in Disinfection Byproducts? Assessing Swimming Pool Water. *Environ. Sci. Technol.* **2006**, *41*, 363–372. [CrossRef] [PubMed]
22. Cruz, M.S.D.; Gago-Ferrero, P.; Llorca, M.; Barceló, D. Analysis of UV filters in tap water and other clean waters in Spain. *Anal. Bioanal. Chem.* **2011**, *402*, 2325–2333. [CrossRef] [PubMed]
23. Loraine, G.; Pettigrove, M.E. Seasonal Variations in Concentrations of Pharmaceuticals and Personal Care Products in Drinking Water and Reclaimed Wastewater in Southern California. *Environ. Sci. Technol.* **2006**, *40*, 687–695. [CrossRef] [PubMed]
24. Schneider, S.L.; Lim, H.W. Review of environmental effects of oxybenzone and other sunscreen active ingredients. *J. Am. Acad. Dermatol.* **2019**, *80*, 266–271. [CrossRef] [PubMed]
25. Lorigo, M.; Mariana, M.; Cairrao, E. Photoprotection of ultraviolet-B filters: Updated review of endocrine disrupting properties. *Steroids* **2018**, *131*, 46–58. [CrossRef]
26. Siller, A.; Blaszak, S.C.; Lazar, M.; Harken, E.O. Update About the Effects of the Sunscreen Ingredients Oxybenzone and Octinoxate on Humans and the Environment. *Plast. Surg. Nurs.* **2019**, *39*, 157–160. [CrossRef]
27. Janjua, N.R.; Kongshoj, B.; Andersson, A.-M.; Wulf, H.C. Sunscreens in human plasma and urine after repeated whole-body topical application. *J. Eur. Acad. Dermatol. Venereol.* **2008**, *22*, 456–461. [CrossRef]
28. Schlumpf, M.; Kypke, K.; Vökt, C.C.; Birchler, M.; Durrer, S.; Faass, O.; Ehnes, C.; Fuetsch, M.; Gaille, C.; Henseler, M.; et al. Corrigendum. *Chim. Int. J. Chem.* **2008**, *62*, 688. [CrossRef]
29. Vela-Soria, F.; Gallardo-Torres, M.; Ballesteros, O.; Díaz, C.; Pérez, J.; Navalón, A.; Vinggaard, A.M.; Olea, N. Assessment of parabens and ultraviolet filters in human placenta tissue by ultrasound-assisted extraction and ultra-high performance liquid chromatography-tandem mass spectrometry. *J. Chromatogr. A* **2017**, *1487*, 153–161. [CrossRef]
30. Schmutzler, C.; Gotthardt, I.; Hofmann, P.J.; Radovic, B.; Kovacs, G.; Stemmler, L.; Nobis, I.; Bacinski, A.; Mentrup, B.; Ambrugger, P.; et al. Endocrine Disruptors and the Thyroid Gland—A Combined in Vitro and in Vivo Analysis of Potential New Biomarkers. *Environ. Health Perspect.* **2007**, *115*, 77–83. [CrossRef]
31. Song, M.; Song, M.-K.; Choi, H.-S.; Ryu, J.-C. Monitoring of deiodinase deficiency based on transcriptomic responses in SH-SY5Y cells. *Arch. Toxicol.* **2013**, *87*, 1103–1113. [CrossRef] [PubMed]
32. Janjua, N.R.; Kongshoj, B.; Petersen, J.H.; Wulf, H. Sunscreens and thyroid function in humans after short-term whole-body topical application: A single-blinded study. *Br. J. Dermatol.* **2007**, *156*, 1080–1082. [CrossRef] [PubMed]
33. Benvenga, S.; Carlé, A. Levothyroxine Formulations: Pharmacological and Clinical Implications of Generic Substitution. *Adv. Ther.* **2019**, *36*, 59–71. [CrossRef] [PubMed]
34. Cairrao, E.; Álvarez, E.; Santos-Silva, A.J.; Verde, I. Potassium channels are involved in testosterone-induced vasorelaxation of human umbilical artery. *Naunyn-Schmiedeberg's Arch. Pharmacol.* **2007**, *376*, 375–383. [CrossRef] [PubMed]
35. Lorigo, M.; Quintaneiro, C.; Lemos, M.C.; Martinez-De-Oliveira, J.; Breitenfeld, L.; Cairrao, E. UV-B Filter Octylmethoxycinnamate Induces Vasorelaxation by Ca2+ Channel Inhibition and Guanylyl Cyclase Activation in Human Umbilical Arteries. *Int. J. Mol. Sci.* **2019**, *20*, 1376. [CrossRef]

36. Schlumpf, M.; Cotton, B.; Conscience, M.; Haller, V.; Steinmann, B.; Lichtensteiger, W. In vitro and in vivo estrogenicity of UV screens. *Environ. Health Perspect.* **2001**, *109*, 239–244. [CrossRef]
37. Sharma, A.; Bányiová, K.; Babica, P.; El Yamani, N.; Collins, A.R.; Čupr, P. Different DNA damage response of cis and trans isomers of commonly used UV filter after the exposure on adult human liver stem cells and human lymphoblastoid cells. *Sci. Total Environ.* **2017**, *593*, 18–26. [CrossRef]
38. Nečasová, A.; Bányiová, K.; Literák, J.; Čupr, P. New probabilistic risk assessment of ethylhexyl methoxycinnamate: Comparing the genotoxic effects oftrans- andcis-EHMC. *Environ. Toxicol.* **2016**, *32*, 569–580. [CrossRef]
39. Cairrão, E.; Santos-Silva, A.J.; Alvarez, E.; Correia, I.; Verde, I. Isolation and culture of human umbilical artery smooth muscle cells expressing functional calcium channels. *Vitr. Cell. Dev. Biol. Anim.* **2009**, *45*, 175–184. [CrossRef]
40. Lorigo, M.; Mariana, M.; Feiteiro, J.; Cairrao, E. How is the human umbilical artery regulated? *J. Obstet. Gynaecol. Res.* **2018**, *44*, 1193–1201. [CrossRef]
41. Mariana, M.; Feiteiro, J.; Cairrao, E.; Verde, I. Mifepristone is a Vasodilator Due to the Inhibition of Smooth Muscle Cells L-Type Ca2+ Channels. *Reprod. Sci.* **2015**, *23*, 723–730. [CrossRef] [PubMed]
42. Morris, G.M.; Huey, R.; Lindstrom, W.; Sanner, M.F.; Belew, R.K.; Goodsell, D.S.; Olson, A.J. AutoDock4 and AutoDockTools4: Automated docking with selective receptor flexibility. *J. Comput. Chem.* **2009**, *30*, 2785–2791. [CrossRef] [PubMed]
43. Benvenga, S.; Di Bari, F.; Vita, R. Undertreated hypothyroidism due to calcium or iron supplementation corrected by oral liquid levothyroxine. *Endocrine* **2017**, *56*, 138–145. [CrossRef] [PubMed]
44. Rosenzweig, P.H.; Volpe, S.L. Effect of iron supplementation on thyroid hormone levels and resting metabolic rate in two college female athletes: A case study. *Int. J. Sport Nutr. Exerc. Metab.* **2000**, *10*, 434–443. [CrossRef] [PubMed]
45. Shakir, K.M.M.; Chute, J.P.; Aprill, B.S.; Lazarus, A.A. Ferrous sulfate-induced increase in requirement for thyroxine in a patient with primary hypothyroidism. *South. Med. J.* **1997**, *90*, 637–639. [CrossRef]
46. Ng, J.M.; Wakil, A.; Dawson, A.; Masson, E.A.; Allan, B.J.; Lindow, S.W.; Krishnan, R.; Wardell, S.; Igzeer, Y. Levothyroxine and iron in pregnancy: Right dose, wrong time? *Endocr. Abstr.* **2009**, *19*, P356.
47. Quan, A.; Leung, S.W.; Lao, T.T.; Man, R.Y. 5-hydroxytryptamine and thromboxane A2 as physiologic mediators of human umbilical artery closure. *J. Soc. Gynecol. Investig.* **2003**, *10*, 490–495. [CrossRef]
48. Lovren, F.; Li, X.-F.; Lytton, J.; Triggle, C.R. Functional characterization and m-RNA expression of 5-HT receptors mediating contraction in human umbilical artery. *Br. J. Pharmacol.* **1999**, *127*, 1247–1255. [CrossRef] [PubMed]
49. Santos-Silva, A.J.; Cairrao, E.; Marques, B.; Verde, I. Regulation of human umbilical artery contractility by different serotonin and histamine receptors. *Reprod. Sci.* **2009**, *16*, 1175–1185. [CrossRef]
50. Santos-Silva, A.J.; Cairrao, E.; Verde, I. Study of the mechanisms regulating human umbilical artery contractility. *Health* **2010**, *2*, 321–331. [CrossRef]
51. Hawley, J.; Rubin, P.; Hill, S.J. Distribution of receptors mediating phosphoinositide hydrolysis in cultured human umbilical artery smooth muscle and endothelial cells. *Biochem. Pharmacol.* **1995**, *49*, 1005–1011. [CrossRef]
52. Santos-Silva, A.J.; Cairrao, E.; Morgado, M.; Álvarez, E.; Verde, I. PDE4 and PDE5 regulate cyclic nucleotides relaxing effects in human umbilical arteries. *Eur. J. Pharmacol.* **2008**, *582*, 102–109. [CrossRef] [PubMed]
53. Alvarez, E.; Cairrao, E.; Morgado, M.; Morais, C.; Verde, I. Testosterone and Cholesterol Vasodilation of Rat Aorta Involves L-Type Calcium Channel Inhibition. *Adv. Pharmacol. Sci.* **2010**, *2010*, 1–10. [CrossRef] [PubMed]
54. Kuo, I.Y.; Wölfle, S.E.; Hill, C.E. T-type calcium channels and vascular function: The new kid on the block? *J. Physiol.* **2011**, *589*, 783–795. [CrossRef] [PubMed]
55. Khan, R.; Sikanderkhel, S.; Gui, J.; Adeniyi, A.-R.; O'Dell, K.; Erickson, M.; Malpartida, J.; Mufti, Z.; Khan, T.; Mufti, H.; et al. Thyroid and Cardiovascular Disease: A Focused Review on the Impact of Hyperthyroidism in Heart Failure. *Cardiol. Res.* **2020**, *11*, 68–75. [CrossRef]
56. Osuna, P.M.; Udovcic, M.; Sharma, M.D. Hyperthyroidism and the Heart. *Methodist DeBakey Cardiovasc. J.* **2017**, *13*, 60–63. [CrossRef]
57. Udovcic, M.; Pena, R.H.; Patham, B.; Tabatabai, L.; Kansara, A. Hypothyroidism and the Heart. *Methodist DeBakey Cardiovasc. J.* **2017**, *13*, 55–59. [CrossRef]
58. Klein, I.; Danzi, S. Thyroid Disease and the Heart. *Curr. Probl. Cardiol.* **2016**, *41*, 65–92. [CrossRef]
59. Barreto-Chaves, M.L.M.; Monteiro, P.D.S.; Furstenau, C.R. Acute actions of thyroid hormone on blood vessel biochemistry and physiology. *Curr. Opin. Endocrinol. Diabetes Obes.* **2011**, *18*, 300–303. [CrossRef]
60. Tian, L.; Ni, J.; Guo, T.; Liu, J.; Dang, Y.; Guo, Q.; Zhang, L. TSH stimulates the proliferation of vascular smooth muscle cells. *Endocrine* **2014**, *46*, 651–658. [CrossRef]
61. Makino, A.; Wang, H.; Scott, B.T.; Yuan, J.X.-J.; Dillmann, W.H. Thyroid hormone receptor-α and vascular function. *Am. J. Physiol. Physiol.* **2012**, *302*, C1346–C1352. [CrossRef] [PubMed]
62. Grais, I.M.; Sowers, J.R. Thyroid and the Heart. *Am. J. Med.* **2014**, *127*, 691–698. [CrossRef] [PubMed]
63. Klein, I.; Ojamaa, K. Thyroid Hormone and the Cardiovascular System. *N. Engl. J. Med.* **2001**, *344*, 501–509. [CrossRef] [PubMed]
64. Kasahara, T.; Tsunekawa, K.; Seki, K.; Mori, M.; Murakami, M. Regulation of iodothyronine deiodinase and roles of thyroid hormones in human coronary artery smooth muscle cells. *Atherosclerosis* **2006**, *186*, 207–214. [CrossRef] [PubMed]
65. Ojamaa, K.; Klemperer, J.D.; Klein, I. Acute Effects of Thyroid Hormone on Vascular Smooth Muscle. *Thyroid* **1996**, *6*, 505–512. [CrossRef]

66. Fukuyama, K.; Ichiki, T.; Takeda, K.; Tokunou, T.; Iino, N.; Masuda, S.; Ishibashi, M.; Egashira, K.; Shimokawa, H.; Hirano, K.; et al. Downregulation of Vascular Angiotensin II Type 1 Receptor by Thyroid Hormone. *Hypertension* **2003**, *41*, 598–603. [CrossRef]
67. Carrillo-Sepúlveda, M.A.; Ceravolo, G.S.; Fortes, Z.B.; Carvalho, M.H.; Tostes, R.; Laurindo, F.R.; Webb, R.C.; Barreto-Chaves, M.L.M. Thyroid hormone stimulates NO production via activation of the PI3K/Akt pathway in vascular myocytes. *Cardiovasc. Res.* **2009**, *85*, 560–570. [CrossRef]
68. Demirel, M.; Gürsoy, G.; Yıldız, M. Does Treatment of Either Hypothyroidy or Hyperthyroidy Affect Diurnal Blood Pressure. *Arch. Iran. Med.* **2017**, *20*, 572–580.
69. Hiroi, Y.; Kim, H.-H.; Ying, H.; Furuya, F.; Huang, Z.; Simoncini, T.; Noma, K.; Ueki, K.; Nguyen, N.-H.; Scanlan, T.S.; et al. Rapid nongenomic actions of thyroid hormone. *Proc. Nat. Acad. Sci. USA* **2006**, *103*, 14104–14109. [CrossRef]
70. Kuzman, J.; Gerdes, A.; Kobayashi, S.; Liang, Q. Thyroid hormone activates Akt and prevents serum starvation-induced cell death in neonatal rat cardiomyocytes. *J. Mol. Cell. Cardiol.* **2005**, *39*, 841–844. [CrossRef]
71. Napoli, R.; Apuzzi, V.; Bosso, G.; D'Anna, C.; De Sena, A.; Pirozzi, C.; Marano, A.; Lupoli, G.A.; Cudemo, G.; Oliviero, U.; et al. Recombinant Human Thyrotropin Enhances Endothelial-Mediated Vasodilation of Conduit Arteries. *J. Clin. Endocrinol. Metab.* **2009**, *94*, 1012–1016. [CrossRef] [PubMed]
72. Zwaveling, J.; Pfaffendorf, M.; Zwieten, P.A. The direct effects of thyroid hormones on rat mesenteric resistance arteries. *Fundam. Clin. Pharmacol.* **1997**, *11*, 41–46. [CrossRef] [PubMed]
73. Ichiki, T. Thyroid Hormone and Vascular Remodeling. *J. Atheroscler. Thromb.* **2016**, *23*, 266–275. [CrossRef] [PubMed]
74. Jain, S.; Murthy, M.; Ramteke, K.; Raparti, G. Thyroid: Disorders, disruptors and drugs. *Int. J. Nutr. Pharmacol. Neurol. Dis.* **2013**, *3*, 87. [CrossRef]
75. Ao, J.; Yuan, T.; Gao, L.; Yu, X.; Zhao, X.; Tian, Y.; Ding, W.; Ma, Y.; Shen, Z. Organic UV filters exposure induces the production of inflammatory cytokines in human macrophages. *Sci. Total. Environ.* **2018**, *635*, 926–935. [CrossRef]
76. Sheikh, I.A. Molecular interactions of thyroxine binding globulin and thyroid hormone receptor with estrogenic compounds 4-nonylphenol, 4-tert-octylphenol and bisphenol A metabolite (MBP). *Life Sci.* **2020**, *253*, 117738. [CrossRef]
77. Ali, M.R.; Latif, R.; Davies, T.F.; Mezei, M. Monte Carlo loop refinement and virtual screening of the thyroid-stimulating hormone receptor transmembrane domain. *J. Biomol. Struct. Dyn.* **2014**, *33*, 1140–1152. [CrossRef]
78. Satpathy, R. Application of Molecular Docking Methods on Endocrine Disrupting Chemicals: A Review. *J. Appl. Biotechnol. Rep.* **2020**, *7*, 74–80. [CrossRef]
79. Gao, L.; Yuan, T.; Cheng, P.; Zhou, C.; Ao, J.; Wang, W.; Zhang, H. Organic UV filters inhibit multixenobiotic resistance (MXR) activity in Tetrahymena thermophila: Investigations by the Rhodamine 123 accumulation assay and molecular docking. *Ecotoxicology* **2016**, *25*, 1318–1326. [CrossRef]
80. Couderq, S.; Leemans, M.; Fini, J.-B. Testing for thyroid hormone disruptors, a review of non-mammalian in vivo models. *Mol. Cell. Endocrinol.* **2020**, *508*, 110779. [CrossRef]
81. Rolfo, A.; Nuzzo, A.M.; De Amicis, R.; Moretti, L.; Bertoli, S.; Leone, A. Fetal–Maternal Exposure to Endocrine Disruptors: Correlation with Diet Intake and Pregnancy Outcomes. *Nutrients* **2020**, *12*, 1744. [CrossRef] [PubMed]
82. Campesi, I.; Franconi, F.; Montella, A.; Dessole, S.; Capobianco, G. Human Umbilical Cord: Information Mine in Sex-Specific Medicine. *Life* **2021**, *11*, 52. [CrossRef] [PubMed]
83. Li, L.-X.; Chen, L.; Meng, X.-Z.; Chen, B.-H.; Chen, S.-Q.; Zhao, Y.; Zhao, L.-F.; Liang, Y.; Zhang, Y. Exposure Levels of Environmental Endocrine Disruptors in Mother-Newborn Pairs in China and Their Placental Transfer Characteristics. *PLoS ONE* **2013**, *8*, e62526. [CrossRef] [PubMed]
84. Chen, M.-L.; Chang, C.-C.; Shen, Y.-J.; Hung, J.-H.; Guo, B.-R.; Chuang, H.-Y.; Mao, I.-F. Quantification of prenatal exposure and maternal-fetal transfer of nonylphenol. *Chemosphere* **2008**, *73*, S239–S245. [CrossRef]
85. Tan, B. Analysis of selected pesticides and alkylphenols in human cord blood by gas chromatograph-mass spectrometer. *Talanta* **2003**, *61*, 385–391. [CrossRef]
86. De Llano, J.J.M.; Fuertes, G.; Torró, I.; Garcia-Vicent, C.; Fayos, J.L.; Lurbe, E. Birth weight and characteristics of endothelial and smooth muscle cell cultures from human umbilical cord vessels. *J. Transl. Med.* **2009**, *7*, 30. [CrossRef]
87. Steinert, J.R.; Wyatt, A.W.; Poston, L.; Jacob, R.; Mann, G.E. Preeclampsia is associated with altered Ca 2+ regulation and nitric oxide production in human fetal venous endothelial cells. *FASEB J.* **2002**, *16*, 721–723. [CrossRef]
88. Gokina, N.I.; Bevan, J.A. Histamine-induced depolarization: Ionic mechanisms and role in sustained contraction of rabbit cerebral arteries. *Am. J. Physiol. Circ. Physiol.* **2000**, *278*, H2094–H2104. [CrossRef]
89. Mallozzi, M.; Bordi, G.; Garo, C.; Caserta, D. The effect of maternal exposure to endocrine disrupting chemicals on fetal and neonatal development: A review on the major concerns. *Birth Defects Res. Part. C Embryo Today Rev.* **2016**, *108*, 224–242. [CrossRef]
90. Glória, S.; Marques, J.; Feiteiro, J.; Marcelino, H.; Verde, I.; Cairrao, E. Tributyltin role on the serotonin and histamine receptors in human umbilical artery. *Toxicol. Vitr.* **2018**, *50*, 210–216. [CrossRef]
91. Tang, Z.-R.; Xu, X.-L.; Deng, S.-L.; Lian, Z.; Yu, K. Oestrogenic Endocrine Disruptors in the Placenta and the Fetus. *Int. J. Mol. Sci.* **2020**, *21*, 1519. [CrossRef] [PubMed]

MDPI
St. Alban-Anlage 66
4052 Basel
Switzerland
Tel. +41 61 683 77 34
Fax +41 61 302 89 18
www.mdpi.com

Biomedicines Editorial Office
E-mail: biomedicines@mdpi.com
www.mdpi.com/journal/biomedicines

www.ingramcontent.com/pod-product-compliance
Lightning Source LLC
LaVergne TN
LVHW070656100526
838202LV00013B/980